Diagnosis, Therapy, and Evidence

Critical Issues in Health and Medicine

Edited by Rima D. Apple, University of Wisconsin–Madison,
and Janet Golden, Rutgers University, Camden

Growing criticism of the U.S. health care system is coming from consumers, politicians, the media, activists, and health care professionals. Critical Issues in Health and Medicine is a collection of books that explores these contemporary dilemmas from a variety of perspectives, among them political, legal, historical, sociological, and comparative, and with attention to crucial dimensions such as race, gender, ethnicity, sexuality, and culture.

For a list of titles in the series, see the last page of the book.

Diagnosis, Therapy, and Evidence

Conundrums in Modern American Medicine

Gerald N. Grob and Allan V. Horwitz

Rutgers University Press

New Brunswick, New Jersey, and London

Library of Congress Cataloging-in-Publication Data

Grob, Gerald N., 1931–
    Diagnosis, therapy, and evidence : conundrums in modern American medicine /
Gerald N. Grob and Allan V. Horwitz.
        p. ; cm. — (Critical issues in health and medicine)
    Includes bibliographical references and index.
    ISBN 978-0-8135-4671-1 (hardcover : alk. paper) — ISBN 978-0-8135-4672-8 (pbk. : alk.
paper)
    1. Social medicine—United States.   2. Diseases and history—United States.   3. Diagnosis.
I. Horwitz, Allan V.   II. Title.   III. Series: Critical issues in health and medicine.
    [DNLM: 1. Medicine—trends—United States.   2. Diagnosis—United States.   3. Disease—
etiology—United States.   4. Therapeutics—trends—United States.   WB 100 G8728d 2010]
    RA418.3.U6G76 2010
    362.1—dc22   2009008097

A British Cataloging-in-Publication record for this book is available from the British Library

Visit our Web site: http://rutgerspress.rutgers.edu

Manufactured in the United States of America

To the memory of our fathers

Contents

Preface

Americans are besieged by advice about the efficacy of medical therapies and drugs as well as behavioral and dietary modifications that will presumably prevent disease, promote health, and extend longevity. Scarcely a day passes without revelations about new medical breakthroughs that will presumably overcome the ravages of age-old diseases. Faith in medical progress leads the United States to spend far more than any other industrialized nation on its health care system. Yet such health care indicators as longevity, infant mortality, access to care, and the effective management of chronic illnesses lag far behind other nations. Indeed, the claim that the United States has the world's best health care system belies the facts.

In this book we have collaborated across disciplinary lines and present a series of case studies to illustrate gaps and weaknesses in the medical care system. One of us (Grob) is a medical historian and the other (Horwitz) is a medical sociologist. Both of us, however, share assumptions and beliefs that transcend disciplinary lines, and we have produced an analytic work that hopefully sheds light on a series of contemporary medical issues. We have found that a substantial part of the contemporary literature dealing with therapeutic efficacy, diagnoses, epidemiology, and evidence ignores longitudinal and historical data, to say nothing about methodological inadequacies and claims that rest largely on faith. Our goal in writing this book, however, is not to denigrate the medical care system. It is rather to call attention to some of its weaknesses and exaggerated claims that lead to dubious therapeutic and behavioral interventions and exacerbate the excessive costs of both care and treatment.

We would like to thank William Rothstein, Janet Golden, and Doreen Valentine, who provided valuable suggestions on an earlier draft of the manuscript. Naomi Breslau and Jerry Wakefield made many astute recommendations regarding the PTSD chapter. Part of the material in chapters 2 and 3 is taken from Grob's "The Rise and Decline of Tonsillectomy in Twentieth-Century America," *Journal of the History of Medicine and Allied Sciences* 62 (October 2007): 383–421, and "The Rise of Peptic Ulcer, 1900–1950," *Perspectives in Biology and Medicine* 46 (autumn 2003): 550–566. Both are reprinted with the permission of Oxford University Press and the Johns Hopkins

University Press, respectively. Some of the material in chapter 6 is adapted from Horwitz's book with Jerry Wakefield, *The Loss of Sadness: How Psychiatry Transformed Normal Sorrow into Depressive Disorder* (Oxford University Press, 2007). We would also like to acknowledge the immense contributions that David Mechanic, the director of the Institute for Health, Health Care Policy, and Aging Research, has made to our research. Horwitz would also like to express his appreciation to Rector Wim Blockmans, the staff, and the fellows of the Netherlands Institute for Advanced Study for providing him with resources, time, and an unparalleled scholarly environment to write a draft of this book during his stay in the 2007–2008 year. He is also grateful to Rutgers University for providing him with a Competitive Fellowship Leave that allowed him the opportunity to visit NIAS.

Gerald N. Grob
Allan V. Horwitz

Abbreviations

ADHD	attention-deficit/hyperactivity disorder
AIDS	acquired immune deficiency syndrome
AMA	American Medical Association
APA	American Psychiatric Association
CDC	Centers for Disease Control and Prevention
CFS	chronic fatigue syndrome
CHD	coronary heart disease
CT	computed tomography
DSM	*Diagnostic and Statistical Manual of Mental Disorders*
ECA	epidemiologic catchment area
FDA	Food and Drug Administration
FAS	fetal alcohol syndrome
GAD	generalized anxiety disorder
GDP	gross domestic product
HDL	high-density lipoprotein
HIV	human immunodeficiency virus
HP	*Helicobacter pylori*
HRR	hospital referral region
ICD	International Classification of Disease
LDL	low-density lipoprotein
MDD	major depressive disorder
MRI	magnetic resonance imaging
NCI	National Cancer Institute
NCS	National Comorbidity Survey
NIMH	National Institute of Mental Health
NSAID	non-steroid anti-inflammatory drug
PSA	prostate-specific antigen
PTSD	post-traumatic stress disorder
RCT	randomized controlled trial
RLS	restless legs syndrome
SSRI	selective serotonin reuptake inhibitor
T&A	tonsillectomy/adenoidectomy
WHO	World Health Organization

Diagnosis, Therapy, and Evidence

Chapter 1

Rhetoric and Reality in Modern American Medicine

Most Americans believe that their health care system is the best in the world. Yet they do not recognize the extent to which many claims about the causes of disease, therapeutic practices, and even diagnoses are shaped by beliefs that are unscientific, unproven, or completely wrong. To so argue is not to condemn American medicine, which admittedly has many strengths, but rather to point to rhetorical claims and practices that rest upon shaky foundations. What we have chosen to do in this book is to present a series of case studies that illustrate the weaknesses of many prevailing beliefs and therapies. In so doing we can not only learn from these examples, but find ways to do better in the future.

The Contemporary American Health Care System

For much of human history death was associated with the infectious diseases that took their heaviest toll among infants and children. Beginning in the late nineteenth century—for reasons that are not clearly understood—infectious diseases began to decline as the major causes of mortality.[1] The reduction in mortality among the young permitted more people to reach adulthood and thus to live longer. Under these circumstances it is not surprising that long-duration illnesses—notably, cardiovascular-renal diseases and a variety of neoplasms—became more prominent elements in morbidity and mortality patterns. These diseases were associated with advancing age; the longer individuals lived, the greater the risk of becoming ill or dying from them. In one sense the increasing prominence of long-duration (or chronic) diseases was in part a reflection of the fact that more and more people were enjoying greater longevity.

To be sure, the decline in mortality from infectious diseases preceded antibiotic drug therapy. Yet the introduction of these and other drugs after World War II reshaped both medical practice and public perceptions. If infectious diseases could be conquered by antibiotic drugs, why could not long-duration diseases also be eliminated by new medical therapies? Slowly but surely Americans, for a variety of reasons, came to believe that the medical care system could play a crucial role in conquering disease and extending longevity.

Yet Americans manifest ambivalent and even contradictory attitudes about their health care system. They take it as an article of faith that a science-based system has the capacity to reduce morbidity and mortality and thereby improve the quality of their lives. They point with pride to a health establishment that in their eyes is superior to that of any other nation. They believe that medical schools turn out the best-trained physicians; that a vast hospital system with its array of imposing technologies provides the most up-to-date therapies; and that pharmaceutical companies have the capacity to develop innovative drugs that both treat and prevent disease.

Beneath the surface, however, there is considerable unease. Constantly rising health expenditures remain a source of concern. Millions of Americans lack health insurance and many are forced into bankruptcy because of huge medical bills resulting from various illnesses. The increasing bureaucratization of the medical care industry has diminished the element of trust between patient and physician, giving rise to fears that doctors do not always act in the best interest of patients. There is concern that insurance companies, in an effort to contain costs, shape treatment protocols in ways that are in their financial interests. Faith in medical therapies is tempered by findings that question their efficacy as well as by the prevalence of iatrogenic diseases (illnesses induced inadvertently by a physician, surgeon, or health care professional, or by any medical treatment or diagnostic procedure, or from a harmful occurrence that was not a natural consequence of the patient's disease). Distrust of the pharmaceutical industry is widespread because of revelations that harmful side effects of drugs are sometimes hidden, that the efficacy of many drugs is exaggerated, and that financial relationships with physicians have adverse consequences for patients. After an explosion of psychotropic drug use during the 1990s and early years of the twenty-first century, controversies have arisen about their effectiveness, negative side effects, dependency potential, and risk of enhancing suicidal tendencies. For these and other reasons the authority of the medical profession has eroded in recent decades.[2]

Despite rising concerns, Americans remain dedicated to their health care system, as is evidenced by the fact that they continue to commit vast resources. Between 1970 and 2006 national health care expenditures increased from $75 billion to $2.1 trillion. During the same period such expenditures as a percentage of the Gross Domestic Product (GDP) rose from 7.2 to 16.0 percent. Changes in per capita expenditures were even more spectacular, rising from $356 to $7,026 in the same period. Nor were the sources of funding unchanged. During these years public funding of health expenditures increased from 38 to 46 percent. Although the rate of increase had begun to slow by the beginning of the twenty-first century, there were predictions that national health care expenditures might at some time in the future account for no less than a fifth of the GDP.[3]

Pride in the American health care system, nevertheless, conceals disquieting elements. The United States spends twice as much on health, compared to the median of industrialized countries. It has the highest percentage of specialized physicians as well as a vast system of hospitals equipped with the latest technology. Yet when compared with other industrialized countries, its health indicators are anything but impressive. In 2002–2003 the United States ranked last among 19 nations in terms of deaths before age seventy-five that were partially preventable or modifiable by timely interventions. Among 23 industrialized nations, it ranked last in infant mortality, with rates more than double the average of the three leading countries (Ireland, Japan, and Finland). It tied for last place on healthy life expectancy at age sixty. Among 192 nations for which data is available for 2004, the United States ranked forty-sixth in life expectancy at birth and forty-second in infant mortality. A 2008 survey of chronically ill adults in Australia, Canada, France, Germany, the Netherlands, New Zealand, the United Kingdom, and the United States found major differences in access, safety, and care efficiency. The study found that American patients "were at particularly high risk of forgoing care because of costs and of experiencing inefficient, poorly organized care, or errors."[4] The situation regarding mental disorders is as bleak; surveys from the World Health Organization indicate that the United States has the highest rates of mental disorders of any of the fourteen countries surveyed despite the fact that it also has the highest rates of treatment for these disorders.[5] On all counts—quality of care, use of health information technology, and costs of administering its health system—the record belies claims that it has the best health care system in the world.[6]

Admittedly, some of these differentials may be due in part to the fact that higher expenditures reflect a greater disease burden and higher rates of disease treatment. In 2004 obesity and smoking rates were much higher in the United States than in ten European nations. Nevertheless, it is difficult to attribute such differentials simply to the burden of disease and disease treatment.[7] Moreover, it is clear that socioeconomic class is an important element in health status. People at the bottom of the income scale have more mental and physical disabilities and die earlier than those above them, partly because of unhealthy behaviors and partly because of relative material deprivation. Yet American social and economic policies—unlike those in many other nations—promote growing disparities between classes, largely because entrepreneurship is valued over equality. Educational, economic, and housing disparities often create unintended health consequences. In terms of equity, the United States—as compared with Australia, Canada, Germany, New Zealand, and the United Kingdom—ranked at the bottom. Individuals with below-average income were much more likely to report not visiting a physician when sick, not getting a recommended test, treatment, or follow-up care, or not filling a prescription. In the 1980s and 1990s those who were already disadvantaged did not experience the gains in life expectancy experienced by the advantaged, and in some areas mortality among the former actually increased. Moreover, physical stature, which in part reflects living standards (including income and medical care), stagnated around 1955 to 1975 despite the fact that incomes were rising. In some ways this was anomalous, since western and northern European heights were increasing during the same period. From the mid-eighteenth to the mid-twentieth century Americans had been among the tallest in the world, but by 2000 had fallen behind many European populations. John Komlos and Benjamin E. Lauderdale have suggested that European welfare states, with their universal safety nets, were "able to provide a higher biological standard of living to their children and youth than the more free-market-oriented U.S. economy, which, at least in this important measure—as well as in life expectancy—has underperformed in affluence."[8]

There are also other reasons to doubt the claims that the American health care system is superior to all others. A study that attempted to measure the quality of medical care in twelve metropolitan areas found severe shortcomings. Taking selected acute and chronic conditions that represented the leading causes of illness, death, and the utilization of health care in each age group, the study attempted to determine the degree to which recommended medical care procedures were delivered to a representative sample of the American population. The results were dismal. "On average," the study found, "Americans receive about half of recommended medical care processes. . . . [T]he gap between what we know works and what is actually done is substantial enough to warrant attention."[9]

It is also not clear that prevailing standards of care are necessarily efficacious. The evidence in support of many widely used therapies (e.g., drugs for decreased bone density, statins for cholesterol reduction, surgery for back pain, and various surgical procedures to treat CHD) is hardly impressive, to say the least. Indeed, when the Centers for Medicare and Medicaid Services offered financial incentives to hospitals to adopt guidelines promulgated by the American College of Cardiology and the American Hospital Association to treat acute myocardial infarctions, it found that the adoption of such guidelines "had limited incremental impact on processes of care and outcomes."[10]

Moreover, many technological innovations come into use even when there is little or no evidence that they will benefit patients. The recent introduction of CT (computed tomography) angiography is one such example. Enthusiasm for the procedure grew rapidly after the sixty-four-slice scanners came to the market in 2005. The scan exposes individuals to high rates of radiation. The Centers for Medicare and Medicaid Services became concerned with the absence of clinical evidence to demonstrate better patient outcomes. In general, patients fell into three broad categories. At one end were the "worried well," individuals who had no symptoms of heart disease and therefore should not undergo the procedure. At the other end were high-risk patients suffering from such symptoms as severe unstable angina. For them cardiac catheterization was the procedure of choice. The middle group was composed of persons who were at intermediate risk because of elevated cholesterol or blood pressure levels. In 2007 Medicare proposed to pay for CT angiography for those falling into this group who had either stable or unstable angina. These patients would be enrolled in clinical trials to determine whether the procedure was more effective than cardiac catheterization. Specialty medical societies representing radiologists and cardiologists were outraged, to say nothing about General Electric (manufacturer of the CT scanner), all of whom had a financial interest. The Society of Cardiovascular Computed Tomography (an organization of 4,700 physician members whose goal was to promote CT angiograms), the American College of Radiology, and

the American College of Cardiology launched a lobbying campaign that succeeded in forcing Medicare to retract its decision even though the procedure
lacked evidence of efficacy for the intermediate group and resulted as well
in high costs. Nor is there conclusive evidence that CT and MRI (magnetic
resonance imaging) scanning for many conditions results in improved health
outcomes. Recent findings indicate that meniscal findings on knee MRIs had
little clinical relevance even though those findings led to arthroscopic surgery that provided no benefit.[11]

Equally striking is the fact that there are regional differences in both
medical therapies and expenditures. Medicare patients living in Rhode
Island undergo knee replacements at a rate of five in one thousand people; in
Nebraska the rate is double. Female Medicare enrollees who are diagnosed
with breast cancer in South Dakota have seven times the chance of undergoing a mastectomy as compared with Vermont. Age-, sex-, and race-adjusted
spending for traditional Medicare in 1996 was $8,414 in the Miami region, as
compared with $3,341 in the Minneapolis region.[12]

Such differences in spending, however, are not due simply to regional
differences in the prices of medical care, differences in disease prevalence, or
socioeconomic status. The evidence strongly suggests that such differences
are a function of the more inpatient-based and specialist-oriented pattern of
practice that prevails in high-cost regions. Neither quality, access to care,
nor outcomes are superior in such regions. Indeed, the more hospitals, physicians, laboratories, and subspecialists in a given geographical area, the more
they are used. An examination of Medicare spending and outcomes of care for
hip fracture, colorectal cancer, and myocardial infarction found that persons
in high-spending regions received 60 percent more care but did not have better quality or outcomes of care. In the 306 Hospital Referral Regions (HRRs)
in 2003, the incidence of hip and knee replacement for chronic arthritis and
surgery for low-back pain varied from 5.6- to 4.8- and 5.9-fold, respectively,
from the lowest to the highest region.[13]

The case of back and neck problems is illustrative. In one survey 26
percent of adults reported low back pain and 14 percent reported neck pain
during the previous three months. Between 1997 and 2005 there was a substantial increase in rates of imaging, injections, use of opiates, and surgery
for spine problems. Total expenditures for these conditions increased no less
than 65 percent, adjusted for inflation, a figure far higher than the increase
in overall health expenditures. Spending for these problems alone was about

$86 billion. Yet there was no evidence that persons with these conditions reported a corresponding improvement in their self-assessed health status. Indeed, lumbar fusion rates accelerated when intervertebral fusion cages were introduced in 1996, even in the absence of any real change in the indications for surgery and despite the fact that this surgery is associated with more complications than discectomy or laminectomy. The relative risk for surgery within a given geographical region also tended to remain constant over time; regions with high rates of surgery remained high and those with low rates remained low. Equally striking was the fact that there were wide disparities within regions. In eight Florida HRRs, for example, surgeons in Bradentown and Orlando performed spine surgery with fusion 2.4 and 1.6 times more frequently than the national average, respectively, while rates in Miami were 60 percent of the national average.[14]

Much the same holds true for cesarean deliveries. The rate for this procedure in the United States is much higher than in other countries. Within the United States there are large geographic variations in cesarean delivery rates, only part of which can be attributed to the characteristics and socioeconomic status of patients. The remaining variations are due to what may be termed the "practice style" of an area. In such areas physicians perform a procedure that is of decreasing medical value to the patient. One hospital cognizant of this fact was able to reduce its rate from 17.5 to 11.0 percent over a two-year period without incurring adverse health outcomes. This reduction followed the introduction of several requirements: a second opinion, provision of objective criteria when such a delivery was indicated, and a review of all cesarean deliveries.[15]

That the rhetorical claims of medical science are overwhelming is obvious. Hardly a day passes without news of some therapeutic advance or behavioral advice derived from epidemiological studies. Equally notable is the proliferation of new diagnoses, which are generally accompanied by the introduction of pharmaceuticals. Unfortunately, little attention is paid to the nature and quality of supporting evidence or the methodologies employed to measure their validity. In offering a critique of exaggerated and sometimes misleading therapeutic and diagnostic claims, we do not wish to denigrate America's health care system, which has impressive achievements to its credit. But for too long many therapies, etiological explanations, and health recommendations have been taken at face value by a receptive public unaware of the shaky foundation upon which they rest and adverse consequences that follow.

The Role of Medicine

In the past the role of medicine was—if possible—to treat the sick person. To be sure, physicians offered advice on how to maintain health, but this advice was generally identified with religious and moral themes. Suffering, sickness, and death were intrinsic to the human condition. Such behaviors as drinking, gambling, taking drugs, smoking, and sexual misbehavior were regarded as vices even though they might have adverse health consequences. Admittedly, there were efforts to medicalize alcoholism in the late nineteenth century, but these were aberrations and generally did not transform attitudes.[16] Vices were rarely converted into medical diagnoses.

Before 1940 the major function of medicine was to diagnose disease; the therapeutic armamentarium, however extensive, was hardly impressive. With the exception of a limited number of medications (digoxin, thyroxine, insulin), immunization for a small number of infectious diseases, and surgical procedures, physicians had few effective means of coping with many infections, cardiovascular diseases, cancer, and many long-duration illnesses. Likewise, efficacious medications for mental illnesses did not emerge until the 1950s. This is not to suggest that physicians were therapeutic nihilists, for such was not the case. Although extensive, there were relatively few effective therapies capable of altering the outcome of most diseases before the 1930s. Nor was there an emphasis on the prevention of disease. Health was simply the absence of disease, and the role of the physician was to treat and care for the sick.

During the latter half of the twentieth century, however, a dramatic perceptual transformation took place. Nowhere was this better expressed than in the constitution of the World Health Organization, promulgated in 1946 and ratified in 1948. "Health," the constitution stated in its declaration of principles, "is a state of complete physical, mental and social wellbeing and not merely the absence of disease or infirmity." Such a definition implied new roles for the medical profession. The care and treatment of the sick and infirm remained part of the physician's responsibility. But to this were added the functions of making people healthy, happy, and socially adjusted. Since health—physical, mental, social—was normal, it followed that sickness, disease, and even distress were not inevitable. Rather they resulted from the operation of a variety of external determinants. Hence the role of medicine was to persuade people to engage in healthy behaviors and thus to avoid the consequences of inappropriate behaviors that resulted in disease and death. The assumption was that medicine had the knowledge to create a disease-free society.

Treatment, care, cure, and prevention, however, were only part of the new face of medicine. Equally significant was its claim that its members, by employing the findings and insights of science, had the power to improve upon nature. Novel interventions seemingly could enhance brain functioning, increase stature, arrest aging, increase longevity, alleviate anxiety, create desirable character traits, maintain high levels of sexual activity, and reshape bodies. Indeed, even the criteria for normality began to undergo frequent changes. Traditionally accepted levels of blood pressure, cholesterol, and glucose were revised sharply downward, thus increasing the population at risk and elevating the rationale for intervention. A coalition of scientists, clinicians, and pharmaceutical companies promoted a variety of interventions (including drugs and surgery) that would presumably enhance both the physical and mental well-being of people, even those who were presumably healthy.[17]

The belief that disease can be both prevented and conquered and nature can be improved reflects a fundamental conviction that all things are possible, that human beings have it within their power to control completely their own destiny. If "developments in research maintain their current pace," according to William B. Schwartz (professor of medicine at the University of Southern California), "it seems likely that a combination of improved attention to dietary and environmental factors along with advances in gene therapy and protein-targeted drugs will have virtually eliminated most major classes of disease." Indeed, Schwartz predicts that in the not too distant future people could enjoy a life expectancy of 130 years or more.[18]

To many Americans disease remains the "enemy" of humanity, and only a war can make it vanish it. As the famous American intellectual Susan Sontag noted in her classic *Illness as Metaphor,* descriptions of cancer are phrased in terms of war. Cancer cells "do not simply multiply; they are 'invasive.'" They "colonize" from the site of origin to far sites in the body, first establishing tiny outposts ("micrometastases"). Medical treatment is also phrased in military language. Radiotherapy is akin to aerial warfare; patients are "bombarded" with toxic rays. Chemotherapy is "chemical warfare, using poisons." That healthy cells are harmed or destroyed is simply collateral damage. The "war on cancer" (a name given to federal legislation in 1971) must be fought to the finish, and the only acceptable outcome is unconditional surrender.[19] Mental health policy has similarly come to emphasize aggressive programs of screening for untreated mental disorders in primary medical care, schools, and the workplace.[20]

The faith that disease is unnatural and can be prevented or conquered, however, rests on a fundamental misunderstanding of the biological world. If cancer is the enemy, then we ourselves are the enemy. Malignant cells, after all, are hardly aliens who invade our bodies; they arise from our own normal cells. The biological world of which we are a part, moreover, includes millions of microorganisms. Some are harmless, while some are parasitic and have the potential to cause infection. Others play vital symbiotic roles that nourish and maintain organic life. Indeed, in the world of nature there is little clarity. Some microorganisms contribute to soil fertility by converting plant debris into humus, while others destroy crops. Some microorganisms cause disease in humans, but others that reside in the gastrointestinal tract play constructive and vital roles. Efforts to destroy pathogenic microorganisms through a variety of drugs are doomed to failure, if only because of their ability to develop resistant properties, which then pose even greater dangers. In the realm of mental health, natural psychological emotions such as sadness and fear are now considered to be depressive and anxiety disorders that psychotropic drugs can suppress.[21]

"Threats to health," Rene Dubos (the distinguished biologist who also played a major role in creating the environmental movement) observed in words that are still as relevant as they were nearly a half century ago, "are inescapable accompaniments of life." Conceding the ability to find methods of control for any given pathological state, he nevertheless insisted that "disease will change its manifestations according to social circumstances" and hence will be an omnipresent part of the human condition.[22] The belief that disease can be prevented or conquered is as much an illusion as Ponce de León's search for the ubiquitous "Fountain of Youth."

Aside from its inability to predict future threats to health—the emergence of Acquired Immune Deficiency Syndrome (AIDS) is one such example—contemporary medical science, disclaimers to the contrary, cannot cure or explain the etiology of many of the long-duration illnesses that account for the bulk of mortality. This is not in any way to denigrate medical science, which has a capacity to manage and alleviate the symptoms of disease and, within limits, to prolong life. Inflated rhetorical claims to the contrary, the etiology of most of our major diseases of our age—cardiovascular disease, cancer, diabetes, mental illnesses—remain shrouded in mystery. These intractable diseases reflect, as David Weatherall (Regius Professor of Medicine at Oxford University) has written, "an extremely complex mixture of nature and nurture, set against the background of aging, which itself may be modified by both genes and environment. They are likely to have multiple causes, and there may be many different routes to their pathology."[23]

The belief that the conquest of disease and the creation of a happy and well-adjusted society are realistic goals, nevertheless, continues to influence the American public in subtle ways. Indeed, the debate over how to provide universal coverage for health care or to find ways of limiting constantly increasing expenditures does not in any way contradict the faith in the redemptive authority of medicine. A variety of groups, including the medical profession and the pharmaceutical industry, fuel this faith. Both benefit by promoting the pursuit of health: the medical profession because it strengthens its legitimacy and its claim on resources, and the pharmaceutical industry because it enhances sales of drugs. The media, both visual and print, contributes to the faith in medical progress by providing coverage of alleged therapeutic breakthroughs and new ways of preventing disease.

Yet reality belies appearances. The appearance of the AIDS epidemic contradicted the belief that infectious diseases no longer posed a significant threat. Laboratory researchers were able to isolate the human immunodeficiency virus (HIV) and develop a diagnostic test to locate its presence in the body. Multi-drug therapy also resulted in the control of the disease. The development of a vaccine to prevent the disease, however, has eluded researchers. Other viral diseases remain a source of concern, especially since ocean and distance no longer serve as protective impediments to the dissemination of old and new microorganisms. Influenza in particular remains a major threat, largely because the virus is constantly undergoing genetic reassortment. Normally, the reassortment is between an animal and human influenza virus. But on occasion there is a direct transmission of an influenza virus from animal and avian species to humans. The 1918 pandemic is one such example. During that pandemic mortality reached unprecedented levels and killed as many as twenty to forty million people worldwide.[24] The ability of microorganisms to develop resistance to medications is omnipresent.

Similarly, medical therapies and drugs are not without risks. Anesthesia, surgery, and sophisticated diagnostic procedures, even when competently undertaken, have the potential to induce iatrogenic illnesses. One study of 815 consecutive patients on a general medical service of a university hospital found that 36 percent had an iatrogenic illness. Perhaps 5 to 10 percent of patients admitted to acute care hospitals acquire one or more infections, and the risk seems to be increasing. Such adverse events affect as many as two million patients and result in some 90,000 deaths. Catheter-related blood-stream infections in intensive care units cause about 28,000 deaths each year and cost the health care system about $2.3 billion. A study by the Institute of Medicine of the National Academy of Sciences concluded that at least 44,000 and perhaps as many as 98,000 Americans die each year as a result of medical errors. Medication errors in both hospitals and community settings are not uncommon, to say nothing about serious side effects caused by drug therapies. Nor are many common surgical procedures without risk. A study of patients undergoing coronary artery bypass found that only 12 percent showed no decline across eight cognitive domains studied; the remainder showed declines in one of more of these domains. Several studies show that children and adolescents who take antidepressants report higher rates of suicidal ideation and/or behavior than those who receive placebos.[25]

To emphasize the deficiencies and shortcomings of the American health care system is not to suggest that its benefits are insubstantial. Even if the goal of cure remains elusive, the treatment of many long-duration illnesses has clearly improved the quality of life and extended longevity. The threat of infectious diseases that have long been the major cause of mortality has diminished sharply. Although infectious diseases associated with childhood had ceased to be a threat to life well before 1940, the widespread use of vaccines after 1945 lessened their prevalence almost to the vanishing point. In 2006 there were no cases of diphtheria, poliomyelitis, and smallpox; and fewer than 100 cases of measles, rubella, and tetanus. Only mumps (6,584 cases and no deaths) and pertussis (15,632 cases and 27 deaths) showed modest prevalence levels. Vaccines developed since 1980 for such infectious diseases as Hepatitis A and B, influenza, varicella, and pneumococcal disease also resulted in sharp reductions in prevalence and mortality.[26] By mid-century the introduction of the steroids (cortisone and its derivatives) transformed a number of medial specialties, made possible the treatment of childhood cancers, and facilitated organ transplantation. The development of psychoactive drugs changed the treatment of severe and persistent mental disorders. Thousands of people who would have resided in inpatient mental institutions in the past are now able to remain in the community. New medications and surgical interventions dramatically increased the ability to manage cardiovascular disease. Technological innovations in laboratory analysis, imaging, and instrumentation also enhanced the ability to manage many diseases that hitherto proved fatal. Potential advances in molecular biology and genetics seem to hold out promise of still greater progress.

Etiology and Therapy

Much has been written about the benefits, risks, and costs of the American health care system. Other issues, however, have been often overlooked even though they may be equally significant. What are the origins of therapies? How is therapeutic efficacy determined? Why do some therapies continue to be a part of medical practice even when evidence about efficacy is either weak or nonexistent? How do diagnoses come into existence and why do many disappear with the passage of time?

Though seemingly arcane, such questions are by no means of minor importance. Consider, for example, the history of therapeutics. In the traditional view the evolution of medicine is a history of progress. Thus such therapies as bloodletting and purging disappeared from the medical armamentarium as newer and more effective ones took their place. Yet the history of therapeutics might also be written in terms of failure or ineffectiveness. In an analysis of a classic medical textbook published in 1927, for example, Paul B. Beeson (a distinguished academic physician who chaired the Yale Department of Medicine and subsequently became the Nuffield Professor of Medicine at Oxford University) noted that most of the recommended treatments of the pre–World War II era had disappeared by 1975. For 362 diseases listed in 1927, 211 therapies were found to be either harmful, useless, of questionable value, or simply symptomatic; only 23 were effective or preventive.[27] In our own time many therapies, initially hailed as breakthroughs, quickly disappear from practice. On the other hand, many therapies—despite the absence of efficacy—persist.

Equally revealing are changing styles of etiological explanations. Historically, human beings have always wanted to know the causes of morbidity and mortality. The explanations offered have varied in the extreme and include the state of the atmosphere, unhygienic conditions, inappropriate diets, immoderate behaviors, to cite only a few. Oftentimes a paradigm that is dominant at a given time becomes the basis for generalized explanations. The specific germ theory of disease, precisely because it provided definitive explanations of some infectious diseases, became an explanatory model for a variety of other diseases subsequently shown to be noninfectious. Researchers in the early twentieth century, for example, sought to find the germs responsible for such diseases as pellagra and cancer. At present the etiology of many long-term diseases is attributed to such risk factors as diet, physical inactivity, smoking, alcohol, and obesity. Unproven explanations that emphasize chemical imbalances have become common reasons for why people develop mental disorders.[28] With notable exceptions, the evidence supporting many contemporary etiological explanations is either weak or nonexistent.

In this volume we offer a variety of case studies to illustrate some of our broad generalizations about the theory and practice of medicine. The history of peptic ulcer in the twentieth century is illustrative. The seeming increase of peptic ulcer after 1900 quickly engaged the attention of physicians. Their understanding and treatment of peptic ulcer was shaped not only by such diagnostic tools as x-rays, but by differences between contesting medical specialties, broad concepts or paradigms current in the larger medical and scientific community, and prevailing social and ideological beliefs. Surgeons and internists, for example, were often at odds over appropriate therapies; each maintained that their personal experiences demonstrated the efficacy of their therapies. The former insisted upon the paramount importance of surgery; the latter argued that diet and regimen were appropriate therapies.

Nor were etiological theories derived from empirical data. The claim that peptic ulcer resulted from focal infections was simply a reflection of the specific germ theory of disease. Other explanations included the role of stress, race, constitutional makeup, psychosomatic factors, diet, and the pressure of modern industrial society. Virtually all were derivative and reflected social and intellectual currents that were common in the larger society of which medicine was but a part. More recently the etiology of peptic ulcer has been attributed to an infection from *Helicobacter pylori* and the use of non-steroid anti-inflammatory drugs. Effective therapies did not come until the late twentieth century, first with the introduction of anti-secretory drugs and then with antibiotics. Paradoxically, the incidence of peptic ulcer declined well before these therapies came into use. Moreover, the debate over pathogenesis remains contested. The history of this disease in the twentieth century provides an illustrative and in many ways a typical case study of shifting explanations and therapies, neither of which were necessarily related.

Tonsillectomy/adenoidectomy (T&A) presents an equally informative although quite different case. Between 1915 and the 1960s, T&A was the most frequently performed surgical procedure in the United States. Its rise was dependent upon novel medical concepts, paradigms, and institutions that were in the process of reshaping the structure and practice of medicine. Initially, the driving force was once again the focal theory of infection, which assumed (but could not be conclusively demonstrated) that circumscribed and confined infections could lead to systemic disease in any part of the body. The tonsils in particular were singled out as "portals of infection," and therefore their removal became a legitimate therapy. Indeed, many physicians believed that all children should have their tonsils removed.

Yet serious questions persisted. What kinds of evidence could prove that tonsils were portals of infection? An inherent difficulty was the absence of any consensus on the criteria that would be employed to judge which children required T&A as well as to measure its efficacy. Yet tonsillectomy persisted despite ambiguous supportive evidence. Although criticisms of the procedure were common by the 1930s, its decline did not begin until well after 1945 and involved debates over the nature of evidence, the significance of clinical experience in the validation of a particular therapy, and the role of competing medical specialties. The decline in the number of tonsillectomies in the last quarter of the twentieth century, however, proved transient. By the 1990s a new justification for T&A had begun to emerge, and the procedure began to be used as a therapy for obstructive sleep apnea disorder. Nor did such traditional justifications for T&A—recurrent throat infections—disappear. T&A is an example of how a therapy is introduced and persists despite the absence of persuasive evidence of efficacy.

Explanations of the etiology of the two most important causes of mortality in contemporary America, namely, coronary heart disease (CHD) and cancer, present equally problematic cases. As late as 1960 most knowledgeable individuals believed that CHD was a chronic degenerative disease related to aging and one that could not be influenced by specific preventive measures. In subsequent decades the focus shifted to the role of risk factors as crucial elements in the etiology of cardiovascular disorders. A series of epidemiological studies, some of which began in the 1940s, transformed the manner in which CHD was understood. The mystery and randomness that had previously characterized explanations of CHD were superseded by the claim that individuals were at increased risk for the disease if they ate high-fat foods, smoked, were overweight, or were physically inactive. Similarly, many cancers were also attributed to a variety of risk factors, of which smoking and diet were most prominent.

Many of the epidemiological studies that explained the genesis of CHD and cancer in terms of risk factors, however, ignored longitudinal data. Between 1920 and 1960, for example, CHD mortality among males in their thirties and forties rose dramatically despite the absence of risk factors and then declined in subsequent decades when behavioral risk factors were on the increase. Moreover, many epidemiologists relied on cohort analysis and observational studies. By monitoring disease rates and lifestyle, they believed that they could identify risk factors. The problem is that the risk factors they identified were at best associations that said nothing about causation. Yet such studies have become the basis of public health recommendations about what individuals should do or not do to prevent disease. Indeed, some recommendations about lifestyle may actually promote rather than prevent disease.

The Creation of Diagnoses

The weaknesses of many etiological explanations (which in turn lead to therapies of dubious efficacy) are by no means unique. The creation of diagnoses poses another equally troublesome problem all too often ignored. The belief in the concept of specific diseases, oddly enough, is of relatively recent vintage. Until the late nineteenth century physicians conceived of disease in individual rather than general terms. Health was a consequence of a symbiotic relationship or balance between nature, society, and the individual. Disease represented an imbalance; its symptoms were fluid and constantly changing as the body attempted to restore a balance. With but a few exceptions (such as smallpox or yellow fever), specific categories were largely absent.[29]

Early efforts to develop some sort of nosological or disease classification system floundered, largely because such systems were based on descriptions of symptoms. François Boissier de Sauvages's opus magnum, published in 1763, is illustrative of the eighteenth-century preoccupation with classification. He listed no less than eighteen kinds of angina, nineteen of asthma, and twenty of phthisis, to cite only a few examples. Subsequent nosologies attempted to differentiate between fevers, which proved equally problematic, if only because fever is a generalized bodily reaction rather than a specific disease. Admittedly, there were exceptions. The work of Richard Bright at Guy's Hospital in London was one such example. He linked albumin in heated urine to renal failure in his classic *Reports of Medical Cases* in 1827.[30]

Toward the middle of the nineteenth century disease began to be reinterpreted in somewhat different terms. Diseases became discreet entities and were equated with specific mechanisms. A disease had both a fixed clinical course and a mechanism. Like plants, diseases could be categorized; the result was an effort to create uniform medical nosologies. The emergence of the specific germ theory of disease represented perhaps the outstanding example of the new reductionist and mechanistic style of modern medicine. It created, at least for infectious diseases, a nosology based on etiology rather than symptomatology. It is true that many noninfectious diseases did not lend themselves to a classification system based on etiology. Nevertheless, the new classification model played a critical role in the transformation of medicine. Hitherto regarded as an art, medicine now became wedded to science and technology. It was no accident that by the early twentieth century the hospital, with its laboratories, elaborate technology, and sophisticated instruments, began to become central to medical practice. Individuals with their idiosyncratic symptoms were no longer of central importance. What was of importance were the objective indicators of disease, which increasingly were expressed in numerical terms (blood pressure, cholesterol and glucose levels, etc.) or portrayed by images initially produced by such innovations as X-ray machines and subsequently by a variety of other scanning machines.

To classify is perhaps inevitable, if only because it facilitates both thinking and communication. Yet classes are neither given nor self-evident; they are created and often have social, political, intellectual, and moral dimensions. Each class embodies a particular point of view, thus implicitly excluding other alternatives. In the early part of the twentieth century, for example, immigrants were categorized by the country from which they came. Those from western and northern Europe were deemed desirable and those from eastern and southern Europe were undesirable. Restrictionist legislation enacted between 1921 and 1924 created quotas based on these categories and thus facilitated the exclusion of the latter. In other words, the creation of classes— which often appear to be neutral—can have a variety of consequences.

The interest in medical classification systems did not occur in a vacuum. In the nineteenth century several currents had converged to give rise to a type of social inquiry whose methodological distinctiveness was a commitment to quantitative research. The seventeenth-century mercantilist concern with population and vital statistics was reinforced by nineteenth-century Baconian science, which tended to identify all of science with taxonomy. To this was added the fascination with *social* problems characteristic of all Western modernized nations. This fascination, in turn, stimulated interest in quantitative methods to a degree where virtually all significant problems were defined and described in statistical terms. Underlying the application of a quantitative methodology was the assumption that social phenomena could be explained in statistical terms. Consequently, mid-nineteenth-century science and medicine were preoccupied with the development of elaborate classification systems capable of ordering a seemingly infinite variety of facts.

While many figures contributed to the effort to explain reality in statistical terms, no one was more important than Adolphe Quetelet. Born in

Belgium in 1796, Quetelet's most enduring and significant work was in the refinement of social statistics. He was a pioneer both in establishing procedures to enhance the accuracy of national censuses and in insisting on the need for accuracy, uniformity, and comparability of data. Deterministic in his outlook, Quetelet maintained that statistical averages depended on social conditions and varied with time and place. The implications of this position were momentous; it meant that causal factors could be isolated, since a change in social conditions would be followed by a change in averages. His goal, in other words, was to reduce ostensibly chaotic social phenomena to statistical laws.[31]

Reliable generalizations, Quetelet reasoned, could only be obtained by the study of many rather than a few individuals. Herein lay the true method for all valid social research. And what could be more important than accurate censuses, which would provide a large body of uniform and comparable data to illustrate social organization and social phenomena. Were these censuses taken at regular intervals and in different places, the result would be a body of material that would ultimately give rise to precise general propositions. Statistically speaking, Quetelet wanted to use these data to determine averages and the limits of variations. The ultimate goal was to measure in a quantitative manner the relationship of two or more variable elements throughout their distribution. To be sure, Quetelet never moved beyond simple statistical averages; the discovery of the correlation coefficient had to await the work of Francis Galton and Karl Pearson at the end of the nineteenth century. Quetelet's method consisted largely of computing averages in different populations. Nevertheless, his work stimulated the collection of data and comparison of averages.[32]

The emphasis on statistical thinking had an equally profound impact upon medicine. Although Pierre Charles Alexandre Louis in 1828 had applied a numerical method to study the effects of bloodletting on pneumonia, his work was simply designed to improve treatment. No individual played a more important role in furthering the statistical analysis of disease than William Farr. In 1838 England created the Office of the Register-General, and the following year appointed Farr as chief statistician, a position he held until his retirement in 1880. In this office he became the primary architect of the British system of vital statistics and a recognized world authority. The collection and analysis of statistics on a population-wide basis, according to Farr, had the potential to uncover the laws governing human life and behavior, thus making possible the amelioration of social and medical problems. He was particularly concerned with population density, unhygienic working conditions, and an impure environment, all of which led to high mortality rates in cities. Morbidity and mortality, in other words, were as much social as medical problems.

Farr made the classification of disease the prerequisite of further medical progress. An accurate nosology made possible the collection and analysis of data on disease, which in turn could illuminate the role of environmental influences and thus explain morbidity and mortality patterns. His nosology had three major divisions. The first consisted of epidemic, endemic, and contagious diseases, including smallpox, plague, mumps, cholera, syphilis, and puerperal fever, all of which he subsumed under the heading of "zymotic." The second division was "sporadic diseases" and included localized ailments arranged under eight organ systems and subdivisions for diseases of unknown etiology and for old age. The last was for deaths by violence. Farr was primarily interested in zymotic diseases that accounted for the bulk of mortality. An understanding of their etiology, he believed, made possible the introduction of remedial measures.[33]

Although receiving some favorable comments, Farr's system also came under criticism. His first category, in particular, aroused the ire of critics. They pointed out that some diseases, including croup, diarrhea, and even cholera, might be epidemic at some times but sporadic at others; their listing under the epidemic class was misleading. Moreover, the mechanism of these diseases was not necessarily the same. The failure to make a distinction between acute and chronic disease posed another problem. In subsequent years Farr revised his nosology, but failed to get other European countries to follow his lead. Indeed, many European countries created their own nosologies. In 1893, however, the French statistician Jacques Bertillon drew up a system that became the International List of the Causes of Death, which in 1900 resulted in the publication of the first ICD (International Classification of Disease).

The creation of the ICD (which in the twentieth century has undergone no less than ten revisions) did not resolve the problem of developing clear and unambiguous diagnostic categories. Indeed, Kerr L. White has noted that there are thousands of "labels" describing the health problems that beset humanity. But there is "no coherent conceptual or organizing theme, to say nothing of theory, and yet this classification and its modifications seek to meet the needs of policy makers, statisticians, third-party payers, managers, clinicians, and investigators of all persuasions and preoccupations in a wide range of socioeconomic and cultural settings around the world."[34]

Because the United States has a divided system of government, the collection of vital statistics followed a somewhat different path. As early as 1639 the Massachusetts General Court mandated that a record be kept of all births, marriages, and deaths. The purpose of this legislation was for preservation of the community's history and for use in legal matters related to probate and responsibility for paupers. In 1842, however, the legislature created a registration system to collect vital statistics. By this time there was widespread concern with health-related issues. John H. Griscom and Lemuel Shattuck—two famous mid-nineteenth-century American sanitary reformers—published reports on conditions in New York City and Massachusetts in 1845 and 1850, respectively, which paralleled Edwin Chadwick's famous survey of the condition of the laboring class in England in 1842. In 1846 the National Medical Convention (which shortly would become the American Medical Association) adopted resolutions urging states to create more effective registration systems and calling upon the medical profession to agree on a nomenclature of diseases.[35]

The preoccupation with the collection of statistical data quickly magnified the importance of the federal government's decennial census. The U.S. Constitution provided for a national census every ten years to determine the size of the population, which then was used to allocate seats in the House of Representatives. In the early nineteenth century the census began to expand the scope of its inquiry to include business and industrial statistics. A major change came in 1850, when the new schedule included the name, age, sex, color, marital status, place of birth, occupation, and date and cause of death of every person who had died during the twelve months preceding June 1, 1850. The census of mortality, however, was fatally flawed because of a nosology that made little sense and because it missed as many as half of the deaths that actually occurred in this time period. Much the same was true of subsequent censuses.[36]

The work of such figures as Louis Pasteur in France and Robert Koch in Germany proved crucial to the emergence of a new kind of nosology. The discovery of diagnostic methods for staining bacteria or employing various specific serum reactions made it possible to establish that a series of diseases were related to the presence of distinct microorganisms. The result was the replacement of a nosography founded on anatomy by one founded on etiology. It was now possible to distinguish between infectious diseases without relying exclusively on shifting signs and symptoms.

Research on infectious diseases clarified their pathology and etiology and thus contributed to the creation of a relatively clear nosology. Most other diseases, however, were unaffected by this development. Functional disorders, for example, could not be categorized in terms of etiology. Nevertheless, they were elevated to distinct disease entities even though they continued to be described in terms of symptoms and signs. Yet symptoms and signs can be ordered in an almost infinite variety of ways. The result is that such diagnostic categories, as Knud Faber noted in a classic history of nosology, "will always be changing and will never be fixed until we know all the various factors which are concerned in producing the morbid phenomena, the external causes as well as the inherited or acquired constitution, and understand how they interact with each other." Indeed, the 1927 edition of Cecil's textbook of medicine had articles on "intestinal sand," "ephemeral fever," "chronic appendicitis," and "gastroptosis," all of which have since disappeared from subsequent medical nosologies.[37]

Consider, for example, how the understanding of blood disorders was shaped by changing technologies, physician identities, and social and political assumptions about patients and diseases. Chlorosis, splenic anemia, aplastic anemia, pernicious anemia, and sickle cell anemia were legitimate diagnostic categories at specific times, but either disappeared or were transformed by changing concepts of blood disorders and by competition among hematologists, surgeons, and oncologists, to say nothing of assumptions of the vulnerability of such groups as women, African Americans, and industrial workers, to cite only a few such examples.[38]

Other diagnoses of relatively recent vintage manifested a similar pattern. It has long been known that excessive consumption of alcohol can have serious consequences for health. Before the 1970s, however, there was little or no awareness of the concept that infants born to women who drink also can have severe health problems and disabilities. Since the 1970s, however, the diagnosis of Fetal Alcohol Syndrome (FAS) has become an accepted part of the medical nosology, and pregnant women are urged to avoid alcoholic beverages. Yet the diagnostic criteria for FAS has often been vague and at the same time expansive, and the evidence linking behavioral and developmental traits in offspring to maternal alcohol consumption is tenuous. There are no biological markers for the syndrome and no laboratory tests, and the reliability of the diagnoses among physicians is not impressive. What began as an obscure diagnosis of a set of severe birth defects among children of chronic alcoholic women during pregnancy soon was transformed into a risk assumed to threaten all pregnant women and to cause many birth defects. As a result, there are exaggerated estimates of both its incidence and the gravity of the problem. Indeed, official estimates from the Institute of Medicine and the Centers for Disease Control and Prevention (CDC) indicate that out of 4 million births per annum as few as 1,200 or as many as 12,000 children are born with FAS every year. The numbers are by no means trivial, but neither do they suggest an epidemic. Nor do they indicate that total abstinence should be the rule rather than the exception. What began as an effort to identify women whose social and physical well-being was compromised by their excessive drinking was transformed by targeting all women who were not at risk, thus neglecting the very real needs of the former.[39]

The case of FAS is by no means unique. Other newly created diagnoses, including fibromyalgia, chronic fatigue syndrome (CFS), restless legs syndrome (RLS), and autism all have similar characteristics. They are of relatively recent vintage and lack clear diagnostic criteria. All have been markedly expansive; the numbers of individuals diagnosed with them have undergone major increases. Fibromyalgia, for example, was given its name by a committee of the American College of Rheumatology in 1990. It was applied to patients who suffered widespread pain and had tender points at various sites. The diagnosis, however, lacked any pathobiology, and subsequent efforts to find one have failed. The diagnosis has appealed to pharmaceutical firms, since the potential market for such drugs as Lyrica and others nearing approval by the Food and Drug Administration (FDA) is huge. Yet Lyrica and similar drugs have severe side effects, to say nothing about long-term health effects. Advocacy groups, however, claim that as many as ten million adult Americans suffer from this disease and thus may require treatment. Dr. Fredrick Wolfe, lead author of the 1990 paper, has all but recanted the diagnosis and considers the condition to be a response to stress, depression, and anxiety. "Some of us in those days thought that we had actually identified a disease, which this is clearly not," he noted. "To make people ill, to give them an illness, was the wrong thing."[40]

Autism, CFS, and RLS, all bear a striking resemblance to fibromyalgia. Their pathobiology remains unknown, and there is little agreement on their diagnostic boundaries. Once given a name, however, the numbers given to each diagnosis have expanded exponentially. Autism is one such example. It was given its classic description by Leo Kanner in 1943. His definition, however, was quite narrow; the determining feature was "aloneness," or an inability to relate to others. Before 1990 the frequency of autism was in the range of 1 per 2,000 to 5,000. At present the CDC estimates that 1 in 150 eight-year-old children are suffering from the disease. Is this increase real, or is the diagnosis now applied to children previously labeled as retarded or learning disabled when such terms have gone out of social favor? Indeed, the concept has dramatically broadened and is now subsumed under the category of "autism spectrum disorders." Shifting diagnostic criteria also conceal from view the fact that there are benefits to parents whose children for one reason or another require special attention. "There is no firm evidence for or against a general rise in the prevalence of 'typical autism' or other autistic spectrum disorders," wrote Lorna Wing, a distinguished British psychiatrist. "The impression that there is a rise could be due to a change in referral patterns, widening of diagnostic criteria for typical autism (which are difficult to apply with precision anyway), and increased awareness of the varied manifestations of disorders in the autistic spectrum (especially those associated with higher IQ)."[41]

CFS and RLS also remain contested diagnoses. Estimates of the incidence of CFS vary in the extreme, largely because the symptoms to identify the syndrome are vague. In some surveys the CDC estimated that more than a million Americans had the illness; their more recent survey in the state of Georgia found that one in forty adults ages eighteen to fifty-nine met the diagnostic criteria—an estimate six to ten times higher than earlier rates. Another study surveyed over sixteen thousand adults over the age of eighteen and concluded that clinically significant RLS is both common and under-diagnosed. Its authors concluded that it has a prevalence rate of 2.7 percent and a significant effect upon sleep and the quality of life. Yet the diagnostic criteria for RLS are hardly specific, and some critics have argued that pharmaceutical companies have deliberately blurred the diagnostic boundaries of this syndrome in order to expand dramatically the market for their drugs. That such syndromes as CFS and RLS exist may be true, but their constantly expanding prevalence rates raise serious doubts.[42]

Nor have older diagnoses avoided being transformed by an expansion in their boundaries. The case of osteoporosis is illustrative. Before the 1990s osteoporosis was a category reserved for patients with painful fractures not associated with trauma. Since that time this category has been combined to include asymptomatic individuals with low bone density. The results of changes in the definition were dramatic. The new threshold increased the number of women ages sixty-five or older requiring treatment from 6.4 to 10.8

million and from 1.6 to 4.0 million among women ages fifty to sixty-five. The net cost of treating these additional women was $46 billion. Yet the claim that treatment (i.e., drugs) would reduce the number of fractures was hardly persuasive. The result is that more persons are diagnosed and more are treated, thus exposing them to the potential harms of treatment, to say nothing about increasing expenditures.[43]

The creation of new diagnoses and expansion of the boundaries of others have also been accompanied by the enlargement of medical jurisdiction in a variety of areas. Male aging, baldness, and sexual performance are now conditions that can presumably be treated by surgery and drugs. Attention-deficit/hyperactivity disorder (ADHD)—a diagnosis that became popular during and after the 1960s—is yet another example of a category that lacks any biopathology. Indeed, this diagnosis was originally limited to allegedly hyperactive children but was soon extended to include adults and now comes in different subtypes. Increasingly, numbers and scales become the definition of disease. Prior to World War II blood pressure readings of 120/80 were regarded as normal, and it was assumed that such readings rose with age. A half century later hypertension was redefined in terms of a broader syndrome, and a reading of 140/90 became the threshold for treatment. Indeed, pharmaceutical companies have recently promoted a new category of "prehypertension," defined as a reading of 120/80 or more. Similarly, desirable cholesterol levels have constantly been lowered. Shifting numbers, of course, result in a dramatic expansion of the population requiring treatment, supposedly to prevent a series of other related conditions.[44]

More recently some physicians and scientists have begun to argue in favor of a nosology that defines disease not in terms of symptoms or physiological measurements, but rather in terms of the genes associated with them. "Recent progress in genetics and genomics," according to a group of scientists, "has led to an appreciation of the effects of gene mutations in virtually all disorders and provides the opportunity to study human diseases all at once rather than one at a time." Such an approach, they concluded, "offers the possibility of discerning general patterns and principles of human disease not readily apparent from the study of individual disorders."[45]

Nowhere is the creation of diagnoses better illustrated than in the specialty of psychiatry. Although debates dealing with the classification of mental disorders are phrased in scientific and medical language, they are shaped by a multiplicity of factors: the ideological, political, and moral commitments of psychiatrists; their desire for status and legitimacy; the characteristics of their patients; the nature and location of their practices; the organization and structure of the specialty; broader social, intellectual currents; and the economic elements prevalent at a given time. These generalizations are illustrated in the creation and subsequent revisions of the *Diagnostic and Statistical Manual of Mental Disorders,* better known as the *DSM.* The first edition appeared in 1952, and it has undergone fundamental revisions in succeeding decades. Although its diagnostic categories are widely accepted, a careful analysis suggests that many of them have a slippery foundation without much evidence to support their existence.

In psychiatry, as in medicine, classification systems play a crucial role. They represent the prevailing consensus within the profession and facilitate communication with patients. Equally important, they play a critical part in the collection and analysis of quantitative data, which presumably leads to greater knowledge and understanding of diseases and therapy as well as the social and physical environment and human behavioral patterns. Yet classification systems are neither inherently self-evident nor given. On the contrary, they emerge from the crucible of human experience; change and variability, not immutability, are characteristic. Indeed, the manner in which data are organized at various times reflects specific historical circumstances. Empirical data, after all, can be presented and analyzed in seemingly endless ways.

The history of psychiatric classification offers a fascinating case study of how diagnoses come into existence. In nineteenth-century America alienists (the name that existed before the term "psychiatrist" came into use) were for the most part uninterested in elaborate nosologies. They identified mental disorders by observing external signs and symptoms. In their eyes elaborate classification systems were of little utility and could not encompass the protean symptoms of insanity. Moreover, they believed that therapy was independent of any nosological system and had to reflect the unique circumstances presented by each person. Occasionally, psychiatrists debated the validity of specific categories such as moral insanity (a condition in which there was a morbid perversion of the emotions but little or no impairment of the intellect), but this was the exception rather than rule. Isaac Ray, the most influential psychiatrist of that era, denied that any classification could be "rigorously correct, for such divisions have not been made by nature and cannot be observed in practice." At best, he wrote, insanity could be divided into two groups. The first—idiocy and imbecility—was composed of individuals with congenital defects. The second encompassed those in whom lesions had impaired the functioning of the mind and included mania and dementia.[46]

If psychiatrists recognized that nosology was not critical to clinical practice, they were cognizant of its role in the collection of statistical data. In the nineteenth century a number of concerns had given rise to a new type of social inquiry whose methodological distinctiveness was a commitment to statistical research. Underlying the commitment to quantification was the assumption that such a methodology could illuminate and explain social phenomena. The collection of such data, of course, required categories. Most of the psychiatric categories employed dealt with the demographic characteristics of patients as well as admission and discharge rates; nosology occupied a distinctly subordinate position.

The intellectual and scientific constraints that inhibited the development of psychiatric nosology persisted for much of the nineteenth century. When Pliny Earle, another major figure in American psychiatry, was queried in 1886 about the possibility of developing a universally accepted classification of mental diseases, he replied in negative terms. "In the present state of our knowledge," he wrote, "no classification of insanity can be erected on a pathological basis . . . [since] the pathology of the disease is unknown. . . . [W]e are forced to fall back on the symptoms of the disease—*the apparent mental condition,* as judged from the outward manifestations." The traditional categories of mania, monomania, dementia, and idiocy, therefore, still sufficed.[47]

Toward the end of the nineteenth century interest in psychiatric nosology reawakened as clinicians began to shift their attention to the course and outcome of mental disorders. Emil Kraepelin, the famous and influential German psychiatrist, in particular, singled out groups of signs as evidencing specific disease entities such as dementia praecox and, later, manic depressive psychosis. Dealing with a large mass of patient data, he sorted out what individuals had in common, and thus diverted attention away from their unique circumstances toward more general and presumably disease entities.[48] In so doing he was simply emulating a distinct trend in medical thinking, where the specific germ theory had led in part to the creation of an etiologically based nosology.

The Kraepelinian emphasis on nosology was not immediately accepted in the United States; nosological uncertainty persisted. Both Henry J. Berkley and Stewart Paton, in their psychiatric textbooks, conceded that classification in psychiatry and medicine differed; the former specialty could not create an etiologically based system. Moreover, a classification based on clinical symptoms was unsatisfactory because the indications of one form of disease overlapped others. Indeed, the growing preoccupation with classification led Charles G. Hill in 1907 to observe that there was little room for addition "unless we add 'the classifying mania of medical authors.'"[49]

The American Medico-Psychological Association (subsequently renamed the American Psychiatric Association) in collaboration with the National Committee for Mental Hygiene in 1918 issued the first standardized psychiatric nosology. Oddly enough, the driving force behind its publication was the Bureau of the Census, which had earlier begun to expand its collection of statistics pertaining to insanity. The bureau found that a lack of psychiatric diagnostic categories hampered its work. The publication of the *Statistical Manual for the Use of Institutions for the Insane* reflected the belief that mental disorders had a biological foundation. It divided mental disorders into twenty-two principal groups, of which only the psychoneuroses and neuroses were not in the somatic category.[50] This *Statistical Manual* guided psychiatric classification in the United States until the development of the first *DSM* in 1952.

To be sure, the adoption of a uniform psychiatric nosology was not without critics. Adolf Meyer, one of the most prominent psychiatrists of the early twentieth century and a member of the Committee on Statistics, refused to be identified with the nosology and thought that the published statistics were worthless. Samuel Orton was equally critical and he argued that the *Statistical Manual* was too narrow, illogical, and inconsistent.[51] Nevertheless, the *Statistical Manual* became the definitive nosology of the interwar years and went through no fewer than ten editions between 1918 and 1942. The first seven editions incorporated minor changes; the latter three had more extensive modifications. The tenth edition made provision for the psychoneuroses and primary behavior disorders in children but continued to emphasize the somatic viewpoint.[52]

World War II marked a major watershed in the history of American psychiatry and mental health policy. Many found that psychiatric disorders were a more serious problem than had previously been recognized, that environmental stress associated with combat contributed to mental maladjustment, and that early and purposeful treatment in noninstitutional settings produced favorable outcomes. These beliefs became the basis for postwar claims that early identification of symptoms and treatment in community settings could prevent the onset of more serious mental disorders and thus obviate the need for prolonged institutionalization. The war reshaped psychiatry by attracting into the specialty a substantial number of younger physicians whose outlook, molded by their wartime experiences, was based on psychodynamic and psychoanalytic concepts. After the war many of these psychiatrists assumed leadership positions and fought to reorganize and energize the American Psychiatric Association (APA), insisted that their specialty assume an activist role in solving many social problems, and attempted to forge new policies that broke with the traditional consensus on the need for prolonged hospitalization of persons with serious mental disorders.[53]

During the 1940s dissatisfaction with the *Statistical Manual* began to mount. Military and Veterans Administration psychiatrists found themselves using a nomenclature ill-adapted for many of their patients. Minor personality disturbances—many of which were of importance only because they occurred within a military context—were placed in the "psychopathic personality" category. Soldiers suffering from symptoms related to combat stress were placed in the "psychoneurotic" category. There was virtually no recognition of psychosomatic disorders. Indeed, by the end of the war both the army and navy had created their own classification.[54]

The nosological confusion, proliferation of nomenclatures, and shift toward psychodynamic and psychoanalytic concepts led the APA Committee on Nomenclature and Statistics in 1948 to propose changes in its manual. By 1950 it had prepared a revised psychiatric nosology, which was widely circulated in mimeograph form and then presented to the APA Council for approval. In 1952 the APA formally published what subsequently became known as *DSM-I*.[55]

DSM-I reflected the intellectual, cultural, and social forces that had transformed psychiatry during and after World War II and that were characteristic of American society at this time. It divided mental disorders into two major groupings. The first represented cases in which the disturbed mental function resulted from or was precipitated by a primary impairment of brain function. The second encompassed disorders resulting from a more general inability of the individual to adjust, in which brain function disturbance was secondary to the psychiatric illness. In effect, *DSM-I* represented a shift away from a somatic nosology and toward a psychodynamic and psychoanalytic nosology and mirrored the dominance of the latter. By themselves the new diagnostic categories did little to transform the practice of psychiatry. But they did suggest that the original purpose of the *Statistical Manual*—to collect statistical data that would serve as the basis of policy—was being transformed.[56] In subsequent decades, as we shall see, changing diagnostic categories, transformation of the mental health occupations, rise of third-party payers, and growing prominence of pharmaceutical companies would combine to reshape psychiatric practice and therapy.

The *DSM-III,* which the APA issued in 1980, radically changed the nature of psychiatric diagnoses. During the 1960s and 1970s the psychiatric profession had undergone a serious crisis of legitimacy. The psychosocial model of mental illness that was preeminent after World War II and that was embodied in the *DSM-II* did not value precise diagnoses, and its diagnostic categories were very general, cursory, and etiologically based in psychodynamics. Neither clinicians nor researchers could reliably use such definitions. Consequently, psychiatric classifications of mental illnesses were idiosyncratic and varied widely among individual diagnosticians.[57] The unreliability of such diagnostic criteria subjected the psychiatric profession to much criticism and even ridicule.[58] Moreover, the psychosocial model did not provide a solid grounding for why psychiatrists—as opposed to many other professionals, including clinical psychologists, counselors, social workers, or nurses—should have professional dominance over the treatment of mental illnesses. Psychiatrists had no more expertise about social conditions or talk therapy than their many other competitors. Psychiatry, which in the twentieth century had a shaky position within the prestige hierarchy in medicine, was in danger of losing its legitimacy as a scientific discipline.

To deal with this dire situation, a group of research-oriented psychiatrists led by Robert Spitzer of Columbia University's College of Physicians and Surgeons concluded that only clear, precise, and reproducible definitions of the entities it studied, comparable to those studied in other branches of medicine, could serve as the foundation for a truly scientific discipline. They explicitly contrasted their scientific approach, which they claimed was rooted in empirically supported facts, to what they characterized as the unprovable theories of the psychoanalysts who had dominated the earlier *DSM-I* and *DSM-II.*

The empiricists controlled the development of the new edition of the official diagnostic manual, the *DSM-III.* This manual replaced the amorphous conditions of psychodynamic psychiatry with several hundred specific definitions of various types of mental illnesses that relied on the characteristics symptoms of each entity.[59] Because of the empiricists' desire to purge the psychodynamic assumptions from the new manual, a core principle of the *DSM-III* was that these definitions could not assume any particular etiology of symptoms. The *DSM-III* replaced etiologically based diagnoses with symptom-based diagnoses as its central classificatory principle. Symptom-based measures were especially valuable because they could easily produce high reliability—unlike the situation in the previous manuals, different psychiatrists examining the same patient would derive the same diagnosis. Such reliability was seen as a way to silence the critics who claimed that psychiatry was not even able to measure the entities it claimed to study and treat. In addition, this strategy allowed these researchers to claim theoretical neutrality as well as gain support from clinicians who held a broad range of orientations. Since 1980, psychiatric research and practice has focused on the hundreds of specific, symptom-based diagnostic categories that the *DSM-III* first enumerated.

The political dynamics that surrounded the creation of the *DSM-III* required the transformation of anxiety from the key process in psychoneuroses to a variety of narrowly defined and distinct disorders. The new classification system carved anxiety, which had been the central component of all of the psychoneuroses in the *DSM-I* and *DSM-II,* into numerous discrete forms: agoraphobia with or without panic attacks, obsessive-compulsive disorder, simple phobia, social phobia, panic disorder, generalized anxiety disorder, post-traumatic stress disorder, and atypical anxiety disorder. The nature of their symptoms, not any underlying etiological process, defined each of these discrete conditions.[60] The new manual gave psychoneuroses that featured purely somatic symptoms a separate category of somatoform disorders. Likewise, it subsumed depressive symptoms under a distinct category of affective disorders. Subsequently, each of the discrete anxiety disorders became the focus of research, publication, teaching, therapy, and professional careers.

The *DSM-III* was also a major factor propelling depression into the forefront of outpatient diagnoses. Prior to 1980, little consensus existed on how many forms of depression existed, whether endogenous and exogenous conditions were similar or different, if the disorder was continuous or categorical, or how depression was related to other kinds of psychoneurotic disorders.[61] At a stroke, the *DSM-III* swept aside these categories and defined major depressive disorder (MDD) as consisting of at least five of nine specific symptoms, at least one of which must be a depressed mood or an inability to experience pleasure. Anyone who displayed these symptoms for a two-week period was considered to have a depressive disorder, with the exception of bereaved people, as long as their symptoms did not persist beyond two months or were not of extreme severity. Unlike the anxiety category, which was carved into numerous specific entities, MDD was clearly the central diagnosis of the mood disorders. This classification, along with the later development of new classes of psychotropic drugs that were called anti-depressants, paved the way for depression rather than anxiety to become the central condition that the psychiatric profession treated subsequent to the *DSM-III*.

Post-traumatic stress disorder (PTSD) also indicates the power of psychiatric classification to shape, rather than reflect, the nature of patient conditions. Before the *DSM-III* no diagnostic category existed that could encompass the conditions of people who had long-term symptoms that resulted from experiencing traumatic stressors. A group of disgruntled Vietnam veterans and their allies in the psychiatric profession were able to gain control over the process of defining PTSD in the *DSM-III*.[62] The resulting classification, along with the subsequent changes implemented in the *DSM-II-R* (1987) and *DSM-IV* (1994), led to a vast expansion of people with this diagnosis. From its initial conception as a diagnosis that would allow Vietnam veterans with long-standing psychiatric conditions to receive treatment and compensation, it expanded to encompass victims of sexual violence and then to a wide range of natural and human-made disasters. Ultimately, the diagnosis has come to include not just people who have experienced a trauma, but also even those who have heard about or watched a traumatic event on television. PTSD, perhaps more than any other psychiatric diagnosis, has become infused with moral meanings and has been the site of intense disputes between groups of proponents and detractors of this condition.

Despite the great uncertainties that underlie psychiatric diagnoses, they are widely considered to reflect empirical findings and psychiatric knowledge. The chapters on anxiety, depression, and PTSD illustrate the key role of a variety of professional and non-professional interest groups in shaping the classification of disease. The configuration of these groups at any particular time shapes the extent to which symptoms will be defined as natural or as pathological. While the framework of debates regarding these conditions is usually phrased in scientific rhetoric, at bottom the debates reflect ongoing controversies about the nature and causes of human suffering.

Conclusion

To delineate the respective roles of rhetoric and reality is not to denigrate either medicine or the health care system. It is rather to point to factors that both shape and distort the nature and practice of medicine. Etiological theories that have little or no basis in fact, diagnoses that lack reliability or validity, and therapies whose efficacy is at best problematic and at worst dangerous are all too common. Yet they receive considerable publicity and are widely accepted. Responsibility for such a situation rests with a variety of individuals, groups, and organizations: a public all too prone to accept exaggerated claims; a media establishment that publicizes new therapeutic "miracles" without examining the quality of supporting evidence; a pharmaceutical industry intent upon marketing drugs irrespective of their efficacy, to say nothing about questionable ethical practices in providing allegedly accurate information and efforts to co-opt physicians; and a medical establishment that is constantly expanding its jurisdictional domain by pathologizing behaviors and advancing unrealistic claims.

The consequences of such developments are by no means trivial. Many individuals are on drug regimens for diagnoses that are at best problematic or for diseases that they do not have. Recently, the leading organization of pediatricians recommended lifelong regimes of cholesterol-lowering drugs for children as young as eight years old, despite the absence of evidence that such practices in any way lower the risk of future heart disease.[63] Dubious etiological and epidemiological claims lead to behavioral recommendations that have little or no basis in fact. Surgical rates vary in the extreme, depending on the number of specialists in a given geographical area. Moreover, for many surgical procedures evidence of efficacy is lacking. To be sure, the American health care system provides many benefits. Yet the overall record, despite massive expenditures, hardly supports the claim that the United States has the best system.

The case studies in this volume illustrate some of these generalizations. We could have, of course, selected others of a more positive nature. But it is our belief that far greater attention has to be paid to some of the deficiencies and shortcomings of the American health care system while at the same time conceding its strengths. Our goal is not to denigrate but rather to present a constructive analysis that might lead to beneficial changes.

Chapter 2

Medical Rivalry and Etiological Speculation

The Case of Peptic Ulcer

In the early twentieth century peptic ulcer aroused the attention of physicians and, especially, surgeons, many of whom believed that its incidence was on the rise. Initially, surgery became the cutting-edge therapy. But it was quickly followed by claims that diet or psychological intervention could best treat the condition. Rivalry between competing specialties thus became characteristic despite the fact that evidence demonstrating the efficacy of each was weak to nonexistent. At the same time theoretical explanations about etiology that had little to do with therapy proliferated. The history of peptic ulcer in the twentieth century suggests that theories and therapies often had little to do with science.

Dyspepsia—a synonym for indigestion—preceded the diagnosis of peptic ulcer. Before the twentieth century dyspepsia was a broad if somewhat vague category; its symptoms included gastric pain, nausea, vomiting, heartburn, and esophageal reflux. For centuries it was regarded as a byproduct of immoderate diets and gluttony. Dyspepsia thus retained an ambivalent character; it was a behavioral and moral problem as well as a medical diagnosis. In the absence of a technology capable of visualizing the interior of the human body, dyspepsia remained an inclusive diagnosis and was the subject of unending human complaint.

During the nineteenth century, however, dyspepsia slowly receded in importance as more specific diagnoses—one of which was gastric or peptic ulcer—entered the medical nosology. In 1857 William Brinton, an English physician, published one of the early descriptions of stomach ulcer. He was not the first to do so, but his work was by far the most comprehensive ever written to that time. Whereas such figures as William Beaumont in the United States and Johann Eberle and Theodor Schwann in Europe had investigated gastric secretion, Brinton approached gastric ulcer from a clinical perspective. He had performed a substantial number of autopsies and had confirmed his conclusions by comparing his findings with necropsy data of other physicians. Stomach ulcers, he noted, were found in 2 to 13 percent of persons dying from all causes. Accurately describing the lesion, Brinton delineated its symptoms, which included pain, vomiting, and hemorrhage.

Conceding that the etiology of stomach ulcer was unknown, Brinton nevertheless offered his own conjectures. "Old age, privation, fatigue, mental anxiety, and intemperance are such frequent coincidents of its occurrence, that we are fully entitled to regard them as its more or less immediate causes in a large proportion (I think we might say in a majority) of cases." The origins of ulceration, he added in somewhat contradictory terms, remained shrouded in mystery. Brinton was also concerned with treatment. He rejected bleeding, promoted the application of cold by means of ice, favored opiates and bismuth for the relief of pain and diarrhea, and recommended the use of the alkaline carbonates to neutralize "the lactic and other acids developed by gastric decomposition." Diet was also important. He urged sufferers to avoid large meals, meat, hot food or drinks, irritating substances, and recommended instead a bland diet of "soft pulpy" food and milk.[1]

The influence of Brinton's work is difficult to ascertain. Peptic ulcer, his book notwithstanding, aroused relatively little interest among physicians, if only because of its seemingly low incidence. More important, physicians had no means of visualizing the interior of the stomach and thus arriving at an accurate diagnosis. In the first edition of his magisterial text in 1893, Sir William Osler thought that post-mortem data overestimated the incidence of peptic ulcer.[2] The first edition of the *Merck Manual* in 1899 also made no mention of peptic ulcer, but instead included Dyspepsia, Acidity, Biliousness, Flatulence, Gastralgia, and Pyrosis.[3]

After 1900 there was a growing consensus within medicine that the incidence of peptic ulcer was on the rise and that it was far more prevalent than previously believed. Whether or not this claim was accurate is difficult to ascertain; surviving data are unreliable. What is clear is that a series of developments had enhanced the ability to diagnose peptic ulcer, thus making it possible to identify more cases. During the previous half century, knowledge about the physiology of gastric secretion had increased dramatically. New technologies also played a major role. Walter B. Cannon was among the first to make use of the recent discovery of X-rays by Wilhelm Roentgen in 1895. By administering barium sulphate, Cannon was able to study the movements of the esophagus and stomach, and ultimately this technique was employed to assist in the diagnosis of peptic ulcer. Radiology remained the primary means of diagnosis until the mid-1930s, when it was supplemented by endoscopy.[4]

The deployment of such technologies resulted in a sharp increase in the number of people diagnosed with peptic ulcer. In the eighth edition of his text in 1916, Osler conceded that the disease was "much more common than medical and pathological statistics indicate." In 1930 Arthur Dean Bevan, a surgeon who also played an important role in the transformation of medical education, estimated that peptic ulcer occurred in at least 10 to 12 percent of the population.[5] The pioneering National Health Survey of 1935, conducted by the Public Health Service, found that peptic ulcer ranked tenth as a cause of death, twelfth as a cause of days lost from work, and fourteenth as a cause of invalidism. Between 1900 and 1943 mortality from peptic ulcer rose from 2.8 to 6.8 per thousand (although it must be remembered that the data pertaining to the causes of mortality are notoriously inaccurate). Throughout most of the twentieth century, hundreds of articles dealing with peptic ulcer were published annually in medical journals. In a survey conducted in 1946, the American Gastroenterological Association found more than seven hundred research projects, involving more than five hundred investigators, having to do with peptic ulcer.[6]

Peptic Ulcer as a Surgical Disease

The growing concern with peptic ulcer paralleled significant changes in the medical profession. The discovery of anesthesia, the development of antiseptic techniques, and the ability to visualize the internal workings of bodily organisms contributed to a dramatic expansion of surgery. The transformation of medicine and medical education and the emergence of the modern hospital combined to elevate surgery—which historically had a relatively low status in medicine—to a preeminent position in medicine. Indeed, surgical therapies became the cutting edge, and surgeons the elite of the medical profession.

It was no accident that surgeons played a key role in the diagnosis and treatment of gastric ulcer. In 1881 Theodor Billroth developed a surgical technique to obviate pyloric obstruction caused by cancer and, subsequently, applied his procedure to the treatment of peptic ulcer. No individual, however, played a more important role in popularizing surgical intervention than

Berkeley G. A. Moynihan, an English surgeon who helped to define his specialty. The publication of his book *Abdominal Operations* in 1905 gave him an international reputation because, in the words of a colleague, it "literally threw open the abdomen to all surgeons."[7] Moynihan's primary interest lay in the peritoneal cavity, and the focus of his book was on gastric and duodenal ulcers, gall bladder and pancreatic diseases, and hernias. In the past, he wrote, dyspepsia was regarded as a functional disorder of the stomach, duodenum, gall bladder, or appendix. The surgeon's contribution was to demonstrate that derangements of the stomach and other organs were caused by organic diseases.[8] Indeed, Moynihan's redefinition of gastric and duodenal ulcers was perhaps the basis for the claims that the disease was on the increase and constituted a virtual epidemic.

Moynihan devoted about seventy-five pages or 11 percent of *Abdominal Operations* to surgery for gastric and duodenal ulcers. Perforation, he wrote, "is one the most serious and most overwhelming catastrophes that can befall a human being . . . and unless surgical measures are adopted early, the disease hastens to a fatal ending in almost every instance." Of his first twenty-two cases, fourteen recovered and eight died. In cases of hemorrhage, Moynihan offered two recommendations. The first and preferred method was to search for the ulcer and deal with it directly by excision, ligation, or cauterization. The second was to perform a gastroenterostomy (connecting the stomach with the small intestine), which, he claimed, would empty the stomach and permit healing to occur. Moynihan also described several other surgical procedures (including gastroduodenostomy) to deal with chronic gastric ulcer.[9]

One of Moynihan's most important contributions was to call attention to the prevalence of duodenal ulcer. Unlike gastric ulcer, duodenal ulcer had long been neglected, partly because of the difficulty of distinguishing its symptoms from the complaints of the dyspeptic patient. Moynihan correlated symptoms with his observations of the duodenum during surgery and concluded that the symptoms of gastric and duodenal ulcer differed. The latter was characterized by delayed pain, which could be relieved by food, milk, or alkaline salts in water; the former by immediate pain, which could not be easily relieved. In Moynihan's opinion, surgery was the appropriate remedy for both duodenal and chronic gastric ulcer. "I do not know of any operation in surgery which gives better results, which gives more satisfaction both to the patient and his surgeon than gastroenterostomy for chronic ulcer of the stomach," he wrote in 1903. Similarly, he recommended that the treatment of a chronic duodenal ulcer "should always be surgical."

He also reported impressive outcome results. Between 1900 and 1908, 186 patients underwent surgery (overwhelmingly gastroenterostomy). Only four deaths (2.15 percent) were recorded. Follow-up reports from patients or their physicians indicated that 144 were cured. It should be noted, however, that Moynihan's data were not based upon longitudinal follow-up of patients who had undergone surgery.[10]

For nearly two decades gastroenterostomy remained the most common surgical procedure in the treatment of gastric ulcer; failures were attributed to faulty techniques. By the mid-1920s, however, it began to become clear that claims about its efficacy had been grossly overstated. The absence of longitudinal studies concealed the lag between the initial surgery and relapse as well as the failure to reduce acidity. Moreover, gastroenterostomy had serious side effects. Surgeons therefore turned their attention to the pyloric valve and developed a group of operations that would hasten emptying of the stomach and thus presumably promote rapid neutralization of stomach acid. Although gastroduodenostomy had many of the same defects as gastroenterostomy, the shortcomings of these dramatic therapies did not discourage those who believed that gastric ulcer mandated surgery.

During the first half of the twentieth century, numerous other surgical procedures were introduced in the hope of curing or, at the least, managing ulcers by reducing acidity. In 1930 a leading surgical journal published nine articles in a single issue, all of which reported low mortality and high improvement rates following surgical treatment of ulcers.[11]

What kinds of evidence justified claims of therapeutic efficacy? Admittedly, the evaluation of surgical therapies presents formidable methodological problems. For much of the twentieth century, there was no consensus on how to evaluate therapies or what constituted a systematic study, or even a methodology to determine efficacy. At that time the concept of a double-blind randomized controlled trial (RCT) was unknown. Yet the application of RCTs to surgical therapies was and is often problematic. Should a control group be composed of individuals undergoing sham operations (an ethically dubious procedure)? Or should the group be composed of untreated persons? Even at present, the RCT—the "gold standard" by which therapeutic efficacy is measured—has significant problems.

A century ago, the medical world differed in many ways from its contemporary counterpart. There was little or no awareness of the importance of population-based data and their relationship to individual decision making; practitioners weighed evidence overwhelmingly in terms of their own clinical experience. The individualistic culture characteristic of American medicine reinforced the belief that clinical experience was the critical element in determining therapeutic efficacy.[12] Data pertaining to the efficacy of surgical and nonsurgical therapies as well as mortality were generated from the records of individual practitioners. Nor was the concept of observer bias acknowledged. This is not in any way to suggest that clinical experience and anecdotal cases are necessarily worthless or unscientific. After all, penicillin and cortisone entered the medical armamentarium in the absence of RCTs. In surgery, such procedures as appendectomy and others are performed on the basis that they are effective in light of available evidence. Nevertheless, it is clear that clinical judgment, however important, may not be adequate to evaluate all therapies, surgical and others.

By mid-century a growing appreciation of the importance of methodological issues was evident. In a classic summation of knowledge of peptic ulcer in 1950, Andrew C. Ivy and his colleagues identified no less than seventeen different surgical procedures employed in the treatment of peptic ulcer. Yet, as they pointed out, most studies of the recurrence rates of ulcer employed patients "as their own control without giving the recurrence rate of the patient prior to the application of treatment." Nor was there a clear definition of "a recurrence, or a satisfactory or unsatisfactory result."[13]

Even before RCTs came into existence, surgery for peptic ulcer was beginning to come under scrutiny because of its risks and subsequent complications. Indeed, the absence of a consensus on the value of surgery was demonstrated by the existence of sharp differences in the frequency of hospital referrals to surgery. "In some cases," noted Ivy and colleagues, "all ulcer patients are subjected to surgery; in others, only those patients who do not respond well to medical management." Medical facilities often had very different therapeutic styles. The Mayo Clinic in Minnesota—an institution created by brothers trained as surgeons—referred 45 to 65 percent of its patients with gastric ulcer to surgery in the ten-year period beginning in 1935; surgical treatment for duodenal ulcer declined from 26 percent in 1920 to 12 percent in 1944. During the same period, by contrast, 6 percent of duodenal and 19 percent of gastric ulcers were referred to surgery at the Lahey Clinic in Boston. At the Brigham Hospital in Boston only 7 percent were treated surgically. Ivy and his colleagues emphasized that most studies of surgical successes were based on a deeply flawed methodology.[14] "The consensus of opinion," Russell S. Boles remarked at the convention of the American Medical Association (AMA) in 1947, "is that peptic ulcer is a medical problem and that operations should be reserved for the familiar complications of perforation, hemorrhage, obstruction and so-called intractability."[15]

Despite significant mortality rates and postoperative problems that followed gastrectomy, the search for the ideal gastric surgical procedure did not in any way diminish. The introduction of vagotomy in the early 1950s (first in combination with partial gastric resection, then with pyloroplasty, and finally selective vagotomy) appeared to minimize the risks and complications that followed the numerous surgical procedures developed to treat peptic ulcer. Medical treatment for benign gastric ulcer, O. Theron Clagett insisted in 1971, was far more dangerous than surgical treatment. Moreover, disability time was less, and lasting good clinical outcomes were three times more frequent. "It seems obvious," he concluded, "that a majority of ulcerating gastric lesions can be dealt with most effectively by surgical means or indeed will require surgery."[16]

Inertia, combined with the fact that those who entered surgical specialties were predisposed to employ their skills, combined to reinforce the belief in the superiority of surgical treatment. Nevertheless, an element of disquiet persisted. "At present," noted one surgeon, "considerable difference of opinion exists as the choice of operation,"[17] a view shared by others.[18] Nor did the introduction of RCTs resolve differences. In a review of trials dealing with the treatment of duodenal ulcer in the period from 1964 to 1974, three Danish physicians found that many were poorly designed. The contributions to knowledge of the various treatments were "rather small, and the information obtained from the best RCT's has had practically no impact on current therapeutic practice, which is predominantly based on uncontrolled observations."[19] While debates over the relative merits of different forms of surgery continued unabated, its dominant position in the medical armamentarium for nearly three quarters of a century diminished but little until the introduction of alternative means of managing peptic ulcer.

Challenges to Surgical Treatment

The early dominance of surgical treatment of peptic ulcer did not forestall challenges by those who believed that medical treatment and diet could result in more favorable outcomes and thus avoid the trauma and risks associated with surgery. By the latter part of the nineteenth century there was growing interest in the role of gastric secretion in ulcer formation. Studies of digestion, secretion, and emptying of the stomach had led to the realization that extreme acidification of the gastric juice, if not the cause of ulcer, surely played a role in its persistence. Indeed, Karl Schwarz's famous statement in 1910—"No acid, no ulcer"[20]—led to the abandonment of bypass operations and the substitution of partial (or occasionally full) gastrectomy, a procedure that had become the gold standard for surgical treatment of ulcers by the 1930s, but one that created what subsequently became known as "gastric cripples."

If acid reduction or neutralization was a major objective in the treatment of gastric and duodenal ulcer, could not it be achieved by less invasive therapies? One answer to this provocative question was provided by Bertram W. Sippy, a Chicago physician whose name became synonymous with the non-surgical treatment of gastric ulcer. Sippy was not opposed to surgery. Secondary carcinoma, perforation into the peritoneal cavity, pyloric obstruction, perigrastric abscess, and copious hemorrhage, he conceded, required surgical treatment. In the vast majority of cases, however, medical treatment was indicated, and he rejected the practice of indiscriminate gastroenterostomy.[21]

Ulcers, Sippy suggested in a famous paper delivered at the annual meeting of the AMA in 1914, developed when the mucous membrane of the stomach or adjacent duodenum lost its normal resistance to the peptic action of the gastric juice and became digested. His approach was to protect the ulcer from gastric juice corrosion until the ulcer healed. In 1912 he thought that microorganisms played a "very slight" role in the genesis of ulcer. The influence of the specific germ theory of diseases, however, proved irresistible. Hence, several years later he came to the conclusion that a streptococcal infection was probably "the most common factor in the production of the local malnutrition and necrosis." A gastric or duodenal ulcer would normally heal as rapidly as an ulcer located elsewhere, were its granulating surfaces "not subjected to the digestive action of the gastric juice."[22]

From Sippy's perspective, it was clear that treatment had to shield the ulcer from the corrosive effect of the gastric juice. Neutralization of hydrochloric acid required frequent feedings and the use of alkalies. His recommended regimen commenced with three to four weeks of bed rest. Patients drank a mixture of three ounces of milk and cream hourly. Their diet included a variety of such soft and palatable foods as jellies, custards, cream, eggs, cereals, and vegetable purees. Alkalies were taken midway between feedings. In addition, aspiration of the stomach at stipulated intervals and before sleep provided the physician with a guide to treatment and ensured that the patient would not be troubled by excessive acidity. Sippy noted that prevailing therapies and surgical procedures did little to protect the ulcer from gastric acid. Medical management of peptic ulcer, he wrote, "protects the pyloric and

duodenal ulcer from gastric juice corrosion, and thus renders gastro-enteros-
tomy combined with pyloric occlusion unnecessary."[23]

The Sippy regimen was by no means unique. In 1876, W. O. Leube had
proposed bed rest and a circumscribed diet that included no food by mouth
for the first week and a limited diet of 350 and 1,200 calories per day thereafter. Others felt that Leube's regimen weakened the patient and proposed sharp
modifications. Osler believed in "absolute bed rest" and a bland diet, while
noting that medicinal measures were of "very little value." Sippy's approach,
however, differed from previous treatments in two significant ways: the large
amounts of alkalies and the specific timing, dosage, and administration of
food and medications. The underlying theory was that gastric juice, by virtue
of its peptic activity, hindered healing. Hence diet could be employed as a
weapon to eliminate peptic activity by neutralizing the hydrochloric acid in
the gastric juice. A variety of dietary innovations followed, including continuous intragastric milk drip as well as bland diets that presumably were
less "irritating."[24]

In addition to diet and rest, the medical armamentarium included the
use of a wide variety of drugs. Some controlled bleeding; some vomiting;
some alleviated pain and restlessness; and others neutralized acid. They
included such substances as aluminum potassium sulfate, Fowler's solution (potassium arsenite), tannic and carbolic acids, bismuth subnitrate and
subcarbonite, magnesium carbonate, rescorcin, calcium carbonate and phos-
phate, hyoscyamus, phenobarbital, tincture of belladonna, morphine sulfate
and hydryochlorate, cocaine, codeine, and silver nitrate. Some had specific
pharmacological rationales; belladonna, for example, inhibited acid secretion. Some were older drugs that had worked their way into medical practice
a century or more earlier and were used for a large variety of illnesses. Others were more recent additions that grew out of the experience of individual
practitioners who claimed to have found them effective in the treatment of
peptic ulcer. Information about their use was widely disseminated in the
medical press.

Under these circumstances, therapeutic eclecticism remained the rule
rather than the exception. In 1929, C. S. Danzer maintained that gastric ulcer
was a generalized systemic disturbance that resulted from a sluggish capillary circulation. Focal infections merely aggravated such a condition, and
he recommended appendectomy. He also maintained that procedures that
increased capillary circulation, including hydrotherapy, ultraviolet light,
and X-ray therapy, were especially effective. Nor were such recommendations

idiosyncratic. The 1940 edition of the *Merck Manual* listed roentgenotherapy, diathermy, and vaccine therapy as effective remedies for peptic ulcer.[25]

Each of the two therapeutic approaches to gastric and duodenal ulcer treatment—surgery and medical management—had their supporters. At the extremes were those who rejected any therapy except their own and insisted that outcome data supported their position. Indeed, at times the rivalry between surgeons and internists became fierce. Moynihan, for example, believed that medical treatment "has failed in its essential aim, the permanent healing of ulcer." Medical interventions were "too often haphazard and perfunctory," and few patients followed instructions pertaining to rest and diet. Nor could medical treatment prevent recurrences, often in catastrophic form. Indeed, mortality was "far greater than with surgical treatment." Although not ruling out medical treatment, Moynihan concluded that the "successes of surgery are won from the failures of medicine."[26]

In 1930 Frank H. Lahey, one of the nation's most prominent surgeons, called for reforms that would mitigate "the surgical and medical rivalry that has existed in the management of duodenal and gastric ulcer." Both approaches yielded comparable results. The indications for surgery, he added, included "failure to obtain relief under medical management, perforation, hemorrhage in spite of good nonoperative management, nonrelievable pyloric obstruction, and malignant degeneration or suspicion of it on a gastric ulcer."[27] Like Lahey, many physicians were uncomfortable with extremists on either side, and they left room for a combination of surgical and medical therapies. In general, however, surgeons and internists tended to reflect their training: the former were likely to recommend surgery, and the latter to lean toward medical management.

How could the competing claims of therapeutic efficacy be measured? So long as outcomes were measured by the same physicians who treated patients, it was difficult to determine efficacy because of observer bias. The introduction of RCTs after World War II, however, slowly began to transform the means by which many therapies were evaluated. In 1956 Richard Doll (who worked with Austin Bradford Hill in employing epidemiology as a means of establishing a relationship between smoking and lung cancer) turned his attention to gastric ulcers. In a clinical trial he and his associates found that the traditional hospital ulcer diet, as compared with a normal diet, conferred no advantage (although those on the former gained more weight). Nor did the intragastric milk drip promote healing.[28]

The introduction of RCTs, however, did not diminish the introduction of novel therapies based on the application of common sense and rational principles. In 1962 Owen Wangensteen, a distinguished surgeon, introduced gastric freezing as a treatment for duodenal ulcer. The rationale was simple: lowering the temperature of the stomach temporarily reduced acid secretion. The therapy immediately came into wide use; by 1964 the procedure had been used on 10,000 to 15,000 patients. Subsequent RCTs established that the therapy was ineffective. Moreover, endoscopy on those undergoing the procedure revealed serious mucosal damage.[29]

Etiological Speculation

The preoccupation with peptic ulcer was accompanied by etiological speculations. Physicians, after all, traditionally played a dual role: they alleviated the symptoms of illness and provided assurance and comfort to the public by demystifying disease. By advancing explanations that appeared rational and plausible, they could diminish anxiety and justify presumably effective medical therapies and preventive strategies.

To determine the precise etiology of peptic ulcer proved an extraordinarily difficult undertaking. There was virtually unanimous agreement that excess acidification was a primary factor in the genesis of peptic ulcer. But what caused excessive acidification? Some conceded that the cause of gastric and duodenal ulcer was unknown.[30] Experimental animal studies, wrote Lahey, offered no leads. "The variety of methods by which it may be produced in animals and the fact that animal ulcers are not characterized by the same features (intractability) as are human ulcers . . . leave one still at a loss as to the true cause or causes of these lesions."[31]

The absence of evidence that could relate etiology to disease processes, however, did not prove a deterrent. Physicians instead drew upon prevailing medical paradigms and external social and ideological belief systems to develop what appeared to be defensible etiological explanations. Some explanations—notably, focal infection theory—came directly from contemporary medical thinking. Others—including the roles of stress, race, and the pressures of modern industrial society—reflected social and intellectual currents in the larger society of which medicine was but a part.

Initially, focal infection theory, which enjoyed widespread popularity in the early part of the twentieth century, was employed by many to explain the genesis of ulcers. The dramatic successes in demonstrating the etiology of specific infectious diseases such as cholera, tuberculosis, diphtheria, typhoid fever, and various gastrointestinal disorders created a model that dominated early twentieth-century medical thought. The result was a determined search to identify pathogens responsible for a variety of diseases. Indeed, the hope was that all diseases could be traced to microbial pathogens.

Focal infection theory, however, went far beyond a search for the pathogens responsible for individual diseases. Increasingly, clinicians began to argue that circumscribed and confined infections could lead to systemic disease in any part of the body. Edward C. Rosenow of the Mayo Clinic, author of numerous experimental studies, was one of the most important advocates of the belief that many diseases were the result of the dissemination of pathogens through the bloodstream from a local focus.[32] His experimental work was echoed by Frank Billings of the University of Chicago and Rush medical schools, an individual who helped to popularize the focal theory of infection. In a paper delivered before the AMA in 1914, Billings noted that "focal infection is very frequently related to local and general disease [and] is an important factor in some systemic diseases, heretofore unsuspected." When delivering the Lane Medical Lectures at Stanford University Medical School the following year, he listed a large number of both acute and chronic diseases related to focal infections, including, but not limited to, rheumatic fever, endocarditis, myocarditis, pericarditis, nephritis, pancreatitis, chorea, peptic ulcer, appendicitis, and arthritis. Nor was Billings unique. Before Joseph Goldberger undertook his pioneering epidemiological studies on pellagra, researchers sought to identify the causative pathogen of that disease. Henry Cotton, superintendent of the Trenton State Hospital in Jersey, was an ardent spokesperson for the infectious origins of mental illnesses; his views were by no means idiosyncratic.[33] Curiously enough, the theory of focal infection enjoyed its greatest vogue in the United States; in Europe it never met with enthusiastic acceptance. American surgeons, in particular, found the theory especially attractive, since it presumably provided justifications for a variety of surgical therapies. Subsequently, a leading pathologist satirically described a focus of infection as "anything that is readily accessible for surgery."[34]

Moynihan was an early exponent of the idea that focal infections—particularly in the appendix—played a role in the etiology of ulcers. Indeed, in a review of 718 operations for gastric and duodenal ulcers in 1923, he reported that he had removed the appendix in no fewer than 307 cases.[35] Experimental work allegedly confirmed the claim that infections played a role in the etiology of ulcers. The sixth edition of the *Merck Manual* in 1934 noted that "focal infection (teeth, tonsils, etc.) is regarded as a very important etiological factor," a theme that was repeated as late as 1940 in the seventh edition.[36]

The pervasive acceptance of focal infection theory was but a reflection of the successes of modern scientific medicine in demonstrating that specific pathogens caused particular infectious diseases. If pathogens were found in teeth, the appendix, or the tonsils, might not their presence be the cause of pathological states elsewhere in the body? The seeming plausibility and rationality of such a theory made it a popular explanatory model as well as a guide to therapy. Removal of teeth, appendectomies, colostomies, and colectomies were by no means uncommon procedures; they reflected the prevailing belief that focal infections in one part of the body had serious systemic effects.

Yet focal infection theory represented little more than simple correlation or argument by analogy. Nor was anyone able to demonstrate a causal relationship between the presence of pathogens, excess acidification, and ulceration. During the 1930s belief in the role of focal infections declined rapidly because of the failure to identify specific infectious pathogens and to satisfy Robert Koch's postulates. "There is little scientific evidence supporting such a theory," Bevan observed in 1930. "The theory of focal infections has been made to cover too many sins."[37] When the focal infection paradigm disappeared, ironically enough, a potentially effective therapy failed to be accepted as a treatment for ulcers. In 1946 physicians at Mount Sinai hospital found that Aureomycin seemed to be an effective therapy. Yet this finding was largely ignored because it seemed to contradict prevailing medical beliefs about the noninfectious etiology of peptic ulcer.[38]

A variety of other etiological theories both complemented and competed with focal infection theory. Indeed, the absence of evidence that could relate causes to disease processes actually resulted in a dramatic proliferation of etiological claims. By the 1920s gastroenterologists and internists were placing increasing emphasis on the importance of stress and psychic factors in the etiology of peptic ulcer. In many ways the work of Walter B. Cannon played a crucial role. In a series of classic works on digestion, Cannon demonstrated the relationship between such emotional states as "fear, horror, and deep disgust" and the digestive process. The mental state of the individual "may have marked effects on both the motility and the secretion of the alimentary tract." Admittedly, it was erroneous "to assume a predominant importance of the psychic state in the causation of digestive disease." Nevertheless, he concluded, the patient's mental state had to be considered, "for just as feelings of comfort and peace of mind are fundamental to normal digestion, so discomfort and mental discord may be fundamental to disturbed digestion."[39]

Two years later in *The Mechanical Factors in Digestion* Cannon reiterated this theme even though he never specifically alluded to ulcers. "Only as the consequences of mental states favourable and unfavourable to normal digestion are better understood can the good results be sought and the bad results avoided, or, if not avoided, regarded and treated with intelligence." In succeeding decades Cannon published a large number of articles and several classic books elaborating these themes. Influenced by Claude Bernard's concept of the *milieu interieur*, he coined the term "homeostasis" in 1926 to describe the manner in which the body maintained consistency and steadiness "in the presence of conditions which might reasonably be expected to prove profoundly disturbing."[40]

Cannon's work had important implications for physicians seeking an understanding of the etiology of peptic ulcer. During and after the 1920s discussions in the medical literature began to call attention to the causative role of the nervous system. In his section on peptic ulcer in 1927 in Cecil's *Textbook of Medicine,* Thomas R. Brown noted that perhaps peptic ulcer was "not a local but a constitutional disease, and that in its origin and in the recurrence of symptoms psychic factors are important." A year later Emanuel W. Lipschutz claimed that virtually every physician admitted that the neurotic, worrisome, emotional, and hard-working individual was at highest risk to develop peptic ulcer. Similarly, in an article dealing with the present status of peptic ulcer in 1930, Sara M. Jordan noted that it was clear that peptic ulcer was the end product of "repeatedly spastic muscle contraction in the stomach" and a high secretion of hydrochloric acid, both of which could have been caused by "increased nervous tension." That same year Walter C. Alvarez, a major figure in the development of American gastroenterology, published *Nervous Indigestion,* a book that emphasized the importance of case histories to rule out organic causes, the need to understand the psychic roots of the individual's distress, and the importance of the relationship between physician and patient. Harvey Cushing, the distinguished and influential Harvard surgeon, offered a unified explanation of ulcers in 1932 that focused on causation as well as physiological mechanism. He suggested that the interbrain—newly recognized as an important but hitherto overlooked station for vegetative impulses—was "easily affected by psychic influences," including "emotion or repressed emotion, incidental to continued worry and anxiety and heavy responsibility . . . [and] other factors such as irregular meals and excessive use of tobacco."[41]

The assertion that psychic factors played an important etiological role in peptic ulcer did not arise in intellectual or scientific isolation. The declining belief in the role of focal infections left a partial etiological vacuum. Cannon's physiological experiments offered tantalizing possibilities, and the experiences of what was known as "shell shock" during World War I reinforced the belief that psychological factors could have somatic consequences.[42] The claim that peptic ulcer grew out of the stress engendered by the vicissitudes of modern life was especially attractive to physicians, since it integrated psyche and soma in a plausible manner.

To be sure, the claim that there was a relationship between advancing civilization and stress was not novel. Physicians—as well as literary figures, social ideologues and critics, social and behavioral scientists, philosophers, and others—had long argued that the competitiveness and stresses associated with a capitalist society fostered conditions that created a myriad of diseases. Indeed, the idea that the human personality had been adversely affected by the acquisitive values, materialism, and competition that dominated society and undermined established social structures and conventions was a recurring theme in American social thought. In medicine such beliefs fostered racial and gender interpretations of disease susceptibility.

Clinicians dealing with peptic ulcer were no different than their brethren who interpreted disease in racial, gender, and class terms. Physiology and environment, they insisted, made peptic ulcer an understandable consequence of the vicissitudes of modern life. The "ever-increasing rapidity of progress, exacts a toll in the health of those who choose to run in its race," observed Andrew B. Rivers of the Mayo Clinic in 1934. "Throughout the various strata of society," he wrote,

> There seems to be a slightly greater tendency to find among them the better educated, more ambitious and more intensive members of society. Their abilities and their willingness to accept responsibility naturally increase the complexity of their lives far beyond that of those who follow along unperturbedly so long as others guarantee a more or less comfortable existence. . . .
>
> Curiously enough, the desirable virtues of the modern, intensive, aggressive American, the characteristics which have been eulogized and designated as the cardinal marks of American successes, are precisely the characteristics so often replicated in the ulcerous type of patient. Because a premium is paid for these characteristics, an ever-increasing number of persons will acquire them. Consequently, one may expect an increase in diseases having their origin in deranged nervous systems, and undoubtedly peptic ulcer is one of these diseases.

In comparing those individuals at risk for peptic ulcer with a group of two hundred African Americans living in Texas, Rivers also found fundamental differences. The latter were "slow-moving" and "easy-going . . . untouched by aspiration for culture." Despite unbalanced diets, abuse of alcohol and tobacco, irregular sleeping habits, reckless behavior, and unhygienic living conditions, peptic ulcer was absent among them.[43]

Race, of course, had always played a significant role in medical interpretations of disease as well as therapy. In this sense Rivers's claims were by no means idiosyncratic. After evaluating seventy-nine patients with ulcers, Samuel C. Robinson advanced a similar psychogenic theory. Ulcers, he noted, were found largely among susceptible individuals of the white race, usually the long thin type who are given to worry and nervous instability." "The negro race in its evolutionary ascent," he added, "has not, as yet, acquired the habit of worry so peculiar to the white race under pressure of routine civilized living."[44] Such claims were characteristic of pre–World War II decades and were not limited to peptic ulcer. To physicians and others, for example, African Americans were supposedly immune to cancer and other diseases. Living a simplistic existence in the agricultural South, they were less susceptible to the burdens of civilization and its maladies. Indeed, antebellum southern physicians had justified slavery on the grounds that African Americans, precisely because they were still in a state of savagery, were not susceptible to diseases of civilization.

The theory of racial selectivity, however, was not without critics. Frederick Steigmann of the Cook County Hospital and University of Illinois College of Medicine, for example, found no statistical differences in the admission of white and black patients for peptic ulcer. In a study that included eleven hospitals in eight states, he found that nearly 26 percent of 1,306 admissions were African Americans. Steigmann agreed with Otto Kleinberg, whose book *Race Differences* (1935) contradicted the theory of innate race differences and placed primary emphasis on environmental factors. "Environmentally conditioned psychic factors," Steigmann concluded, "play an equally important role in the genesis of peptic ulcer in White and Negro patients." A physician has to deal with "the problem of peptic ulcer in the Negro with the same attitude as he does in the White patient."[45]

Stress and nervous tension, of course, were omnipresent elements that every human being confronted to one degree or another. Why, then, did some individuals develop peptic ulcers while others remained free of this disease? Most clinicians were preoccupied with practical concerns and rarely considered this question. But to a minority the question of vulnerability was important. One answer was provided by supporters of what came to be known as "constitutional medicine." As George Draper, its foremost champion, wrote in 1924, an inherited characteristic, "influenced more or less by environment, . . . determines the individual's reaction, successful or unsuccessful, to the stress of the environment." Such an approach led constitutionalists to offer etiological theories based on the inherited idiosyncratic immune response. Draper identified what he called the "four panels of personality"—morphology, physiology, psychology, and immunity—and suggested that individuals with similar profiles tended to be affected with the same diseases.[46]

In 1932 Draper and an associate applied their findings to peptic ulcer. Individuals with a definite constitutional type, they found, were predisposed toward peptic ulcers. "Ulcer race families" produced a preponderance of long, thin males who displayed "a well marked emphasis on the feminine component of the androgynous mosaic." The man-environment unit disturbance, they concluded, could be corrected permanently by the application of appropriate psychotherapeutic methods, particularly analytic psychology.[47]

Draper's elaborate personal inventory to screen patients and his attempts to develop a taxonomy of "disease races" did not draw much support from gastroenterologists and internists preoccupied with the clinical aspects of peptic ulcer.[48] Yet constitutionalism influenced medical thinking in broad and generalized ways. In 1929 Arthur F. Hurst and Matthew J. Stewart noted that there appeared to be a general ulcer diathesis that rendered the individual susceptible to the development of a chronic ulcer and special diatheses that determined whether the ulcer developed in the stomach or duodenum. Conceding that it was difficult to define the ulcer diathesis, they nevertheless suggested that individuals with short stomachs were prone to duodenal ulcer, while those with long stomachs were likely to have gastric ulcer.[49]

During the 1930s interest in the role of psychogenic factors in physical illness drew the attention of psychoanalysts, many of whom were European émigrés who played important roles in the emergence of psychosomatic medicine. In 1934 Franz Alexander, the leader of the Chicago Institute for Psychoanalysis, reported the results of an ongoing comprehensive investigation of psychic factors in gastrointestinal disorders. The most conspicuous feature of what he termed the "gastric type" (which was characterized by gastric neurosis and duodenal ulcers) was intense receptive and acquisitive wishes "against which the patient fights internally because they are connected with extreme conflict in the form of guilt and sense of inferiority which usually lead to their denial." Stomach symptoms, in turn, were conditioned "by the repressed and pent-up receptive and aggressive taking tendencies which serve as chronic psychic stimuli of the stomach function."[50] Subsequently, Alexander and his colleagues as well as other psychoanalysts elaborated the role of psychodynamic conflicts and personality in the development of peptic ulcer as well as a variety of other diseases, and suggested ways of treating such conditions.

The psychoanalytic interpretation of the genesis of ulcers rested largely on theory rather than empirical findings. In Alexander's study in 1934 the description of the gastric type was based on an investigation of nine cases, three of which involved gastric neuroses and six of which were duodenal ulcers. This extraordinarily small sample, to say nothing about the absence of any objective method of patient selection or control group, raised serious questions about the validity of the study. The psychoanalytic approach to the treatment of peptic ulcer, to be sure, drew little or no support from most nonpsychiatric clinicians. Yet there was little difference between psychoanalysts, on the one hand, and gastroenterologists, internists, and surgeons, on the other, in terms of their respective evaluative methodologies. The very same criticisms levied against the former were applicable as well to the latter.

Alexander's formulation, nevertheless, stimulated interest in the psychosomatic interpretation of ulcer genesis and the role of stress. The experiences of World War II seemed to confirm the claim that stress could have marked physiological consequences. During that conflict high rates of neuropsychiatric symptoms were found among soldiers exposed to extended combat. Indeed, the highest rates were found not among green, untested soldiers, but among combat veterans.[51]

Wartime experiences contributed to the triumph of psychodynamic psychiatry in particular and environmentalism in general, both of which created a milieu in which stress became a near universal explanatory factor for many behaviors and interpersonal relationships as well as an important etiological element in many diseases. In their well-known study of an individual who had undergone a gastrostomy that left him with a hole in the abdominal wall, Stewart Wolf and Harold G. Wolff found that emotional disturbances accompanied profound changes in gastric function. Subsequently, Wolff extended the concept of stress, which he believed to be a significant etiological element in many diseases.[52]

The stress model had many adherents in the postwar decades. It was popularized by Hans Selye, the famous endocrinologist who spent his career in an effort to demonstrate that stress played a role in virtually every disease.[53] A variety of studies involving both humans and animals attempted to demonstrate the existence of such a relationship, although the results remained problematic.[54] During these decades the diagnosis of "stress ulcers" entered the medical nosology. The category referred to an acute erosion of the gastroduodenal mucosa following a major physical or thermal trauma, shock, or sepsis, or the ingestion of such chemical agents as aspirin and alcohol.[55]

Stress was by no means the only element implicated in the genesis of peptic ulcer. For most of the twentieth century physicians speculated that other factors played a significant etiological role, including excessive smoking, mental and physical exhaustion, a large, indigestible diet, inadequate mastication of food, and the ingestion of coffee and spices.[56] These ideas reflected a large and long-standing literature, embodying both religious and secular themes, that offered Americans a guide to proper and improper behavioral patterns. Even people who were skeptical of prevailing explanations of ulcer genesis could not resist the temptation to provide their own explanations. The "cause of ulcer is unknown. . . . The accumulation of observation is tremendous," Heinrich Necheles noted in 1949. "A number of theories on the etiology of peptic ulcer have been brought forward, but none of them have been definitely proven." Nonetheless, Necheles provided his own tentative hypothesis that emphasized an initial disturbance that hastened cell death, which in turn increased acid secretion. Russell Boles, by contrast, questioned the traditional claim that peptic ulcer was due to excessive acid secretion and called for greater investigation of cell resistance. He was especially critical of prevailing therapies and reserved his greatest scorn for surgery, even though he was hostile toward prevailing medical therapies. "In the light of our present knowledge, I believe that we should regard ulcer as an incurable disease, but still recognize that it may be held in abeyance by cultivating a new manner of living."[57]

In 1950, Ivy and his colleagues summarized the many and sometimes conflicting theories of ulcer genesis. The intragastric or intraduodenal theories included such mucosal disturbances as excessive secretion of acid-pepsis and deficiency of neutralizing secretions, mechanical factors (rough food, pressures of organs and clothing, peristalsis), irritants in food and drink, gastritis and duodenitis, inadequate production of mucus, and natural differences in mucosal susceptibility. A second subcategory included anatomic vascular defects (poor blood supply, infarction, and arteriosclerosis) and physiologic disturbances (vasomotor spasm). The extragastric and extraduodenal category comprehended constitutional predisposition, psychogenic factors (occupation, frustration, population density, marital status), infections and toxins, allergic responses, nutritional deficiencies, endocrine gland involvement, and neurotrophic factors. Ivy and his colleagues insisted that, although not mutually exclusive, the "acid factor properly stands first in the list of preferred theories of ulcer formation." Their conclusions were clear and unequivocal. Everyone, they wrote, "looks forward to the day when mutilating operations will be unnecessary." The ideal approach to ulcer therapy was to find two orally active substances, one that would specifically prevent "the parietal cell from forming acid" and another that increases "the resistance of the mucosa to injury and stimulates repair."[58]

In the years that followed the publication of Ivy's book, etiological explanations continued to proliferate. In 1962 Thomas L. Cleave advanced the claim that peptic ulcer was caused by the ingestion of such refined carbohydrates as sugar and white flour. Subsequently, he expanded his theory and played a key role in formulating the influential concept that Western diets with their refined carbohydrates were the cause of many diseases, including coronary heart disease, obesity, and diabetes.[59]

The claim that peptic ulcer was increasing rapidly during the first half of the twentieth century—like the increase in lung cancer and coronary heart disease—was of major concern in the post–World War II decades. Epidemiologists in particular became preoccupied with explaining such increases. Indeed, they were mystified why peptic ulcer rates appeared to be declining after mid-century. Birth cohort analysis—much like focal infection theory in an earlier period—seemed to suggest a new explanatory approach. The detection of birth cohort phenomena in morbidity and mortality suggested that early life experiences had the potential to shape subsequent morbidity and mortality patterns. In a series of studies Melvyn Susser and Zena Stein identified what appeared to demonstrate the existence of clear birth cohort patterns in the rise and decline of peptic ulcer in Britain. This suggested that the determinants of peptic ulcer were to be found in early life experiences. Ultimately, Susser suggested that peptic ulcer had a multifactorial etiology that included diet, alcohol, smoking, emotional strain, personality, and heredity, although he did not rule out the possibility that a single causal factor, as yet unidentified, was responsible.[60]

Birth cohort analysis assumed a new form when peptic ulcer was reconceptualized as an infectious disease related to the presence of the *Helicobacter pylori* (HP) bacterium. To explain the seeming (but questionable) rise of peptic ulcer in the nineteenth century and subsequent changes in the incidence of gastric and duodenal ulcer in the twentieth, such scholars as J. H. Baron and A. Sonnenberg have pointed to two opposing time trends—a declining infection rate (largely due to increasing hygienic standards) and a shift in the initial acquisition of HP infection toward older ages. They also point to the increase in publications dealing with gastric and duodenal ulcer, which demonstrates that gastric ulcer increased during the nineteenth century, but declined after 1900 as the incidence of duodenal ulcer rose. They therefore conclude that such trends imply that exogenous risk factors shape the course of both gastric and duodenal ulcer and that the presence of HP provides only a partial explanation of the epidemiology of peptic ulcer.[61]

Yet empirical data to validate the numerous etiological claims, whether based on clinical, observational, or epidemiologic methodologies, remain problematic. The increase in publications dealing with peptic ulcer, for example, cannot justify claims about the alleged statistical increase in incidence, if only because the diagnosis prior to the development of surgery did not exist. If the statistical increase in incidence remains unproven, the etiological claims become equally questionable. "Theories about the etiology of peptic ulcer range from the formulas of physiology . . . through hardheaded studies of the mucosal barrier and its integrity . . . to the fantasies of psychiatry. . . . [But] we have only speculations," Howard M. Spiro, a noted Yale gastroenterologist, observed in 1971. "The physician," he wrote in the third edition of his *Clinical Gastroenterology,* "must remain an agnostic when it comes to the cause of duodenal ulcer." Others echoed Spiro's skepticism.[62]

Etiological and Therapeutic Change

Toward the end of the twentieth century both etiological theories and therapies underwent significant changes. The dominant point of view was that peptic ulcer was due in part to the use of non-steroidal anti-inflammatory drugs (NSAIDs) and infection with HP, the latter accounting for more than three-quarters of duodenal and gastric ulcers, and the former for the bulk of the remainder. Aspirin, which had come into use by the beginning of the twentieth century, had long been known to cause dose-related gastric ulcers in rats and bleeding in humans. The introduction of other NSAIDs in addition to aspirin and their widespread use led to the conclusion that they played a major role in the epidemiology of peptic ulcer by inhibiting mucosal prostaglandin synthesis and disrupting mucosal defenses.

The first major change in peptic ulcer therapy came in the 1970s when James Black and his colleagues developed the histamine H_2 receptor antagonists, which led to the introduction of several drugs, including cimetidine (Tagamet), ranitidine (Zantac), famotidine (Pepcid), and nizatidine (Axid). These agents reduced acid secretion and promoted healing. Subsequently, proton pump inhibitors, including omeprazole (Prilosec) and lansoprazole (Prevacid), also proved successful in suppressing acid secretion. These drugs seemed to confirm the traditional belief that ulcer healing was dependent upon the tight control of acid. Aside from providing an effective therapy, they further undermined the central role that surgery had occupied for nearly three-quarters of a century. Elective surgical treatment became rare and was employed only when pharmacologic therapy did not work. Emergency surgery for perforation, bleeding, and gastric outlet obstruction remained unchanged. Antacid drugs, however effective in controlling the symptoms of ulcers, did not cure the disease; recurrence was common.[63]

The second major therapeutic innovation involved the introduction of antibiotic therapy. In the early 1980s Barry J. Marshall and Robin Warren stained a gastric biopsy specimen and noted the presence of mucosal bacteria subsequently identified as HP. The former successfully treated a patient with gastritis and gastric bacteria with tetracycline. In 1982 the bacilli was cultured, and Marshall subsequently suggested an association with peptic ulceration after experimenting on himself by swallowing the bacilli and then treating the ensuing dyspepsia with antibiotics. Initially, his findings were ignored or treated with skepticism. Since the 1990s, however, the association between HP and peptic ulcer and type B gastritis has been incorporated into the medical lexicon and treated with a variety of antimicrobial agents.[64]

That there are major differences between the early twentieth-century theories of peptic ulcer genesis and those of the present is clear. Therapies, moreover, are now far more effective and less invasive. Yet there are scientists who concede that a full understanding of the etiology of peptic ulcer (as with many long-term diseases) remains somewhat enigmatic. The role of gastric hydrochloric acid in peptic ulcer, for example, is still murky. Why do high concentrations burn a crater in a confined section of the stomach or duodenum in some individuals and not in others? Why does the concentration of acid vary so much in individuals and why do some develop a peptic ulcer when acid levels are not high? Moreover, the causal relationship between NSAIDs and peptic ulcer is by no means as clear as some would claim. Less than 4 percent of patients taking such drugs develop gastrointestinal disorders, raising the fascinating question of why the remaining 96 percent do not.[65]

The role played by HP in peptic ulcer as well as in the pathogenesis of gastric cancers is not entirely clear. HP is one of the most common infections in the world. The prevalence among middle-aged persons in developing countries is over 80 percent, as compared with 20 to 50 percent in industrialized nations. Only a small proportion, however, develop duodenal or gastric ulcer; the lifetime risk of an infected person in the United States is 3 percent. In India the infection is nearly universal even though peptic ulcer is rare. The clinical course of HP may be influenced by the interaction of microbial, host, and other as yet unknown factors. Indeed, in 1995 Marshall conceded that Koch's postulates had not been fulfilled because "no human or animal experimental model has produced peptic ulcer after inoculation with H. pylori," although the author of a more recent review insisted that the postulates had been "fulfilled substantially." Those who believe in the infectious etiology point note that the disease can be cured by eliminating the microorganism—a fact that offers powerful evidence that the microorganism causes the disease. Those who are not persuaded note that only a minority of infected individuals ever develop an ulcer, suggesting that a variety of host factors—genetic, iatrogenic, nutritional, behavioral, psychological—may be involved.[66]

Those who prefer physiological and reductionist explanations also reject stress as an etiologic agent. Stress, after all, is a protean concept. What precisely constitutes the elements of stress and how can it be measured? Is stress environmental, psychological, or both? Why do some individuals respond positively and creatively to stress, and others negatively? Since all humans experience stress in one form or another, why do a few develop ulcers and most do not? Nevertheless, there are those who continue to believe in stress as a significant etiological agent. The author of a recent analysis concluded that the evidence supported the conclusion "that stress contributes to the etiology of between 30% and 65% of peptic ulcer cases," a view endorsed in part by Spiro.[67]

At present there is overwhelming agreement that HP plays the crucial etiological role. Yet dissenters are by no means absent. Indeed, clinical trials have demonstrated that the identification of an ulcer through endoscopy may have little clinical significance, a finding that is true for a large number of other diseases. Should a person with such an ulcer be regarded as having the disease and requiring medical or surgical treatment? In recent years, moreover, the very diagnosis of peptic ulcer has come into question. As Spiro

noted in 1974, it is difficult "to avoid the conclusion that dyspepsia, duodenitis, and duodenal ulcer are part of the same spectrum." "We should be a little
less certain," he added, "about what we mean by the diagnosis of duodenal
ulcer."[68] Growing agreement "that 'peptic ulcers' are multifactorial in origin,"
he wrote in 1991, "means that there is no more reason to think that an ulcer
crater signifies a specific disease than finding edema of the leg certifies a specific cardiac disorder."[69] Moreover, some, including Baron and Sonnenberg,
insist that as yet unidentified endogenous factors are involved in the etiology
of peptic ulcer.

An understanding of the pathogenesis of a disease, however, is not necessarily a prerequisite for therapy. In the case of gastric and duodenal ulcer,
treatments that involve combinations of a proton-pump inhibitor, an antibiotic, and a nitroimidazole yield a cure rate of about 80 percent. Although prophylactic and therapeutic vaccination has been successful in animal models,
effective human vaccines have not been developed, partly because knowledge about the immunology of the stomach is not well understood.[70]

Conclusion

The history of peptic ulcer in the twentieth century (as well as other diseases)
offers some sobering lessons. Neither medical explanations nor therapies flow
from rational scientific discovery; often they reflect divisions between specialties, prevailing paradigms, ideological beliefs, and personal convictions.
A realistic understanding of medicine requires a recognition of the contingent character of both etiological explanations and therapies.

Chapter 3

How Theory Makes Bad Practice

The Case of Tonsillectomy

For much of the twentieth century tonsillectomy (generally with adenoidectomy) was the most frequently performed surgical procedure in the United States. Despite the fact that relatively little was known at that time about the precise function played by this organ, theoretical speculation served as a justification for a procedure for which there was little persuasive evidence. Moreover, despite intense criticism, it took decades before tonsillectomy rates began to decline, only to begin a modest increase in recent years. The checkered history of tonsillectomy provides a cautionary lesson and suggests that the enthusiasm that often accompanies new therapies should be weighed in the light of evidence of efficacy.

The history of tonsillectomy also illustrates the individualistic foundations of clinical medicine and the absence of barriers to inhibit therapies whose efficacy is at best unclear. Indeed, the enthusiasm for tonsillectomy was shaped by broad concepts and paradigms current in the larger medical and scientific community. Neither etiological theory nor prevailing practices grew out of a body of empirical data. Tonsillectomy provides an instructive if cautionary case study of the complexities and difficulties posed by the introduction and persistence of new therapies into clinical practice. It reflects as well the role of inertia and tradition in the persistence of a surgical therapy that came under increasing criticism in the decades following its introduction.

Late Nineteenth- and Early Twentieth-Century Practice

The removal of tonsils dates back to ancient times. Two thousand years ago Celsus wrote in his *De Medicinâ* that "indurated tonsils" resulted from inflammation. They could be enucleated with fingers or excised with a mechanical device. In succeeding centuries the removal of enlarged tonsils was incorporated into the medical armamentarium, particularly after the dread of hemorrhage diminished. After 1700 surgeons began to ligature the tonsils and excise the projecting portion. Soon thereafter, specific instruments, including a variety of guillotines, came into use.[1]

Until the early twentieth century, however, tonsillectomy was uncommon. The medical literature suggested that a sense of uncertainty was characteristic, particularly in view of the fact that the function of the tonsils remained shrouded in mystery. "I think the very fact that we do not know the physiology of the tonsil ought to make us a little chary about doing needless operations," remarked one Kentucky physician.[2] Nor was surgery necessarily recommended for alleged structural abnormalities. In an examination of the nose and throat of over two thousand children in 1888, W. Franklin Chappel found over 1,200 abnormalities, including 279 enlarged tonsils. He urged that children between the age of six and fourteen should be examined, but omitted mention of tonsillectomy.[3]

The prevailing consensus at that time was that hypertrophy of the tonsil and the accompanying "catarrhal inflammation of the throat, soreness and painful swallowing" justified tonsillectomy. Nevertheless, physicians conceded that the decision to remove the tonsils was neither easy nor obvious. That the procedure was not dangerous, wrote Adolph O. Pfingst, "in no way justifies an indiscriminate removal of [enlarged] tonsils." He urged that "a conservative stand [be] taken" and the operation undertaken only when it was determined that "the presence of the tonsils is a detriment to the welfare of the patient." Ernst Danziger, a New York City physician, warned against making tonsillectomy a "routine operation," if only because he regarded the tonsils as a defensive organ that inhibited the passage of bacteria into the digestive tract, a view that was echoed by others.[4]

Late nineteenth and early twentieth century medical texts were equally conservative in their approach. In the early editions of their famous and influential textbooks, William Osler and L. Emmett Holt took similar positions. Both agreed that acute tonsillitis required medical treatment with such medications as salol (a derivative of salicylic acid). Osler thought that exposure to wet and cold and a poor hygienic environment were significant etiological factors. Chronic tonsillitis was often related to enlarged tonsils. He recommended tonsillectomy, but only if the enlarged tonsils threatened the general health of the child. Similarly, Holt—one of the founders of the specialty of pediatrics—believed that chronic hypertrophy of the tonsils was a source of continued danger and increased susceptibility to diphtheria and scarlet fever. Iodide of iron administered in large doses over several months was the sole internal remedy, although in most cases it was ineffective. Tonsillectomy was virtually mandatory where the tonsils were nearly or quite in contact. In the majority of cases, however, surgery was not indicated.[5]

Specialists in laryngology echoed Osler and Holt. Cornelius G. Coakley divided the etiology of acute tonsillitis into predisposing and exciting causes. The most important predisposing cause was the "rheumatic diathesis;" the most exciting cause was wet feet or sitting in a "cold draught." He recommended bed rest in a warm room and the use of such drugs as calomel and salol. The causes of chronic hypertrophic tonsillitis were unknown, but tonsillectomy was the only effective therapy. St. Clair Thomson, an eminent London physician whose text was published in an American edition, enumerated a variety of reasons for removal, including interference with respiration and voice, a chronic condition of ill-health attributed to tonsillar infection, and frequent attacks of tonsillar inflammation. He believed that the septic state of the tonsils, rather than size, was the critical factor.[6]

The Expansion of Tonsillectomy

After 1910 medical attitudes toward tonsillectomy began to undergo a significant transformation, and its use expanded dramatically. Within decades it became the most common surgical procedure in the United States. Yet this change was not the result of new pathological or epidemiological findings. On the contrary, the rise of tonsillectomy was dependent on novel medical concepts, paradigms, and institutions that were in the process of reshaping the structure and practice of medicine. Indeed, surgical therapies became the cutting edge of medical practice and the symbol of the successes of modern scientific medicine. The introduction of anesthesia and antisepsis diminished the risk of infection and expanded the world of surgical opportunities. At Johns Hopkins, William Halsted pioneered in developing the radical mastectomy, thus making breast cancer a "surgical disease." Halsted's residency training program contributed toward the professionalization and expansion of American surgery. Similarly, Berkeley G. A. Moynihan's work made gastric and duodenal ulcers conditions that required surgery. At the same time Sir Arbuthnot Lane, the most important interpreter of autointoxication (a belief that constipation led to self-poisoning), popularized both the ileosygmoidostomy and colectomy.[7] The elevated status of surgery thus contributed to the heightened interest in tonsillectomy.

Perhaps the most important development in promoting the widespread expansion of tonsillectomy was the appearance of focal infection theory, which in the early twentieth century became the dominant paradigm in American medicine. This theory also became a guide to therapy. If infectious pathogens gained entrance to the body from the mouth, nose, and throat, it followed that the elimination of portals of infection was crucial. The ease with which tonsils could be accessed, when combined with the belief that tonsillectomy posed relatively few dangers, were also important factors in promoting its use.

A somewhat more aggressive view toward tonsillectomy was already evident in the first edition of William A. Barrenger's laryngology text in 1908. Barrenger conceded that the tonsils were a limited "barrier against the invasion of microörganisms." Yet such pathogens gained entrance into the system through the tonsils, thus necessitating their removal under certain conditions. Nasal, ear, and pharyngeal infections, hypertrophy of the tonsils, tonsillitis, and recurrent acute articular rheumatism all justified its removal. "Clinically," Ballenger noted, "there is little to show evil effects from its removal, whereas there is much evidence to show the good resulting from its removal, especially its complete removal." Nor was hemorrhage a major risk, and he agreed with a prominent surgeon's observation that the tonsil was of greater importance than the appendix and "causes more suffering and more deaths."[8]

What kinds of evidence could validate the claim that tonsils were portals of infection and that tonsillectomy was an appropriate therapy? To those who performed surgery the answer was clear; the personal case series of the individual practitioner were the vehicle by which therapies were judged. In other words, clinical experience was the crucial element in the determination of whether a therapy was or was not effective. For much of the twentieth century there was no established methodology that could evaluate therapeutic efficacy, especially when it came to surgical procedures. Physicians weighed evidence overwhelmingly in terms of their own clinical experience. Hence the supposed alleviation or disappearance of symptoms after tonsillectomy was taken as proof that diseased tonsils were the cause. In a similar vein, studies that purported to demonstrate that rheumatism and other diseases frequently followed an episode of tonsillitis proved the existence of a probable causal relationship. To be sure, clinicians attempted to measure efficacy by collecting aggregate data. Yet there was no consensus on how to gather or even to analyze epidemiological data. For obvious reasons, most studies of tonsillectomy outcomes resulted in favorable findings. One Massachusetts General Hospital physician polled 992 patients, and 143 responded by reporting in person. The survey found an improvement in general health of the children and less susceptibility to illness. These results were echoed in other surveys. "In view of these reports and the attitude of the most prominent pediatricians and health officers in the country," noted Daniel W. Layman, "should we not seriously consider the removal of the tonsils as a wise prophylactic measure in early childhood in many more cases than formerly?"[9]

Most discussions about tonsils and their relationship to systemic disease concealed an underlying contradiction that was rarely addressed. The belief that the function of the tonsil was unknown was accompanied by a claim that it possessed a pathogenic character. In a book devoted exclusively to the tonsils, Harvard laryngologist Harry A. Barnes conceded that knowledge of the function of the tonsils was uncertain. Nevertheless, he noted that the concept that many systemic infections had their origin in the entrance of pathogens into the tonsillar crypts was "now almost universally admitted." An often-cited study of one thousand tonsillectomies by three members of the Johns Hopkins Hospital's Department of Laryngology echoed this assertion. "It is our opinion, as yet unproven by any large series of cases, that during the early stage of an acute tonsillitis there is a general bacteriaemia. . . . If the organism happens to be of low virulence, or one to which there is a sufficient degree of immunity, it is quickly killed off. . . . If, on the other hand, it chances to be a viridans, or one of the streptococci that E. C. Rosenow has shown may have a specific affinity for certain organs, then serious metastatic infections occur." Like Barnes, the Hopkins investigators concluded that focal infections could give rise to acute rheumatic fever, endocarditis, septicaemias due to various organisms, arthritis, nephritis, neuritis, arteriosclerosis, general debility, and neurasthenia.[10]

The growing acceptance of focal infection theory was evident in the 1916 edition of Osler's influential textbook. By then the conservatism that marked the first three editions in the 1890s had largely disappeared. "The tonsils, swarming with saprophytic and pathogenic germs," Osler wrote, "are the main gates through which the invaders try to storm the gates. . . . Too often the enemy gains entrance, and streptococci, staphlococci, pneumenococci, etc., pass to distant parts and cause arthritis, endocarditis, and serious membrane inflammations." He was therefore far more aggressive in his endorsement of tonsillectomy.[11]

By the early 1920s reports about the benefits of tonsillectomy proliferated in medical journals. "The importance of the tonsils in the acute infections as a point of attack and as a portal of entry for infections . . . is so much a matter of common experience as to require no demonstration here," wrote Edwin H. Place. He presented data from his hospital demonstrating that T&A shortened the duration of scarlet fever. A study by the Public Health Committee of the New York Academy of Medicine found that the Bureau of Child Hygiene of the New York City Department of Health had determined that between 10 and 19 percent of schoolchildren had hypertrophied tonsils and adenoids. In 1920, 47,000 operations were performed, whereas the number needing surgery was 55,000. The committee urged an expansion of hospital-based facilities to facilitate tonsillectomies.[12] Others added their voice in the support of tonsillectomy as a weapon in the struggle against infectious diseases and provided data from their own private and institutional practice supporting the beneficial effects of the procedure. In a book addressed to a general audience in 1926, Martin Ross wrote that "no finer breeding place for bacteria exists in the entire body than in diseased tonsils. . . . From this excellent bacterial hothouse, the organisms, or the poisonous products resulting from their activity, are readily absorbed and carried to distant parts of the body." Five years later Robert H. Fowler, a well-known New York City laryngologist, summed up the indications for tonsillectomy. They included frequent colds and sore throat, otitis or sinusitis, rheumatism, endocarditis, neuritis, and enlarged tonsils. "The tonsil operation is a useful and important surgical procedure," he added, but "it would be a pity to overdo it."[13]

Such claims led parents, particularly those from more affluent and educated backgrounds, to have their children undergo tonsillectomies. In *Cheaper by the Dozen* two of Frank and Lillian Gilbreth's children recalled the day when their family physician observed that the kids had "really ugly tonsils," thus leading to frequent sore throats. Frank, a pioneer in scientific management, then suggested that the physician come to their home and extract the tonsils of no less than six of the twelve offspring. At the same time he arranged to have a photographer take motion pictures in order to ascertain the most efficient means of performing this surgical procedure. The experiment failed because the photographer forgot to remove the lens cap of the camera! Shortly thereafter Frank had his own tonsils removed. The story illustrates the widespread belief both in the efficacy and safety of tonsillectomy.[14]

To be sure, the emerging paradigm that emphasized the pathogenic character of the tonsils had its critics. In a survey of sixteen San Francisco laryngologists who had performed tonsillectomies on more than ten thousand children between 1905 and 1915 (three-quarters of whom were under the age of fourteen), Sanford Blum found that most of his colleagues had determined that the tonsils were the source of a large number of "functional disturbances, developmental derangements, and diseases of the entire human economy." This provided a rationale for tonsillectomy. Blum, however, found the claim unpersuasive. Any local infection could be the source of systemic infection. He therefore concluded that "the practice of tonsillectomy in children should be restricted." In another study S. E. Moore of the University of Minnesota's medical school found that the complications and fatalities from tonsillectomy were sharply underestimated and that the pathogenic character of the organ had been exaggerated. "The tonsil," he added, "has become the germ of medical hysterias, and by the indiscriminating and immoderate employment of tonsillectomy this operation has blossomed into the jester of therapeutic measures, and the clown of surgical procedures—but a prince of financiers nevertheless." In an experimental study in 1928 Paul S. Rhoads and George F. Dick found that in 73 percent of cases tonsillectomy failed to rid the body of tissue harboring bacteria because of incomplete removal of tissue even by established surgeons. The following year W. Lloyd Aycock and Eliot H. Luther of the Department of Preventive Medicine and Hygiene of the Harvard Medical School noted that there was a correlation in a small number of cases between tonsillectomy and the subsequent occurrence of poliomyelitis.[15]

Nor did Holt follow the prevailing paradigm. The differences between the first (1897) and sixth (1914) editions of his influential text were minimal. He did not allude to the tonsils as portals of infection, and his approach to tonsillectomy was cautious. In the fifth edition of his standard text on diseases of the nose and throat in 1914, Cornelius G. Coakley took an equally conservative approach. Neither figure alluded to focal infection theory or recommended routine tonsillectomies.[16]

In the 1920s there was a literal explosion in the number of articles dealing with the tonsils and tonsillectomy. In a review Arthur W. Proetz estimated that between four and five articles appeared weekly. "The great majority of these communications," he added, "do not contribute anything to the sum of knowledge." The efforts to justify or condemn tonsillectomy by employing the tools of epidemiology resulted in a variety of findings, some of which were contradictory. A five-and-a-half-month follow-up study of five hundred tonsillectomies at the New York Hospital concluded that the results were "good." A study of colds among Cornell University undergraduates in the early 1920s found that tonsillectomies did not result in a reduction in the frequency of colds. One analysis found that tonsillectomy and adenoidectomy in cases of tonsillitis conferred an advantage, whereas another found no advantage in

reducing a variety of chronic ailments. A critic of indiscriminate tonsillectomy insisted that alternative therapies—including the use of the X-ray and
radium to shrink the tonsil—were valuable alternatives.[17]

At about this time Albert D. Kaiser at the University of Rochester Medical
School began a pioneering follow-up study of children who had undergone
tonsillectomy; this quickly established his credentials as the leading figure
on this subject. In 1920 Kaiser became involved with a community-wide program in the city that made it possible for all children designated by examining physicians as suffering from diseased tonsils to have their tonsils and
adenoids removed at a local clinic. No less than ten thousand children had
their tonsils and adenoids removed in a five-month period. In order to ascertain the effects of the operation, Kaiser decided to observe a subset of these
children for a period of ten years and to compare their growth and development with children whose tonsils and adenoids had been recommended for
removal but for one reason or another had not had the operation. The numbers
of children studied in his decade-long and subsequent studies were substantial and ran to well over twenty thousand. In the decade following the inau-
guration of the study Kaiser published a series of articles that culminated in
1932 with the appearance of his book *Children's Tonsils In or Out: A Critical
Study of the End Results of Tonsillectomy.*[18]

Nowhere was the problem of employing epidemiology to determine the
efficacy and outcomes of tonsillectomy better illustrated than in Kaiser's
indefatigable labors. As a later admirer of Kaiser pointed out, an ideal clinical
trial to determine the effectiveness of a surgical procedure would involve the
random assignment of patients and a double blind procedure, which would
require sham operations.[19] Given the fact that the double blind clinical trial
was unknown at that time (to say nothing about the problems of conducting
such a trial even at present), Kaiser's approach to determine the efficacy of
T&A was understandable. He was acutely aware of the problems involved in
evaluating the requirements for tonsillectomy. The absence both of knowledge of the function of the tonsil and laboratory tests to determine pathology
forced investigators to fall back on clinical investigations. Such investigations
had major shortcomings because of the numerous variables and the fact that
many studies employed different methods. "The beneficial results following
tonsillectomy in selected cases," he wrote in 1940, "inspired this procedure
on a large percentage of children often without a good cause."[20]

Kaiser's findings, which remained more or less consistent over the course
of his study, were relatively cautious and conservative. He noted that the real

value of tonsillectomy and adenoidectomy could not be established in a few years. Indeed, apparent benefits during the few post-operative years were less evident over a ten-year period. Surgery contributed to the reduction of tonsillitis and sore throat, middle ear infections, and cervical adenitis. But the incidence of such respiratory infections as laryngitis, bronchitis, and pneumonia actually increased in tonsillectomized children. First attacks of rheumatic manifestations occurred less often in tonsillectomized children, but recurrent attacks did not change. In the ten-year study the only benefits were "in the reduction of sore throats, cervical adenitis, otitis media, scarlet fever, diphtheria, rheumatic fever and heart disease." Tonsillectomy offered no benefits insofar as the incidence of sinusitis, colds, chicken pox, mumps, measles, tuberculosis, asthma, and hay fever was concerned.[21]

At about the same time that Kaiser was undertaking his studies, Selwyn D. Collins and Edgar Sydenstriker of the Public Health Service were collecting epidemiological data dealing with respiratory diseases.[22] In 1927 they published a monograph dealing with tonsillitis and related throat conditions. Much of their data came from their twenty-eight-month study of illness in Hagerstown, Maryland, as well as material gathered by clinicians and pathologists. They found that the highest percentage of tonsillectomies was in urban areas. Acute tonsillitis and sore throat were more than twice as high among schoolchildren with defective tonsils as compared with those who had their tonsils removed. Children with normal tonsils had the lowest incidence. Other respiratory diseases were also somewhat more frequent among children with defective tonsils than among those with normal or removed tonsils. The incidence of rheumatism, heart conditions, cervical adenitis, and ear conditions was lowest among children with normal tonsils, higher among those with defective tonsils, and highest among the tonsillectomized. Children who had their tonsils removed had the highest rates of measles, whooping cough, chickenpox, and mumps. The two statisticians also found that during the previous fifteen years rates of tonsillectomy had increased dramatically. In the families of medical officers in the army, navy, and Public Health Service, 50 percent of children in the five- to nine-year-old group and 60 percent in the ten- to fourteen-year-old group had their tonsils removed.[23]

Doubters and Critics

During and after the 1930s many of the commonly accepted rationalizations previously employed to justify tonsillectomy slowly began to be questioned. What had previously passed as proofs now came to be regarded with skepticism, if not outright rejection. The epidemiological studies purporting to demonstrate the benefits of tonsillectomy came under increasing criticism. In 1928 an editorial in the *Journal of the American Medical Association* pointed out that there was little agreement on what constituted "diseased," "enlarged," and "normal" tonsils; there were wide variations in the reports of examiners. Although data indicated that tonsillectomy was "a useful and justifiable procedure," the benefits were not so evident when compared with a large control group. Three investigators found no statistical relationship between tonsillectomy and rheumatic heart disease. More importantly, they were critical of many of the early epidemiological studies. Few included an adequate sample, uniform criteria for rheumatic infection and diseases of the tonsils, complete enucleation of the tonsils, an extended duration of observation, and control groups not operated on and matched to the treated cases. Three years later their criticisms were echoed by Theodore K. Selkirk and A. Graeme Mitchell. Little or no attention, they wrote, had been paid to "age, sex, race, heredity, financial class, season, effect of adenoidotomy alone, length of observation after operation, source from which the history and other data are obtained, incidence of tonsillectomy in the community at large and the suitability of the control group." The neglect of such factors "often invalidated the conclusions." Kaiser, clearly the most careful investigator, admitted as much in 1934. He noted that the "desired relationship between the tonsils and the various infections in childhood is not as clear today as it seemed 10 years ago. Statistical and controlled clinical studies have obliged us to modify or even change our views on this relationship. Not so many infections can be prevented or modified by the removal of the tonsils as was prophesied in the early days of enthusiasm for the treatment of diseased tonsils." Six years later he continued to question the "real value" of many epidemiological studies.[24]

Slowly those who studied tonsillectomy (with and without adenoidectomy) became increasingly disenchanted with the procedure. The faith in focal infection theory that had played such a significant role from 1915 to 1930 no longer claimed the allegiance of most clinicians and researchers. In 1938 Russell L. Cecil and D. Murray Angevine called "for a complete reevaluation of the focal infection theory," which in their view was nothing more than a "fetish." In a clinical lecture the following year reviewing the extant literature Hobart A. Reimann and W. Paul Havens insisted that focal infection theory was unproven and lacked clinical and experimental support, and that the routine extraction of teeth and tonsils was not justified. They suggested that in many cases financial considerations played a role, if only because tonsillectomy among children from more affluent backgrounds was two or three times more frequent than among the poor. The theory continued to be strongly defended because, quoting Kant, "certain things repugnant to the reason find acceptance among rational people simply because they are spoken of." That same year *Scientific American* published an article entitled "The Great American Rite." Its author summarized many of the studies that questioned the widespread popularity of tonsillectomy and urged laypeople to cease trying to persuade physicians to perform an operation that in most (but not all) cases was unnecessary.[25]

The criticisms of tonsillectomy were popularized in novelist Kenneth Roberts's *It Must Be Your Tonsils*. In a satirical manner he described how a series of both American and British physicians had attributed his arthritic symptoms in his knee to infected tonsils. As the knee grew worse, he consented to undergo a tonsillectomy. As time passed, his knee continued to give him trouble. One day on the golf course he had to quit after the fourteenth hole. A friend with whom he had been playing and who was involved with collegiate athletics examined the knee and determined that the problem was a pulled cartilage. He suggested that Roberts wear an elastic bandage, which resolved the problem. So much for infected tonsils![26]

The growing criticisms of tonsillectomy in the United States, interestingly enough, echoed those in Great Britain. In 1938 the Medical Research Council published data from a five-year statistical study of epidemics in schools that found no evidence that tonsillectomies resulted in a diminished incidence of infections. Its conclusion was simple: "there is a tendency for the operation to be performed as a routine prophylactic ritual for no particular reason, and with no particular result." J. Alison Glover, an English pediatrician whose work was known in the United States, also insisted that the number of tonsillectomies was "excessive," and had little value as a prophylactic measure.[27]

The abandonment of focal infection theory as a justification for tonsillectomy was accompanied by growing skepticism and doubts about the efficacy of the procedure in general. Aside from the question of its role in improving health, there was evidence that many operations were poorly performed. During the first third of the twentieth century there was a vigorous debate that dealt with both instrumentation and technique that often involved competing points of view. By then there were more than half a dozen different operations even though there was little or no effort to evaluate their relative merits.[28] Regardless of the technique employed, questions over quality persisted. One study of 887 first-year female students at the University of

Pennsylvania between 1936 and 1938 found that 77.3 percent of the 621 who had undergone tonsillectomy had remnants of tonsillar tissue in the fossae. Another study found residual tonsil tags in 68 percent of 1,000 tonsillecto-mized patients, suggesting that the procedure was a failure.[29]

More importantly, the standards that presumably were the basis for medi-cal decisions to recommend for or against tonsillectomy remained extraordi-narily variable. A sampling of 1,000 New York City schoolchildren in the early 1930s found that 61 percent had undergone tonsillectomies. The remaining 39 percent were then examined by a group of school physicians, who selected 45 percent for surgery. The rejected children were examined by a second group of physicians, who recommended 46 percent of those remaining for surgery. The rejected children were examined a third time, and 44 percent were selected for tonsillectomies. After three examinations only 65 out of the 390 children remained; they were not examined again because the supply of physicians had been exhausted.[30] Such variability was a reflection both of the individu-alistic character of medical practice and the difficult problem of determining what constituted evidence to validate a particular therapy.

Between the late 1930s and 1950s an extended controversy grew out of the claim that high rates of poliomyelitis, particularly the bulbar form, fol-lowed T&A. In following up Aycock's observation a decade earlier, Albert B. Sabin—soon to become one of the premier poliomyelitis researchers—noted that the tonsillopharyngeal region appeared to be more sensitive to the virus and that perhaps nonemergency operations on the throat and mouth ought not to be done in the summer and early autumn when poliomyelitis was most prevalent. At precisely the same time two Harvard Medical School pediatricians who studied 418 consecutive patients with acute poliomyelitis admitted to the Infants' and Children's Hospitals of Boston came to the same conclusion as Sabin.[31]

Given the inability to isolate a causal mechanism between poliomyeli-tis and T&A—assuming that one existed—investigators again resorted to clinical epidemiological studies. Nevertheless, they faced the same meth-odological problems that had plagued earlier attempts to correlate surgery and specific diseases. As three public health physicians from the New York City Department of Health observed, the problem was beset by the low inci-dence of the disease, poor reporting, and incomplete data on the population at risk, to say nothing about the need to correct for such variables as age, monthly incidence, and time of operation. Moreover, the selection of dif-ferent types of control groups and statistical techniques gave rise to mixed results. Otolaryngologists obtained their data from patient surveys, physicians, hospitals, and health departments, which tended to point to the rarity of poliomyelitis following tonsillectomy. Other studies reported an increase in incidence following surgery. When data from an otolaryngological study showing no relationship was reaggregated using a different statistical methodology, the results showed twice the incidence of the bulbar form of the disease in those who had tonsillectomies within the previous two months. Indeed, Charles K. Mills's review of more than two dozen studies in 1951 found that opinion was divided between those who found and those who did not find a relationship between tonsillectomy and poliomyelitis. A majority, however, agreed that if poliomyelitis followed T&A, there was a likelihood that it would be the bulbar form. One investigator presented data showing that surgery done many years before still increased susceptibility to the bulbar form.[32]

The debate did not end until the introduction of the polio vaccine rendered the issue moot. Although the relationship between poliomyelitis and tonsillectomy was never resolved,[33] the controversy revealed subtle differences between pediatricians and laryngologists. The former were more prone to believe that the hazard was a real one; the latter, while conceding that the increased susceptibility to the bulbar form of poliomyelitis required sober judgment, also pointed out that nonremoval of tonsils could even be more hazardous. "When properly done under the right indications," noted one laryngologist, "surgical removal of these organs is one of the most gratifying procedures in medicine. Its benefits greatly outweigh any possible dangers, including a theoretically increased susceptibility to bulbar poliomyelitis." "It is my personal belief," wrote Lawrence R. Boies, "that when the facts are all in we will not regard the tonsil and adenoid operation as predisposing to poliomyelitis." For many clinicians, however, the ambiguous data presented them with a serious dilemma in weighing surgery. James L. Wilson, who believed there was a causal relationship, noted that even if the issue was unsettled it implied a risk. Rather than await definitive evidence, he added, "I can only ask what the risk is of postponing the tonsillectomy and then try to weigh one risk against the other."[34]

Over time the differences over tonsillectomy between laryngologists and pediatricians widened. Boies was a staunch defender. In 1948 he wrote that tonsillectomy "should be a worn-out subject." Nevertheless, the number of published papers remained high; between 1942 and 1946 an average of over one hundred papers per year had appeared. Moreover, lay periodicals aired and emphasized the negative aspects of the procedure. Having performed more than three thousand tonsillectomies, Boies insisted that the procedure was justified in cases of repeated attacks of tonsillitis, hypertrophy, and evidence of persistent chronic infection. Nor were the claims about less than adequate surgery or the alleged risks of the procedure justified. The following year he repeated his beliefs in the first edition of his *Fundamentals of Otolaryngology* (a standard work in the field) and restated them in the next two editions.[35]

The Persistence of Tonsillectomy

Changes in medical practice often do not follow new findings or evidence to the contrary. The doubts in the medical literature concerning tonsillectomy did not lead to immediate change. A survey sent to 10,200 pediatricians in 1956 by Irving J. Wolman, editor of the *Quarterly Review of Pediatrics,* was revealing. Nearly 90 percent of the 3,441 replies noted that they referred the surgery to others, although this was less true of those who practiced in rural areas. There was as yet little overt opposition to surgery, but the poll demonstrated a growing conservatism among pediatricians. There was unanimous agreement that recurrent or chronic otitis media required adenoidectomy, usually with tonsillectomy. A majority also recommended such intervention for mouth breathing, recurrent or chronic tonsillitis, and for early hearing impairment. But fewer than 10 percent deemed size alone as requiring surgery. Wolman concluded that the survey revealed disagreement rather than consensus. The absence of definitive data, therefore, led pediatricians "to make decisions on an empirical basis, tinged with a high degree of probability."[36]

Yet parents continued to be receptive toward tonsillectomy. Admittedly, there were publications that presented the procedure in a highly favorable light. In a child's book directed as well toward parents, Ellen Paullin emphasized the ease and benefits of tonsillectomy while ignoring any potential risks.[37] Yet periodicals that often provided medical advice rarely extolled the virtues of tonsillectomy or suggested that all tonsils be removed. The *Reader's Guide to Periodical Literature*—a publication that included, with some exceptions, magazines addressed to a general audience—averaged only 12.6 entries a decade between 1920 and 1980. Indeed, during the 1950s when rates of tonsillectomy remained high, most of the articles urged caution and insisted that tonsils should only be removed when there were specific and justifiable reasons. The idea that tonsils should be removed, noted Dr. Robert L. Faucett in an article in *Good Housekeeping,* developed at a time when diseases that afflicted children "were poorly understood." Although the need for tonsillectomy has decreased, "many parents still submit their offspring to this frightening operation without understanding how and why it is done." The first edition (1946) of Benjamin Spock's manual of baby and child care—soon to become the most popular book of its kind in the nation—was relatively restrained in his discussion of the tonsils. He believed that the size of the tonsils was unimportant and that tonsillectomy should be considered only in cases of chronic infection or an attack of quinsy sore throat (an abscess behind the tonsil). The likelihood that tonsillectomy would reduce the frequency of colds, rheumatism, and chorea was doubtful. In subsequent editions Spock was even more forceful in his belief that tonsillectomy was rarely justified.[38] High rates of tonsillectomy, therefore, cannot be attributed to favorable publicity.

Parental enthusiasm for tonsillectomy was largely driven by medical advice that began in the 1920s and persisted among practitioners in subsequent decades despite growing conservatism among elite practitioners. "Parents continue to press strongly for the operation," complained Harry Bakwin, a pediatrician at New York University's College of Medicine. "There is still a widespread impression among the laity that it is, in some way, a desirable health measure and that it protects against colds." His concern was shared by other physicians. Parents, according to Robert A. Furman, labored under two misconceptions: "first, that the tonsils' only function is to be removed surgically; and, second, that any respiratory illness is a tonsillitis." There was a pressing need, he added, for "educational efforts to combat misconceptions about surgery." Socioeconomic class remained a significant element. In a study of two New York State communities, Jane C. Mertz found that in each age group there was a higher proportion of tonsillectomies in the professional and managerial class than in the clerical, skilled, semi-skilled, or unskilled groups. Higher socioeconomic groups were more aware of and had greater faith in medicine and more frequent contact with physicians, creating a receptivity toward interventionist therapies. The rapid spread of voluntary health insurance plans after World War II also played a role. In their study of family medical costs and health insurance in 1956, Odin W. Anderson and Jacob Feldman found that the tonsillectomy rate among insured children was more than three times that of uninsured children.[39]

In 1958 Bakwin published an exhaustive review of the epidemiological studies dealing with tonsillectomy and adenoidectomy. From the outset he made it clear that in the overwhelming majority of cases the procedure was "useless." He drew on a variety of cross-national studies, all of which demonstrated that, in spite of evidence to the contrary, tonsillectomy not only remained at high levels, but had few benefits. The overwhelming majority of children had their tonsils removed for one or more of three reasons; parental pressure, large tonsils or adenoids, and frequent upper respiratory infections. Nor was the operation a minor procedure. The number of deaths from those undergoing the surgery ranged from a high of 346 in 1952 to 220 in 1955, to say nothing of the risks of other complications. Neither were the costs of this surgery negligible. Assuming 1,500,000 tonsillectomies per year—which meant that 40 percent of the population had undergone tonsillectomies and adenoidectomies—the cost to the nation as a whole was $150,000,000 (a not inconsiderable sum considering the level of medical expenditures at that time). Bakwin thought that few physicians were motivated by pecuniary considerations, since the children of physicians were operated on as often as the children of others. Given the paucity of evidence to support such high levels of surgery, the continuance of the procedure in his eyes was "indeed an enigma" for an era which considered itself "scientific."[40]

During the 1960s and 1970s both pediatricians and laryngologists continued to debate the efficacy of tonsillectomy and adenoidectomy and to attempt to arrive at definitive answers by clinical epidemiological studies that paid more attention to methodological concerns. These studies began to narrow the range of conditions and to separate tonsillectomy and adenoidectomy, which hitherto had run hand in hand. Kaiser's studies in the 1920s and 1930s had included nearly two dozen diseases. The clinical and epidemiological studies undertaken between the 1960s and 1980s, by contrast, were much narrower; they included fewer conditions and began to separate the differential consequences of tonsillectomy and adenoidectomy. A five-year investigation of the effect of tonsillectomy on the incidence of streptococcal respiratory disease of nearly seven thousand young airmen found that those who had undergone tonsillectomies were neither more nor less susceptible to such infections.[41]

Between 1963 and 1970 three investigations, two in Great Britain and one in New Zealand, aroused considerable interest. The first by W.J.E. McKee was a two-part study. The first part measured the benefits of tonsillectomy/adenoidectomy, and the second the role of adenoidectomy in the combined procedure. McKee did not rely on parent or physician reports, but followed up both the operated and the control group by home visitations. He found that the principal benefit of surgery was relief from throat disorders and a reduction in otitis media; respiratory or other disorders were not affected.

Adenoidectomy played little role in the reduction in throat disease but was important in the reduction in otitis media. Five years later a study by Stuart R. Mawson, Peter Adlington, and Mair Evans came to somewhat different conclusions. There was a noticeable reduction in the frequency of sore throat, tonsillitis, cervical adenitis, and colds, but no change in the incidence of otitis media. The third by Noel Roydhouse (conducted in New Zealand, but also published in an American Medical Association journal in 1970) concluded that children with a marked susceptibility to respiratory tract infection benefited from the combined operation, especially by a reduction in throat illness.[42]

In 1971 Jack L. Paradise and colleagues at the Children's Hospital and the University of Pittsburgh School of Medicine began a prospective, controlled clinical trial to determine the indications for tonsillectomy and adenoidectomy; two years later the National Institutes of Health agreed to provide funding. Paradise was cognizant of the flaws in previous clinical trials, and that the reporting of attacks of tonsillitis by parents was unreliable. His study was not completed until 1982, and the results were published in 1984. The 147 children included were selected because of the frequency of severe and recurrent throat infection; children with other conditions (e.g., extreme hypertrophy of the tonsil) were excluded. At the completion of the study the investigators concluded that the incidence of throat infections during the first two years of the follow-up was significantly lower in the surgical than the nonsurgical group. The investigators emphasized that tonsillectomy was warranted in children meeting their stringent eligibility criteria, which they conceded were atypical. For children with less severe throat infections there was room for nonsurgical treatment. Hence, decisions had to be made on an individualized basis.[43]

Differential epidemiological findings reflected a generalized confusion about the efficacy of tonsillectomy that became characteristic during and after the 1960s. An author of a *Lancet* annotation observed that the data from the McKee and Mawson studies demonstrated that the greatest benefit occurred in the twelve months following the surgery. Under such circumstances the "improvement could conceivably be due to *an* operation rather than *the* operation!" In reviewing these and other studies, Hugh G. Evans was highly critical. McKee, he pointed out, failed to subtract the number of days lost in the hospital and during convalescence from the total number of days "saved" in the operated group. The net result was a trivial "savings." Similarly, Mawson's results were inconsistent. "There are as yet no categorical indications for tonsilladenoidectomy other than intrinsic disease such as quinsy or suspected malignancy." Short-term benefits might accrue to four- to six-year-old children with documented histories of severe concurrent tonsillitis, but precise identification of such children was impossible. "There is still no compelling evidence of any long term benefit from T and A," concluded Evans, and the burden of proof of the efficacy of such surgery had to rest with those who urged the operation. Subsequent evaluations of evaluative studies of tonsillectomy also found severe methodological and substantive shortcomings.[44] And even the Paradise study seemed problematic because it included only children with severe and recurrent throat infections.

Indeed, by the late 1960s tonsillectomy was coming under sharp attack in the medical press. In a letter to *Pediatrics* in 1968 A. Frederick North Jr. referred to "an epidemic unchecked." The epidemic in question was caused neither by a pathogen, an environmental contaminant, nor a genetic defect, but by a medical procedure that was unsafe and ineffective. The procedure, he added, should at best be considered "experimental and have the status of an experimental drug." Clinical studies had to "determine whether tonsillectomy and/or adenoidectomy is actually treatment or really a more severe health problem than any of the conditions it purports to cure." The following year Robert P. Bolande described tonsillectomy (along with circumcision) as "ritualistic surgery" performed on a "nonscientific basis" in order to fulfill parental need.[45]

Given such conflicting evidence and claims, how did physicians in active practice deal with tonsillectomy with and without adenoidectomy? In 1968 the editors of *Modern Medicine* attached a questionnaire to the April issue that went to over 200,000 physicians. They received 13,495 responses; 27.0 percent had performed surgery within a fifteen-day period, and 18.5 percent had recommended the operation during that period (but had not operated). Those responding were distributed in the same pattern as all physicians in the nation. Of those performing surgery, 58 percent were general practitioners, 23 percent otolaryngologists, and 12 percent general surgeons; only 3 percent were pediatricians. As a group, otolaryngologists were the most active; they performed more than eighteen surgeries during the period; the overall average was 8.4 per operating physician. The survey also suggested the presence of a generational divide. The older the physician, the more operations performed. The average number of operations reported were ten for each physician fifty or older; seven for ages thirty-five to forty-nine, and five for each younger than thirty-five. There was general agreement on the indications for surgery. Over 90 percent of all respondents believed that chronic infections, tonsillitis, adenoiditis, pharyngitis, upper respiratory infection, adenopathy, lymphadenopathy, and bronchitis required surgery; more than 60 percent included hypertrophy of tonsils or adenoids. Nearly 80 percent of otolaryngologists and pediatricians accepted recurring otitis media, ear infections, hearing problems, and obstruction of the eustachian tubes as indications for surgery. The contraindications for surgery were relatively few and included bleeding problems, hemophilia, anemia, and clotting defects.[46]

The results of the survey were followed by an article by Joseph Lubart from New York City's Albert Einstein Medical College. Citing both the work of Kaiser and others questioning the efficacy of tonsillectomy, Lubart nevertheless argued that the pendulum had swung too far the other way. There were "many chronically ill children today who have been denied the benefits of a carefully and adequately performed adenotonsillectomy." Citing the National Health Survey, he noted that there were nearly six million persons whose defective hearing could have been prevented or alleviated by surgery.[47]

The survey, however unrepresentative, indicated the existence of a gap between practice and the growing doubts about the efficacy of tonsillectomy that were appearing in medical journals. There was some (but not conclusive) evidence of a generational gap between those who favored surgery and those who were opposed. Physicians who entered practice before World War II, many of whom were in general practice but performed tonsillectomies, generally accepted the paradigm that tonsils and adenoids were responsible for a variety of diseases that plagued both children and adults and that surgery was both an efficacious and safe therapy. In subsequent decades their practice continued to reflect what they had been taught. As both physicians and human beings, it was also natural for them to judge their clinical interventions in a highly favorable light; the concept of observer bias was absent. The pervasiveness of tonsillectomy and adenoidectomy in the face of mounting doubts of their effectiveness, nevertheless, raises a fascinating issue, namely, the extent to which findings that appeared in the medical literature affected the daily practice of physicians. To what extent were ordinary practitioners familiar with the medical literature dealing with tonsillectomy? Although evidence to answer this question for the most part is lacking, the persistence of tonsillectomy in the face of growing doubts suggests that many of those who had entered practice in earlier decades were less familiar with more recent findings; they practiced as they had been taught.

In the early 1970s Mary Ann Sullivan, a physician and a faculty member at the Johns Hopkins School of Medicine, undertook a more representative micro study of physician attitudes toward tonsillectomy and adenoidectomy in Allegheny County, Pennsylvania (which included the metropolitan area of Pittsburgh). Questionnaires were sent to otolaryngologists, pediatricians, and general practitioners (general surgeons were included in the survey, but they were excluded from the analysis because their responses indicated a lack of contact with the problem). Otolaryngologists were far more disposed to favor surgery and performed on average 235 per year. Pediatricians and younger general practitioners tended not to do surgery. There were large variations in physicians' attitudes toward tonsillectomy and adenoidectomy, and there was little agreement on what constituted the criteria for the diagnosis of tonsillar disease or the indications for surgery. The survey revealed that complications were by no means infrequent and that the mortality rate was considerably higher in that geographical area than rates in the general medical literature.[48]

The manner in which medical practice was structured clearly assisted in the persistence of tonsillectomy. Tonsillectomy rates were in part a function of geographical location. There were much higher rates in urban than rural areas, largely because the latter tended to have fewer physicians and hospital facilities. The experience of World War II also hastened medical specialization; and, increasingly, these specialties (with some notable exceptions) tended to be surgical in nature. As John Bunker pointed out in 1970, the United States, when compared with England, had twice as many surgeons in proportion to the population and performed twice as many operations. Fee-for-service, solo practice, and a more aggressive therapeutic approach also contributed to the greater number of operations in the United States.[49]

By the 1970s it had become clear that the scientific evidence of the benefits of tonsillectomy was at best questionable. The randomized trials that had been done were difficult to interpret, given variable results and the multiplicity of factors. In 1975 the Rand Corporation undertook a study for the Department of Health, Education, and Welfare that attempted to measure the quality of medical care assessment using outcome measures for eight conditions. The study pointed out that there was a better understanding of the natural history of conditions for which surgical procedures had been performed. Many of these conditions—upper respiratory infections, otitis media, hypertrophy of the tonsils and adenoids—could be managed successfully either with antibiotics or, in the case of otitis media, with lesser surgical procedures, including myringotomy with or without the insertion of ventilation tubes (a therapy that subsequently would itself come under question). The panel also expressed concern about the possible roles of tonsils and adenoids in the immune system and the potential negative consequences that might follow their removal. Although members defined three categories ("certain or absolute indications," "reasonable indications, for which evidence of benefit is uncertain," and "contraindications") as well as standards by which to measure outcomes, the differences among them in arriving at their conclusions was striking and added little to resolving the indeterminacy that was characteristic of the surgery. Seven years later two Mayo Clinic otolaryngologists conceded that "a well-designed prospective study concerning the indications for and results after these operations has not been presented."[50]

The uncertainty about the efficacy of tonsillectomy was evident as well in the deliberations of a group of leading physicians attending a workshop in 1975. The problems included inadequate knowledge, a failure of communication and education, and a lack of concern in finding solutions. Those attending found it difficult to agree and urged that high priority consideration be given to prospective investigations in order to define approaches to the optimal management of diseases of the tonsils and adenoids. They also emphasized that additional studies of the pathogenesis, pathophysiology, and epidemiology of these disorders were required in order to identify basic mechanisms that were so essential to the solution of therapeutic problems.[51]

The Decline and Persistence of Tonsillectomy

The mounting doubts about tonsillectomy in the post–World War II decades did not immediately lead to a reduction in tonsillectomy rates. Between 1915 and 1950 the frequency of this surgical procedure increased. Selwyn D. Collins, in a study covering about nine thousand families between 1928 and 1931, found that the adjusted rate for all ages was 38 per thousand, with a peak of 68 at age six. He estimated that tonsillectomy constituted nearly one-third of all surgical operations, of which about 60 percent were performed in hospitals and the remainder in offices, clinics, or homes. By mid-century perhaps 1.5 to 2 million individuals (overwhelmingly children) had their tonsils removed each year. In a careful longitudinal study of three age cohorts (born before 1910, 1910–1929, 1930–1948) in two New York State communities, Jean Downes found a marked increase in the risk of tonsillectomies in the decades between 1880 and 1949. In the first group only 4 percent of males had their tonsils removed by age five. The comparable figures for the next two groups were

18 and 42 percent, respectively. By age nineteen 67 and 61 percent of males in the latter two groups, respectively, had undergone surgery. In Rochester, the urban area where Kaiser had conducted his epidemiological studies, between 33 and 40 percent of all admissions of children to hospitals in the 1960s were for the removal of tonsils and adenoids. A decade later it remained the most common surgical procedure in the United States and the main reason for the hospitalization of children.[52] Data from the National Health Survey in 1965 indicated that 1,215,000 tonsillectomies (with and without adenoidectomies) had been performed. Thereafter tonsillectomy began a slow albeit uneven decline and by 1986 had fallen to 281,000.[53]

Despite increasing skepticism about the need for and efficacy of tonsillectomy, it persisted in medical practice. What accounted for the growing discrepancy between theory and practice? Why did not doubts about this surgical procedure result in immediate changes in the behavior of physicians? The answers to these questions shed much light on the structure and nature of medical practice.

The slow decline of tonsillectomy was *not* due to conclusive evidence that it did not result in the benefits claimed by its advocates. Admittedly, it is difficult, even at the present time, to measure many therapeutic outcomes with any degree of precision. Clearly, the absence of an agreed upon method to determine efficacy played a role in the persistence of tonsillectomy. Most epidemiological studies had encountered formidable methodological problems that made it extraordinarily arduous to establish causal relationships. Results changed from study to study, and the criteria employed were so variable that the findings were at best highly problematic. Hence, physicians, whatever their specialty, could find data that purportedly supported the manner in which they practiced. As Michael Bloor pointed out, even otolaryngologists who were aware of the scientific standards that presumably governed their practice demonstrated consistent variations in their clinical assessments. The very nature of medical knowledge, he suggested, provided for these differences, if only because the theoretical construction of a disease entity was often arbitrary and value-laden. Indeed, any disease entity was in effect a general designation and could refer to a wide variety of different conditions.[54]

Although the early faith in focal infection theory and the claim that tonsils were portals of infection had long since passed, the belief that tonsillectomy had clear benefits persisted. Physicians who had received their training in medical schools prior to World War II accepted tonsillectomy as a legitimate therapy. Their reading of medical journals, given the demands of clinical practice, was probably confined to their own specialty, and they may have been unaware of dissenting views that appeared in other specialty publications. Nor were many trained in either epidemiology or statistical analysis, and therefore were not in a position to evaluate in a critical manner the studies they encountered. Hence, their clinical approach continued to reflect their training. The fact that solo practice was the norm resulted in a quasi-professional isolation that insulated them from the growing skepticism about the procedure. The absence of therapeutic norms and standards and professional regulation meant that practitioners were free of institutional constraints.

Perhaps the most important elements in reducing tonsillectomies were the change in the nature of specialty training and practice and a growing skepticism in medical school departments of pediatrics about the efficacy of the surgery. After World War II, specialty training became more common. Those who selected pediatric internships had little opportunity to learn surgical techniques and, hence, did not—as those who came to confine their practice to children in an earlier era—perform tonsillectomies. Wolman's survey in 1956 revealed that younger pediatricians were less likely to perform tonsillectomies or to refer them to their older colleagues. The widespread use of antibiotics also persuaded many that surgery was unnecessary.[55] In addition, the number of tonsillectomies performed by general practitioners dropped precipitously. Unlike the pre–World War II generation of general practitioners, their postwar successors found that they had lost their surgical prerogatives as medicine was increasingly divided by specialty. As hospitals became central to medical practice, home and office surgical procedures virtually disappeared.

If pediatricians were less prone to recommend tonsillectomy, the same was not true of otolaryngology, which remained a specialty in which surgery played a major role. The growing differences between the two were already evident in a symposium in 1953, which was published the following year in the *Journal of the American Medical Association*. Conservatism was evident in the presentations by Theodore L. Badger, a Harvard Medical School internist, and R. Cannon Eley, from the Harvard Department of Pediatrics. The former expressed his belief that "too many tonsils are still being taken out." The latter observed that most pediatricians "view the tonsil and adenoid question with respect, but they also view the general health of their patients with a great respect and in selected instances and under proper circumstances advocate the removal of these lymphoid tissues." Boies, one of the nation's most eminent laryngologists, took a more activist position and expressed his belief that in many cases nonremoval of the tonsils could be more hazardous than removal.[56]

That pediatricians were becoming dubious about the efficacy and benefits of tonsillectomy was clear. During and after the 1970s pediatric texts manifested considerable conservatism in their approach to surgery and greater appreciation of the immune role of the tonsils. In the sixteenth edition of *Pediatrics* in 1977 (the successor to Holt's *Diseases of Infancy and Childhood*), Robert J. Ruben devoted only two paragraphs to tonsillectomy. The procedure, he noted, "should be reserved only for those children who have four or more repeated episodes of bacterial pharyngitis associated with tonsillitis and in whom the immunologic systems were felt to be adequate." In the sixteenth edition of *Nelson Textbook of Pediatrics* in 2000 Margaret A. Kenna was even more restrained. For children with recurrent throat infections (seven in the past year, five in each of the past two years, or three in each of the past three years or more), tonsillectomy decreased the number of infections in the subsequent two years as compared with no tonsillectomy. But children who met these criteria and who did not have tonsillectomies also experienced a decline in the number of throat infections. Conceding that chronic or recurrent tonsillitis or adenotonsillar hypertrophy were often given as justifications for tonsillectomy, she nevertheless wrote that the only absolute indications were the presence of a tumor or severe aerodigestive tract obstruction. Kenna rejected virtually all of the claims that had served as a justification for the surgery for nearly three-quarters of a century.[57]

Yet the decline in the number of tonsillectomies proved transient. By 1996, 383,000 tonsillectomies were performed, and a decade later the number exceeded 400,000.[58] The resurgence of the procedure reflected both a change in the structure of medical specialties and a new concern with sleep-related breathing disorders. In earlier decades pediatrics and otolaryngology were distinct specialties. Toward the end of the twentieth century departments of pediatric otolaryngology had become more common. Pediatric otolaryngologists, unlike pediatricians, were somewhat more aggressive in recommending surgery for a variety of conditions even though supportive evidence remained problematic.

To be sure, otolaryngologists, like their pediatric brethren, employed drugs and antibiotics. Yet their proclivity to recommend surgery, albeit less aggressively, remained constant. The changed perspective of otolaryngologists was evident in the 1978 revision of the classic Boies textbook, which listed only chronic airway obstruction, peritonsillar or parapharyngeal abscess, hypertropy sufficient to cause respiratory distress, or a suspected malignancy as indications for surgery. Yet the editors of the revised Boies textbook were still inclined to give credence to older justification.[59]

In the 1990s a new justification for tonsillectomy and adenoidectomy emerged. During this decade concern with sleep disorders began to mount. Although such disorders had a long history, the diagnosis of obstructive sleep apnea disorder (which applied to both children and adults) aroused interest. In the case of children the consensus of opinion was that this disorder was caused by adenotonsillar hypertrophy and therefore constituted a definite indication for surgery.[60] Moreover, many older justifications for T&A (e.g., recurrent throat infections) persisted as well.

Nevertheless, the problem of what constituted adequate evidence to support tonsillectomy persisted. To be sure, standards for RCTs had become more formal and rigorous. Similarly, statistical analysis was based on more sophisticated techniques. Yet the results of RCTs were at best ambiguous. A meta-analysis of studies to determine the efficacy of tonsillectomy in children under the age of eighteen concluded that the procedure provided a small reduction of sore throat episodes, days of sore throat associated school absences, and upper respiratory infections compared to watchful waiting. Jack L. Paradise, who had spent his career in an effort to determine efficacy, was critical of the meta-analysis. Its major shortcoming, he noted, was its failure, "by considering only pooled risk differences across studies, to relate the outcomes of individual randomized trials to the stringency of the indications used in determining trial eligibility." Paradise's own studies, which used criteria that were more stringent than the criterion in current official guidelines, had concluded that "the degree of benefit conferred by either operation [tonsillectomy and adenoidectomy] was modest, and appears not to justify the inherent risks."[61] Perhaps the comments of an individual in Oxford, United Kingdom (also associated with the Cochrane Collaboration), are revealing. Parental decisions to opt for surgery, he observed, were made independently of any evidence. "In many quarters the 'word on the street' is still this—'if you're having trouble with your throat, you should have your tonsils out.' Fashions may change capriciously; tenets in popular culture are harder to dispel."[62]

Conclusion

The checkered history of tonsillectomy offers a sober and cautionary lesson. Its initial introduction grew out of the popularity of the specific germ theory

of disease, which gave to medicine a powerful explanatory tool that held
out the promise of new therapies. Yet what had been an empirically based
theory was quickly extended in a manner that ignored evidence. The focal
theory of infection was based on analogy, which then served as a justification for the claim that tonsils were portals of infection and thus should be
removed. Inertia also played a role. Once introduced into the therapeutic
armamentarium, tonsillectomy persisted for decades and was widely hailed
for its alleged successes.

The absence of a consensus on how to design systematic studies to validate its efficacy led physicians to justify tonsillectomy on the basis of their
own clinical experience. Clinical experience, however, has two very different forms. The first is a somewhat intangible but indispensable entity. Unlike
the practice of science, the practice of medicine involves radical uncertainty.
Whereas scientific research is intended to give rise to generalizations, medical practice, by contrast, seeks particularization. Thus, physicians must
negotiate between these two extremes in an effort to understand the nature of
the patient's distress. They employ scientific knowledge, but such knowledge
is insufficient if only because each individual case must be studied holisti-
cally and not subsumed under unambiguous regularities of scientific laws.[63]
The second is quite different. Clinical judgment is a sine qua non of medical
practice. Nevertheless, it does not necessarily enable a physician to arrive at
an informed judgment about the efficacy of a particular therapy. Physicians
deal with individual cases, and their personal experiences cannot always be
used to establish acceptable standards of practice. Observer bias, after all, is
a perennial element in human behavior and often leads individuals to come
to faulty judgments. This is especially true of tonsillectomy. That this surgery
is useful and even mandatory in specific instances is clear. More problematic has been its widespread and indiscriminate deployment for much of the
twentieth century.

Too often the history of medicine is presented as the story of inevitable
progress. Yet there is a side to medicine that is often overlooked, namely,
the introduction and persistence of therapies such as tonsillectomy that rest
largely on analogy and faith. Were one to undertake a comparable analysis
of other therapies during the last half of the twentieth century, the results
would not be fundamentally different. To be sure, it is undeniable that bio-
medical science has much to offer in controlling and alleviating disease. Yet
the history of tonsillectomy as well as other therapies provides a cautionary
lesson as well. Therapeutic enthusiasm must be tempered by sober realism

and a recognition that the evaluation of therapies is a complex undertaking that requires attention to both methodology and clinical experience. It is also wise to remember that even the best-designed studies to evaluate therapies (including the RCT) do not necessarily yield conclusive or reliable results. Finally, in an ideal system there should be a way of ensuring that therapies of questionable efficacy are excluded from the medical practice.

Chapter 4

How Science Tries to Explain Deadly Diseases

Coronary Heart Disease and Cancer

In contemporary America cancer and coronary heart disease are the two leading causes of mortality. They arouse fear and anxiety among many, and there are perennial calls for "wars" to conquer them. A variety of groups—physicians, scientists, epidemiologists, and others—provide bewildering and ever-changing explanations of the causes of these two diseases. These explanations shape surgical and medical therapies as well as preventive interventions. Scarcely a day passes without new behavioral and dietary advice that presumably will lessen the risk of developing cancer and CHD. Yet, as we shall see, many of the claims about the etiology of these diseases are frequently not based on hard empirical data or sound epidemiological analysis. On the contrary, they often reflect broad social and intellectual currents that perceive of disease as the result of changing social and environmental conditions or inappropriate lifestyles.

That cancer and heart disease are now the major causes of mortality is a relatively recent development. In 1900 infectious diseases accounted for 56 percent of total mortality; cardiovascular-renal diseases and malignant neoplasms accounted for only 22 percent. In 2004, by contrast, diseases of the heart accounted for 27 percent of all deaths, malignant neoplasms 23 percent, and cerebrovascular diseases slightly over 6 percent. Of the fifteen leading causes of death, pneumonia and influenza (2.5 percent) were the only ones that fell, at least directly, into the infectious group, and they often took their greatest toll among individuals suffering from a variety of other serious health problems. The remainder included such varied categories as chronic lower respiratory diseases (5 percent), accidents (5 percent), and diabetes mellitus (3 percent).[1]

What accounts for the increasing importance of heart disease and cancer as the major causes of mortality in the last hundred years? Medical as well as social scientists have provided a variety of theories that presumably account for changing epidemiological patterns of mortality and morbidity. Whether or not supported by empirical data, such theories serve to alleviate anxiety and provide assurance to a broad public by demystifying disease. Moreover, explanatory theories often justify prevailing medical and preventive interventions. Admission of etiological ignorance, by contrast, would clearly diminish medical and scientific legitimacy.

Yet etiological explanations, however plausible and rational, often rest on a slippery foundation. What kinds of evidence can be employed to validate them or illuminate basic physiological mechanisms? Indeed, questions of what constitutes evidence are by no means self-evident. The cases of heart disease and cancer in many ways illustrate the problematic character of many contemporary explanatory theories.

The Checkered Epidemiology of Coronary Heart Disease

That part of the increase in heart disease and cancer mortality is related to the changing age distribution of the American population is obvious. In 1900 infectious diseases resulted in high death rates among infants and children. The slow decline of infectious diseases as the major cause of mortality after 1900 (which had relatively little to do with the introduction of new therapies) meant that more individuals survived to old age. Consequently, the incidence and prevalence of cardiovascular diseases and malignant neoplasms rose as the population grew older. Diseases of the heart (which included a variety of subcategories), for example, took an increasingly higher toll among the various age groups. In the twenty-five to thirty-four age group in 2004 the age-adjusted mortality rate was 8 per 100,000; in each of the next six age groups by decade the comparable figures were 29, 90, 219, 542, 1,506, and 4,896, respectively. Malignant neoplasms manifested a similar pattern. In the twenty-five to thirty-four age group, mortality was 9 per 1,000; the greatest increases were in the next six age groups: 33, 119, 333, 755, 1,280, and 1,653.[2]

Yet age by itself cannot explain these changes, if only because patterns of morbidity and mortality have not remained static. The fact of the matter is that there were important if not clearly understood changes in their patterns over time. The checkered history of these two diseases in the last hundred years suggests that many cherished etiological explanations as well as preventive strategies are based on questionable evidence.

In the early twentieth century the most common form of heart disease was rheumatic heart disease. The disease, which affected children and young adults, was associated with the Group A streptococcus. Exposure to this organism created antibodies that cross-reacted with heart tissue. The result was impairment of the mitral valve. Thickening of the valve reduced blood flow, which often resulted in congestive heart failure and death. Even in the absence of effective therapeutic or preventive measures and for reasons which are not completely clear, mortality from rheumatic fever declined steadily during the first half of the twentieth century and by the 1980s the disease had largely disappeared.[3]

The decline in mortality from rheumatic heart disease was accompanied by a steady rise in age-specific mortality from CHD among all age groups. Admittedly, changes in terminology add an element of complexity. In the early part of the century "diseases of the heart" was the diagnostic category. Subsequently, heart diseases came to include such categories as ischemic heart disease, coronary heart disease, and arteriosclerotic heart disease, all of which are basically the same. They denote the clinical symptoms of atherosclerosis, which is the obstruction of the flow of blood through the arterial network and, specifically, the coronary arteries.

At the beginning of the twentieth century CHD was relatively uncommon. To be sure, "organic heart disease" was a common cause of death. But this category was quite different and included valvular diseases related to rheumatic fever and infections that impaired the heart and kidneys (which led to congestive heart failure). In the 1920s, however, an upward trend in CHD mortality began and continued unabated for more than thirty years. Male death rates for CHD far exceeded those for females. The ratio was highest among the younger age groups and decreased with advancing age. To Paul Dudley White, one of the nation's most prominent cardiologists, this was a mystery. "Why should the robust and apparently most masculine young male be particularly prone to this disease?" he asked in 1944. Interestingly enough, the increase in CHD was not confined to the United States, but was international in scope and occurred in more than two dozen countries.[4]

Beginning about 1950, age-specific death rates for all major cardiovascular-renal diseases began to fall. Between 1960 and 2005 age-adjusted mortality rate for all heart diseases fell from 559 to 211 per 100,000. Virtually every age group shared in the decline. The aging of the population was not a factor in the increase in mortality from heart disease, if only because a larger proportion of people within each age group perished from heart disease in 1950 than in 1900. The pattern for CHD followed a similar path. Mortality began to decline somewhere in the 1960s. Between 1970 and 1993 mortality among men ages forty-five to sixty-four dropped by more than 60 percent, a decline far greater than the decline in overall mortality rates. Women experienced a similar decline even though their rates were far lower than those of men. As a result, CHD became largely a disease of the very old.[5]

The decline in cardiovascular mortality had a significant effect upon life expectancy. Between 1962 and 1982 the death rate from all cardiovascular diseases dropped about 36 percent. By 1982 this translated into five hundred thousand fewer deaths than would have occurred based on 1963 rates. The improvement in cardiovascular mortality (a category that accounted for nearly half of all deaths) played a major role in the increase in life expectancy during these years. The decline in CHD mortality was an important component in the overall mortality decline and assisted in reversing the trend of greater longevity of women.[6]

What explains the irregular trend of mortality from CHD in the twentieth century? The answer to this seemingly obvious question is anything but simple. As late as the 1950s many researchers and clinicians believed that what is now known as CHD was a chronic degenerative disease related to aging and could not be influenced by specific preventive measures. The Commission on Chronic Illness, created in the 1950s to study the problems of chronic disease, illness, and dependency, noted that the "causes of the most significant cardiovascular diseases—rheumatic fever, arteriosclerosis, and hypertension—are known only in part. . . . In the present state of our knowledge then, prevention of cardiovascular disease is largely confined to the prevention of complications." Atherosclerosis, it conceded, "is not preventable at the present time."[7]

By the 1960s the focus had shifted to the role of risk factors as crucial elements in the etiology of cardiovascular disorders. A series of epidemiological studies, some of which began in the 1940s, transformed the manner in which CHD was understood. Ancel Keys, head of the Laboratory of Physiological Hygiene at the University of Minnesota, was a key figure in developing the argument that risk factors explained the rise in mortality from CHD. He began with the observation that CHD was the dominant cause of mortality among males ages forty through fifty-nine; the disease caused 40 percent of all deaths in this group within a five-year period. Keys was among the first to claim that dietary fat raised serum cholesterol and led to atherosclerosis.

In the 1950s, with support from the Public Health Service, Keys launched his Seven Countries Study that included Italy, Yugoslavia, Greece, Finland, the Netherlands, Japan, and the United States. The initial results appeared in 1970 and then at five-year intervals. The conclusion was simple: the three critical variables in the genesis of CHD were age, blood pressure, and serum cholesterol. The study also found that weight, smoking, and physical activity appeared to play no role in the disease.[8]

So confident was Keys in his findings that he and his wife published a book in 1959 entitled *Eat Well and Stay Well.* Designed for both physicians and the lay public, it included a laudatory introduction by Paul Dudley White. CHD, according to the Keys, was a major problem among populations with high cholesterol levels. Such elevated levels were largely a result of a diet high in meat and diary fat, margarine, and hydrogenated shortenings, which in turn produced clogged arteries. In the past, carbohydrates played a much more important role in the American diet. In most parts of the world 60 to 75 percent of food calories came from carbohydrates. In the American military, by contrast, barely 40 percent came from this source, and the whole population had gone almost as far in replacing carbohydrates with fats. The moral was clear; a low-fat diet would prevent CHD, and the book offered dietary advice as well as a series of recipes.[9]

At about the same time that Keys was developing his theory, the famous Framingham study was launched in 1948. The study enrolled over five thousand residents free of CHD in the early 1950s and tracked them for years. They received comprehensive physical examinations and were re-examined every two years. In 1961 the study identified three characteristics associated with the development of CHD; elevated serum cholesterol levels, hypertension, and the electrocardiographic pattern of left ventricular hypertrophy. Over time the study seemed to indicate that high blood pressure, obesity, cigarette smoking, and a family history of heart disease played crucial roles in CHD.[10]

The seven-country and Framingham studies were followed by a variety of other studies that emphasized similar themes. The monograph on cardiovascular diseases sponsored by the American Public Health Association, published in 1971, accepted the claim that behaviors peculiar to modern industrialized society explained the high rates of CHD. As Menard M. Gertler and Paul Dudley White noted in 1976, the idea of identifying individuals at risk for CHD was "becoming firmly established." To be sure, "unanimity is lacking on the question of which risk factors should be used." Nevertheless, they believed that "this matter will be resolved eventually."[11]

During the 1970s and 1980s there was a rising crescendo of claims that high fat diets and obesity were linked to heart disease as well as cancer. The Senate Select Committee on Nutrition and Human Needs, chaired by George McGovern, pushed the diet-heart hypothesis in its hearings; the result led to the publication of the U.S. Dietary Guidelines, which was revised every five years. In 1983 a twenty-six-year follow-up study of participants in the Framingham Heart Study concluded that obesity was an independent risk factor for cardiovascular disease. Dieting and slimness, to be sure, had been a cultural ideal since the early twentieth century. By the 1980s, however, the virtues of slimness had been transformed into an article of faith that was seemingly supported by the objective findings of medical science.[12]

Taken as a group, most studies rejected the older degenerative hypothesis and substituted in its place the claim that CHD was related to a series of behaviors peculiar to the industrialized world. Such an interpretation gave meaning to CHD in the sense that it identified those who were presumably at greatest risk and suggested ways of decreasing that risk. The mystery and randomness that had previously characterized explanations of CHD were superseded by the claim that individuals were at increased risk for the disease if they ate high-fat foods, smoked, were overweight, or were physically inactive. That such a theory emerged in the postwar decades is understandable. The emphasis on behavioral risk factors mirrored a belief that each individual was responsible for health as well as a faith that medical science and epidemiology could illuminate the behavioral etiology of CHD. Many chronic diseases, including CHD, various forms of cancer, diabetes and other conditions, Lester Breslow noted in 1960, reflected the availability of rich and abundant foods, alcohol, smoking, less physical activity, and other "good things" associated with the modern industrialized world.[13]

In summing up their findings of the Alameda study, Lisa F. Berkman and Breslow concluded that health and disease "arise mainly from the circumstances of living."

Rural communities with poor sanitation located in areas heavily infested by parasites, mosquitoes, and other disease agents and vectors are afflicted with one pattern of health, disease, and mortality. Urban communities starting on the path of industrialization but affected by crowding, inadequate food, and poor sanitation have another pattern. Modern metropolitan communities with advanced industrialization and reasonably good sanitation, but low physical demand coupled

with access to plenty of fatty foods, alcohol, and cigarettes, have still
a third kind of health, disease, and mortality pattern. . . . In the latter
part of the twentieth century, their [infectious diseases] place has been
taken by coronary and other cardiovascular diseases, lung cancer, and
other forms of noninfectious respiratory disease.[14]

Studies of the decline in mortality from CHD in the United States emphasized two elements, namely, improvements in treatments and reductions in
risk factors. Clinical trials to identify risk factors posed methodological difficulties, however, particularly because such trials were generally of relatively short duration. Hence, observational studies were employed to provide
evidence supporting the causal association between risk factors and CHD.
The likelihood of causation, according to a task force of the American College of Cardiology in 1996, was strengthened under the following conditions.
First, the stronger the association, the more convincing that the relationship
was causal. Second, exposure to the risk factor had to antedate the onset of
disease. Third, the association had to be dose-dependent. Fourth, the relationship had to be consistently demonstrated under diverse circumstances
(e.g., various populations). Fifth, the association was biologically plausible.
Finally, the association was specific in that the risk was associated with a
particular disease.[15]

Another task force then specified interventions for specific risk factor
categories. The first included risk factors for which interventions proved to
reduce the incidence of CHD (cigarette smoking, LDL cholesterol, hypertension, and thrombogenic factors). The second were those that were *likely* to
reduce the incidence of CHD (diabetes, physical activity, HDL cholesterol,
obesity, postmenopausal status). The third were those that *might* reduce CHD
incidence (psychosocial factors, triglycerides, Lp(a), homocysteine, oxidative
stress, and alcohol consumption). Finally, it identified risk factors that could
not be modified (age, gender, family history). The task force conceded that
diet was important but had not been included since diet reacted with different factors at many different levels. If diet had been included, however, it
would have been placed in the first category.[16]

Another study explaining the decrease in CHD mortality from 1980 to
2000 attributed 47 percent of the decrease to a variety of specific treatments,
including initial treatments for myocardial infarction or unstable angina,
secondary preventive treatments after myocardial infarction, treatments
for heart failure, revascularization for chronic angina, and other therapies.

Approximately 44 percent of the decline in mortality was attributed to changes in risk factors, including reductions in total cholesterol, systolic blood pressure, and smoking, as well as increased physical activity. The latter reductions, however, were partially offset by increases in body-mass index and prevalence of diabetes, which accounted for an 18 percent increase in the death rate.[17]

The emphasis on risk factors as major elements in the etiology of CHD, however, is not entirely persuasive. Why, for example, did CHD mortality rates rise especially among younger men in their thirties and forties from the 1920s to the 1950s? If a causative factor is responsible for atherosclerosis, a latency period of perhaps twenty years must be subtracted from the time when the mortality curve initially began its rise. Such was not the case. Risk factors did not begin to be an important element until the late twentieth century, whereas CHD mortality began to rise in the early part of the century. Dietary change came after World War II. If the more recent switch from saturated to unsaturated fats and the decrease in serum-cholesterol played a role in the last quarter of the twentieth century in declining CHD mortality, why did this not occur as well during the depression of the 1930s when most Americans could not afford rich diets? Death rates for heart disease in general did not follow dietary changes.[18] Similarly, cigarette smoking—whose health effects generally take several decades to appear—first became prominent in the 1920s, when the increase in mortality from CHD was already underway. Much the same holds true for the claim that diminished physical activity was a crucial factor. Like cigarette smoking, the use of automobiles was not common until the 1920s and during the depression of the 1930s remained a luxury. Nor did physical activity diminish during World War II; if anything, military service and factory labor resulted in increased physical activity. To be sure, life for most Americans became more sedentary in the latter part of the twentieth century. Similarly, saturated fat consumption, generally associated with CHD, increased during decades during which mortality from CHD was declining. In a careful analysis of the major variables associated with CHD, Reuel A. Stallones observed that "hypertension does not fit the trend of the mortality from ischemic heart disease at all; physical activity fits only the rising curve, serum cholesterol fits only the falling curve and only cigarette smoking fits both. In no case is the fit as precise as one would like."[19]

Comparative data from other countries also failed to sustain the claim that risk factors such as high-fat diets explained CHD mortality. Throughout southern Europe, for example, heart disease death rates steadily declined while animal fat consumption rose because of increasing affluence. Some epidemiologists, as a matter of fact, have suggested that national differences may reflect the availability and consumption of fresh produce year round. Scotland and Finland have high rates of CHD; its citizens eat high-fat diets but consume relatively little fresh vegetables and fruits. Mediterranean populations, by contrast, consume large amounts of fresh produce year-round. To University of Cambridge epidemiologist John Powles, the antifat movement that has gained such prominence in recent decades was founded on the notion that "something bad had to have an evil cause, and you got a heart attack because you did something wrong, which was eating too much of a bad thing, rather than not having enough of a good thing."[20]

Although epidemiology has become a major discipline during the second half of the twentieth century, many of its methodologies and explanations of disease etiology raise serious problems. Some epidemiological studies rely on cohort analysis and observational studies. In employing this methodology, investigators monitor disease rates and lifestyle factors (e.g., diet, physical activity, among others) and then infer conclusions about the relation between them. Thus they identify risk factors, such as high-fat diets, which presumably cause cardiovascular disease. The problem is that risk factors are at best associations and do not necessarily explain changes in epidemiological patterns in time and space. At best, cohort analysis can generate hypotheses, but say nothing about causation. The danger is that associations between disease and behavior become the basis of public health recommendations about what individuals should do to prevent disease. There are numerous examples of observational studies that have proven erroneous. The claims that hormone replacement therapy or beta-carotene consumption protected against cardiovascular disease and that fiber intake protected against colon cancer were all discredited by subsequent RCTs. Indeed, David L. Sackett has written about what he termed the "arrogance of preventive medicine." "Without evidence from positive randomized trials (and, better still, systematic reviews of randomized trials) we cannot justify soliciting the well to accept any personal health intervention. There are simply too many examples of the disastrous inadequacy of lesser evidence as a basis for individual interventions among the well."[21]

Numerous epidemiological studies are also severely limited by methodological inadequacies and often fail to shed light on pathological mechanisms. In surveying some of this literature, Alvan R. Feinstein found that "56 different cause-effect relationships had conflicting evidence in which the results of at least one epidemiologic study were contradicted by the results of another. About 40 more conflicting relationships would have been added if the review had included studies of disputed associations between individual sex hormones and individual birth defects." Indeed, Americans are besieged by behavioral advice that seems to change daily. They are first told that margarine is better than butter, and subsequently learn that the former may lead to clogged arteries. They exercise because it is good for their heart, but soon are told that it increases the risk of sudden death. They are told that vitamin E and beta carotene help prevent cancer, only to learn that both were no better and possibly worse than a placebo.[22]

Changes in disease incidence and prevalence may have little relationship to risk factors. The decline of rheumatic heart disease offers a contrasting example. Risk factors and even antibiotic therapy played minor roles at best in its disappearance, which may have followed the lessened virulence of the Group A streptococcus. Changing disease concepts, moreover, complicate the problem of measuring variations in incidence and prevalence. Advances in diagnostic technology, for example, have led to overestimation of the prevalence of many diseases and increased interventions of dubious benefit. Sophisticated imaging and laboratory technologies have determined that about a third of adults have evidence of papillary carcinoma of the thyroid, 40 percent of women in their forties may have ductal carcinoma in situ of the breast, and 50 percent of men in their sixties have adenocarcinoma of the prostate. Yet most of these individuals will not develop clinical forms of the disease, and treatment in such cases can result in harm.[23]

The emphasis on risk factors as a major element in CHD morbidity and mortality has had a major impact upon medical practice. By the 1970s the asymptomatic treatment of hypertension—one of the risk factors identified by both Keys and the Framingham study—had become standard medical practice. High cholesterol, by contrast, could not be treated nor was it yet regarded as a significant factor in CHD etiology. The introduction of pharmaceuticals (notably, the statins) in the 1980s to control cholesterol levels, however, led to dramatic changes in medical thinking and practice. Cholesterol reduction, fueled by the introduction of a variety of statins, became an important goal. In other words, the availability of statins was accompanied by the creation of a new disease category. Elevated cholesterol, however, is a disorder of pure number, and the number is largely a function of the negotiating process between pharmaceutical companies and consensus committees that set numbers, often in an arbitrary manner. Whether elevated cholesterol level is a disease in the conventional sense of the term or simply a number that has been reified is open to question. At best, the evidence that cholesterol reduction medications prevent cardiovascular disease is hardly conclusive. Yet the sale of statins remains at high levels (nearly $29 billion in 2004), thus creating a financial incentive to define pathology in terms of a numerical scale from "normal" to "abnormal."[24]

The faith in risk factor explanations also has had a major impact on the dietary and behavioral advice given Americans in the late twentieth century. Since high saturated fat allegedly played an important role in CHD genesis, such prestigious organizations as the American Heart Association and the AMA, as well as others, have urged Americans to reduce their intake of saturated fat by eating less meat, eggs, butter, and cheese, all of which play a role in elevating cholesterol, clogging arteries, and adding weight. Similarly, they have been urged to cease smoking. That Americans have heeded this advice is clear. Fat intake, cigarette smoking, hypertension, and cholesterol levels all declined in the last quarter of the twentieth century. Yet there is little evidence that the incidence of heart disease has declined. Moreover, obesity levels and diabetes have at the same time risen dramatically. Between 1960 and 1980 age-adjusted prevalence of obesity of men between the ages of twenty and seventy-four increased from 11 to 30 percent; the rise among women was from 16 to 34 percent. Weights of children and adolescents increased correspondingly. The number of new cases of diabetes rose from 493,000 in 1980 to 1,440,000 in 2005; the age-adjusted incidence increased from 3.5 to 7.5 during the same period.[25]

Indeed, the emphasis on low-fat diets has led to a corresponding rise in carbohydrate consumption. Between 1971 and 2000 there was a statistically significant increase in caloric intake and the percentage of calories from carbohydrates. The percentage of calories from carbohydrates increased from 42.4 to 49.0 percent among men and from 45.4 to 51.6 among women. The percentage of calories from total fat decreased among the former from 36.9 to 32.8 percent and among the latter from 36.1 to 32.8. Survey data suggest that these developments were due in part to consumption of food away from home as well as from salty snacks, soft drinks, pizza, and increased portion sizes.[26]

The relationship between a high-carbohydrate diet and disease is complex. The more carbohydrates consumed, the greater the need for insulin to send the glucose from carbohydrates to the cells to be used as fuel. If blood sugar is higher than normal, resistance to insulin-stimulated glucose develops, which is characteristic of persons with either insulin-dependent or non-insulin-dependent diabetes mellitus and impaired glucose tolerance. Resistance to insulin-stimulated glucose is common, and the compensatory response is to excrete more insulin. The other side of the equation, however, is that excess insulin leads the liver to secrete triglycerides for storage in the fat tissue with all of the corresponding risks. The ensuing state of hyperinsulinemia often prevents the development of diabetes but increases the risk of developing hyperlipidemia and hypertension, which in turn heightens the risk of developing CHD. Indeed, Gerald M. Reaven, who has made major contributions to our understanding of the critical role of insulin in a variety of diseases, has pointed out that a low-fat/high-carbohydrate diet did not modify the basic defect in insulin-resistant persons (estimated to be about one-third of the American population) and actually accentuated all of the undesirable metabolic manifestations, including CHD.[27]

In recent years, insulin resistance, hypertension, high triglycerides, and low high-density lipoprotein cholesterol levels have become known as the *metabolic syndrome,* a designation that has aroused considerable debate about whether it is or is not a distinct entity. There is general agreement, however, that central obesity, particularly upper body (as contrasted with lower body) obesity, is one of the most important causes of insulin resistance. Other factors include both diet and a sedentary lifestyle. "Insulin," according to one authority, "is at the root of the metabolic syndrome," a syndrome that plays a crucial role in causing cardiovascular events. Two studies, one in the United States and the other in Germany, found that a significant proportion of the population who were either overweight or obese were metabolically healthy. In other words, insulin resistance appeared to be a far more important variable than weight. Indeed, the CDC and NCI have found that overweight individuals have longer life expectancies than so-called normal weight persons.[28]

Nevertheless, the National Institutes of Health's National Cholesterol Education Program, created in 1986, continued to promote the claim that high LDL cholesterol—the result of high saturated fat diets and cholesterol— was the major cause of heart disease, a position seconded by most prestigious medical organizations. Yet such claims were not confirmed by a recent study that placed over three hundred obese subjects on three diets (low-fat, restricted-calorie; Mediterranean, restricted-calorie; low-carbohydrate, non-restricted-calorie) and followed them for two years. The low-carbohydrate group (which also had the highest consumption of saturated fat) lost the most weight and had the highest reduction in the ratio of total cholesterol to HDL.

The study, in other words, did not confirm the prevailing consensus on the deleterious role of saturated fats.[29]

That the hold of the risk factor hypothesis remains powerful is clear. In discussing declining cardiovascular mortality, William B. Kannel and Thomas J. Thom admitted that "no one has yet established a convincing fit of trends for any risk factor with cardiovascular mortality trends." Nor was it possible to "directly associate specific improvements in cardiovascular disease prevention and treatment with the mortality decline." Conceding that the influences of altered behaviors, medical treatment, and prevention were "incomplete, indirect, and equivocal," they nevertheless suggested that these elements had "indeed contributed to the decline in mortality."[30] Although the etiology of CHD has by no means been resolved, it seems clear that the risk factor theory, despite its popularity and widespread acceptance, has severe gaps and shortcomings. If this is the case, it may very well be that many of the dietary standards promulgated by government and private organizations may not be valid and in some instances actually harmful.

The risk factor theory is by no means the only explanation of the rise of CHD after 1900. In England David Barker was puzzled by the fact that CHD was a common cause of death among men who had low risk characteristics. He ultimately pioneered the concept that fetal undernutrition during critical periods of development in utero and during infancy led to permanent damage which increased susceptibility to CHD, stroke, hypertension, and type 2 diabetes in later life. He found that areas with the highest rates of neonatal mortality in the early twentieth century also had the highest rates of low birth weights. Barker then suggested that impaired fetal growth among those who had survived infancy predisposed them to such diseases in later life. Low birth weight infants, moreover, were at increased risk for hypertension, lung disease, and high cholesterol. The search for the causes of "Western" diseases, Barker noted, focused on the adult environment and ignored the childhood environment. He attributed this in part to the fact that most environmental models had their origin in the epidemiological studies dealing with the effects of cigarette smoking. CHD, he suggested, "may turn out to be the effect of the intrauterine or early postnatal environment."[31]

Barker's thesis has stimulated considerable work by others. In a review of the literature several researchers noted that there was evidence from a variety of disciplines to support the belief that "environmental factors acting during development should be accorded greater weight in models of disease causation." They conceded that molecular epidemiology has to date "failed to define strong genetic determinants of developing metabolic disease," but expressed the hope that "epigenetics will provide some explanations of how subtle early-life influences can produce long-term functional and structural changes." Developmental plasticity, they added, "could contribute an adaptive model that includes the effects of environmental factors during early development."[32]

The theory that adult disease may have fetal origins is intriguing, but the mechanism is unclear and conclusive supportive evidence is lacking. Barker has offered several suggestions about the ways in which undernutrition might operate, such as adversely influencing the formation of cells and hormone production or introducing vulnerabilities to adverse environments in later life. Nevertheless, other researchers have found that periods of famine had only modest effects on later health. Moreover, undernutrition is related to socioeconomic status, which also plays a significant role in health.[33]

Recent research on CHD has also begun to focus on the possible role of early life infections, which is compatible with the developmental model of disease causation. It has long been known that individuals with atherosclerosis and its clinical complications of unstable angina, myocardial infarction, and stroke have elevated markers of inflammation. At a time when the focal theory of infection was popular, William Ophüls, who was involved in more than three thousand autopsies in San Francisco hospitals during the first quarter of the twentieth century, found that lesions associated with early life infections were quite common. He collected evidence that included disease histories as well as age at death, class, race, and sex. Though dealing with an unrepresentative population, he compared individuals with a history of infectious diseases with those who did not. Ophüls found that aging alone could not explain the differences between the two groups; the former had far greater arterial and aortal damage. "The development of arteriosclerosis," he concluded, "is closely connected with injury to the arteries from various infections." Rheumatic chronic infections in particular seemed "to play the most important role." Moreover, arterial lesions reached "their full development after the active infectious process had long subsided." In recent years this older claim has reappeared in a new version. Researchers now believe that increased levels of the inflammatory biomarker high-sensitivity C-reactive protein predict cardiovascular events.[34]

Whether or not chronic inflammation is a cause or result of atherosclerosis remains unknown. Nevertheless, there are some indications that certain chronic infections caused by *Chlamydia pneumoniae* and cytomegalovirus (as well as other infectious agents) may be etiological factors. Potential mechanisms may include vessel wall contamination, which could result either in direct damage or indirect damage by initiating an immunologic response. Chronic infection may also assist in the development or destabilization of atherosclerotic plaques. Although it may be a coincidence, according to some, the decline in atherosclerosis-related deaths corresponded with the introduction of antibiotic therapy after 1945. Whether or not infections play a role in the etiology of CHD remains a provocative but as yet an unproven theory.[35]

That CHD may be related to infections is not as novel as first appears. Until the 1980s peptic and duodenal ulcers were attributed to gastric acidity, stress, smoking, alcoholic consumption, and genetic predispositions even though in 1946 it was successfully treated at Mount Sinai and the New York Hospital by an antibiotic (Aureomycin). But for unknown reasons—perhaps because of the prevailing paradigm that peptic ulcers was a noninfectious disease—a successful empirical treatment never entered clinical practice.[36] In the 1980s the *Helicobacter pylori* bacterium was identified as one of the causal agents. Though initially disregarded by clinicians, this finding ultimately led to a partial reconceptualization of peptic and duodenal ulcer and to the use of antibiotic as well as traditional therapies. Whether research on CHD will follow a similar path is as yet unclear. At present it is possible to diagnose and manage CHD by such means as bypass surgery, angioplasty, stents, and drugs (although their effectiveness remains controversial). In general, these medical technologies improve the quality of life even if they do not always extend it. The etiology of CHD, however, remains shrouded in mystery. In noting the decline in heart disease mortality, Lewis Thomas admitted,

> No one seems to know why this happened, which is not in itself surprising since no one really knows for sure what the underlying mechanism responsible for coronary disease is. In the circumstance, everyone is free to provide one's own theory, depending on one's opinion about the mechanism. You can claim, if you like, that there has been enough reduction in the dietary intake of saturated fat, nationwide, to make the difference, although I think you'd have a hard time proving it. Or, if you prefer, you can attribute it to the epidemic of jogging, but I think that the fall in incidence of coronary disease had already begun before jogging became a national mania. Or, if you are among those who believe than an excessively competitive personality strongly influences the incidence of this disease, you might assert that more of us

have become calmer and less combative since the 1950s, and I suppose you could back up the claim by simply listing the huge numbers of new mental-health professionals, counselors, lifestyle authorities, and various health gurus who have appeared in our midst in recent years. But I doubt it, just as I doubt their effectiveness in calming us all down.[37]

The Enigma of Cancer Epidemiology

Like CHD, cancer presents similar enigmas. In 1900 malignant neoplasms accounted for perhaps 4 percent of all deaths and ranked sixth as a cause of mortality. The proportion of deaths from cancer began a gradual rise, and by 1940 cancer was ranked second and accounted for 11 percent of mortality. In 1960, 1980, and 2004, the figures were 16, 21, and 23 percent, respectively. Of 2.39 million deaths in 2004, about 554,000 were from malignant neoplasms. Between 1950 and 1993 cancer death rates rose. In 1950 the rate was 140 per 100,000; by 1993 it had risen to 206. At that point there was a modest decline in cancer mortality. Between 1993 and 2002 the decrease was 1.1 percent per year. The decrease then accelerated; between 2002 and 2004 the decline was 2.1 percent.[38] Like heart disease, mortality from cancer was related to age. The increase in the number of cancer deaths was in part a reflection of the fact that far more individuals survived infancy and youth and lived a relatively long life. Yet age alone cannot explain cancer epidemiology.

Statistical data, however, revealed little about a disease that has aroused profound fears and anxieties. Cancer, of course, was not a new disease; it was found in mummies. Despite its ancient lineage, it remained somewhat of a mystery. For precisely this reason, paradoxically, competing theories about its nature and etiology were plentiful in the early twentieth century. Some argued that it was a contagious disease caused by germs; some insisted that it was inherited; some thought it related to the rise of industrial civilization; some suggested that it was caused by emotional or mental stress; and others believed that various forms of irritation predisposed tissue to cancerous growth. The seeming inability of physicians to treat most forms of cancer also led to a proliferation of therapies. In 1913 the American Society for the Control of Cancer (later the American Cancer Society) was created to educate the public about the importance of early detection and surgery.[39] Nearly a quarter of a century later a congressional act created the National Cancer Institute, which after World War II enjoyed phenomenal growth. Indeed, by the late 1960s a powerful lobby had declared "war" on cancer, leading to the passage of the "war on cancer" act of 1971.[40]

Cancer has also received more publicity than almost every other disease. The disease, according to Keith Wailoo, "has long been a barometer of social difference, an index of social roles and relations, a vital indicator of inequalities, a marker of fundamental differences among people, and a vehicle for expressing anxieties about change and social status." Speculation about its etiology has involved a myriad of competing theories. Heredity, microbes, viruses, irritations, occupation, behavior, diet, environment, and such psychological factors as stress were all advanced as causal elements in cancer genesis. Nor were race, ethnicity, class, and gender excluded. In the early twentieth century, for example, cancer was regarded as a "white disease," and white women were most at risk because they had rejected their traditional roles as mothers. African Americans, by contrast, had low rates, partly because they lived in a simpler stress-free environment and thus did not develop diseases of civilization. To demonstrate such differences, experts relied on statistical data despite their severe shortcomings. In the late twentieth century, by contrast, cancer had crossed the racial divide even as the older categories of white and non-white were replaced by such new categories as Hispanic and Asians, which proved equally complex because of the divisions within each of these groups.[41]

As the research effort into the mysteries of cancer multiplied exponentially after 1945, explanations continued to proliferate. There were, of course, precedents to draw upon. In 1775 Percivall Pott noted that young English chimney sweeps often developed scrotal cancer, which he attributed to inflammation caused by soot. In 1910 Peyton Rous demonstrated that chicken sarcoma could be reproduced by a filterable virus. The major emphasis in postwar America, however, was on the effect of carcinogens, including radiation, air pollution, occupation, food additives, exposure to sunlight, and various chemicals. At the same time risk factor explanations that emphasized diet and smoking proliferated. The therapeutic armamentarium also multiplied, and surgical intervention was augmented by chemotherapy and new forms of radiation that were effective against certain types of cancers.

What is cancer? Like many other long-duration illnesses, it is much easier to describe its pathology than its etiology. Recent work in molecular biology has begun to unravel some (but not all) of the mysteries of cancer. The mammalian genome contains tumor suppressor genes as well as proto-oncogenes. The latter are essentially accelerators and the former brakes in cell growth. Excessive cell growth can result from a defect in either. An inherited cancer syndrome or a genetic accident—either random or induced by a carcinogen—transforms the function of tumor suppressor genes or proto-oncogenes and thus distorts the normal process of cell growth and differentiation. It is also becoming increasingly clear that human cancers are biologically heterogeneous and that future therapies will have to take this into account.[42]

Contrary to popular belief, the genesis of cancer is a slow process; decades pass before the disease becomes symptomatic. The progression of lung cancer (which is associated with cigarette smoking) is relatively slow. In general, a person has to smoke for three decades before a single cell becomes malignant. In reports of doubling times for primary lung cancer (n = 228) it took approximately 102 days for the malignant cell to double. Thus a single cell became a tumor of 1 mm. in diameter after doubling twenty times. A further ten doublings produced a tumor of 1 cm. in diameter and after ten more doublings it had a diameter of 10 cm. It took 8.4 years (thirty doublings) to grow to 1 cm. (the earliest stage at which the tumor could be diagnosed) and 9.8 years to reach 3 cm. (the time when the usual diagnosis was made). Death followed when the tumor reached 10 cm. (11.2 years). In other words, lung cancer is diagnosed about 10 years after the initial malignant stage, at which time it reached seven-eighths of its total size.[43]

The example of colorectal cancer (a significant factor in cancer mortality) is equally instructive. The natural progression of the disease is slow, often taking between twenty and forty years. At the outset epithelial cells lining the bowel wall proliferate excessively. In the second stage they thicken. Subsequently, these thickenings protrude into the cavity of the colon, resulting in small polyps. These growths are not life threatening, but later some evolve into true malignant cells, obstruct the colonic tube, invade the underlying muscle wall, and eventually metastasize to other parts of the body. Recent research has revealed that each stage is accompanied by a genetic change. Early polyps follow the loss of a tumor suppressor gene. The appearance of mature colorectal carcinomas is dependent on several genetic changes plus mutant forms of another gene.[44]

Unlike CHD, cancer mortality rates did not fluctuate radically during the past century. Yet the overall cancer mortality rate is not necessarily an accurate barometer. Rates for specific cancers have changed dramatically over time. Moreover, there are considerable variations in mortality based on sex, ethnicity, race, class, age, and geographical location. Such variations make it extraordinarily difficult to make definitive statements about the etiology of what may be very different kinds of diseases even though they are all subsumed under a single general category.[45]

Between 1930 and 1965 age-adjusted mortality rates from all cancers increased. Pancreatic cancer, particularly among those age forty-five or older, showed a decided increase, as did cancers of the urinary organs, kidney, ovaries, intestine, and, especially, the lung. Cancer of the prostate declined for those under sixty-five and remained stable or increased for those over sixty-five. Breast cancer mortality among women remained more or less stable, while increasing among African American females. The data on the relationship between race and neoplasms, however, did not take socioeconomic class into account, thus limiting their usefulness.[46]

Mortality from lung cancer among males, which was relatively unknown before 1930, began a spectacular rise after that date. Between 1960 to 1962 and 1990 to 1992 mortality among this group increased 85 percent from 40 to 74 per 100,000; after 1992 a slight decline became evident. Female rates leaped from 6.0 to 32.3, an increase of 438 percent. Indeed, overall mortality from cancer would have shown a slight decline had it not been for the increase in lung cancer. Mortality from melanoma of the skin also showed large percentage increases, but the number of cases was relatively small. At present, lung and bronchus cancer account for 31 percent of mortality among males and 26 percent among females. Prostate cancer mortality, which doubled between 1930 and 1990 and remains the second leading cause of death among males, then began a period of decline. Breast cancer, the second leading cause of mortality, began to decline about 1990 and accounts for 15 percent of deaths among women. Colorectal cancer mortality averages between 9 and 10 percent and has also been declining during the past two decades. Stomach cancer by far experienced the greatest mortality decline since 1930.[47]

To be sure, overall cancer mortality rates have continued to decline since the early 1990s. Yet the changes were by no means evenly distributed. Of the fifteen leading causes of cancer deaths, rates decreased for these cancer sites: colorectum, stomach, kidney, brain, non-Hodgkin lymphoma, and myeloma in both men and women; lung, prostate, and oral cavity and pharynx in men; and breast, uterine cervix, and bladder in women. On the other hand, deaths from esophageal cancer in men, pancreatic cancer in women, and liver cancer in both men and women increased. Complicating the picture even further is the fact that there are wide variations in mortality rates by state and region.[48]

What accounts for overall cancer mortality as well as changes in the rates for particular neoplasms? As in the case of CHD, the answer is by no means self-evident. There is general agreement that certain cancers have external

causes. Lung cancer, for example, is clearly related to smoking even though
other co-factors may play a role. In general, lung cancer was not significant in
the early twentieth century when tobacco consumption was low. In 1880, for
example, the average cigarette smoker consumed 0.047 pounds of unstemmed
tobacco (before the removal of stems). There was a gradual rise in usage, but
as late as 1914 consumption was 0.82 pounds. Shortly thereafter consumption
began a steady rise; the first peak in usage came in 1953 when the average
cigarette smoker over the age of fourteen consumed 10.46 pounds or 3,558
cigarettes per annum. In 1979 the average smoker age eighteen and over
consumed 33.5 cigarettes per day. The lag between the time that cigarette
smoking became common and the increase in lung cancer mortality is understandable, for the health effects of the habit take many years to appear.[49] Only
after World War II did epidemiological data and pathological evidence began
to confirm the association between smoking and lung cancer even though the
precise mechanism was unknown. That other substances and behaviors are
involved in specific cancers is also clear. Asbestos, certain industrial chemicals, prolonged exposure to sunlight, and ionizing radiation all have carcino-
genic qualities, although the numbers of people exposed are far smaller than
the number of cigarette smokers.

The etiology of most cancers and the changes in prevalence and mortality rates, however, remain somewhat of a mystery. Consider the case of gastric
cancer. Prior to World War II gastric cancer was the leading cause of cancer
mortality in males and the third in females. But by 1930 a decline in mortality appeared that persisted for the rest of the century. In 1960 it had fallen to
sixth place, and in 1992 it ranked ninth. Between 1962 and 1992 the number
of deaths fell from 19,378 to 13,630 even though population had increased.
Other industrialized nations experienced a comparable decline, although
there were considerable variations in rates.[50]

What explains this dramatic decline? There is no evidence that new treatments played a role; surgery remained the only option and was effective only
if the tumor was confined to the mucosa and submucosa. Nor was there any
change in survival rates after diagnosis. Since the decline in mortality from
gastric cancer was international, the assumption of those who have studied
the disease is that the major etiologic influences were environmental rather
than genetic and that changes in referral, diagnosis, and treatment played no
role. Of all environmental factors, diet was the focus of most attention. High-
carbohydrate diets, nitrates and nitrites, and salt were implicated as potential etiologic factors, whereas the consumption of vegetables and fruits (and

therefore an increased intake of vitamins C, E, and A) were associated with a decreased risk. More recently the emphasis has been on bacterial infection with HP in conjunction with previously cited risk factors. The highest rates of gastric cancer are found in Japan. In that nation age-standardized mortality rates in 2002 were 24.1 per 100,000 for men and 9.6 for women, as compared with 3.4 and 1.7, respectively, in the United States. Despite the claim that HP infection and dietary factors were the major risk factors leading to high rates in Japan, researchers have been unable to quantify their effect with any degree of accuracy. Indeed, the persistence of wide variations and changes in mortality rates and diets between countries render many etiological explanations problematic at best. More significantly, the decline in mortality antedated dietary change, which in any case would have taken at least two decades to make its influence felt. Like the decline in mortality from CHD, the decline in mortality from gastric cancer remains a puzzling enigma that epidemiological studies have failed to explain.[51]

The striking relationship between smoking and lung cancer, as well as evidence that exposure to a relatively small number of chemicals and radiation can also result in malignancies, fostered the emergence of an explanatory model that emphasized an environmental and behavioral etiology for most cancers. Yet the evidence to demonstrate such linkages in many cases was hardly persuasive. Virtually all of the epidemiological studies that emphasize such factors as diet and lifestyle in cancer genesis suffer from the same defects as similar studies of the etiology of CHD.

Richard Doll, who played a significant role in illuminating the risks of smoking, extended the environmental interpretation of cancer etiology in dramatic fashion. Cancer, he and Richard Peto wrote in 1981, "is largely a preventable disease." More than two-thirds (and perhaps more) of all cancers were due to smoking and diet, while occupational hazards, alcohol, food additives, sexual behavior, pollution, industrial products, and medical technology played very minor roles. The two men gathered comparative data that revealed differential incidence rates for specific cancers in various countries. Only diet and lifestyle, they insisted, could explain such differences. Their study, which originally appeared in the *Journal of the National Cancer Institute,* was also published separately in book form and was cited in countless journal articles.[52]

For a variety of reasons the belief that cancer was a preventable illness continued to prevail. In 1996 the *Harvard Report on Cancer Prevention* included a table listing the estimated percentage of total cancer deaths attributable to established causes of cancer. Tobacco and adult diet/obesity each accounted for 30 percent of mortality. A sedentary lifestyle, occupation, family history, biologic agents, and perinatal factors each accounted for 5 percent; the remainder were divided among reproductive factors, alcohol, socioeconomic status, environmental pollution, radiation, prescription drugs/medical procedures, and salt and other food additives. Cancer, the report concluded, was "indeed a preventable illness." It offered a variety of suggestions: a reduction smoking and consumption of alcoholic beverages; dietary modifications involving increased consumption of vegetables, fruits, bread, pasta, and cereals; reduced consumption of red meat, animal fat, salt, and refined carbohydrates; greater use of plant oils; avoidance of obesity in adult life; increased physical activity; and avoidance of exposure to radiation and environmental hazards. A recent report by the World Cancer Research Fund came to similar conclusions and argued for a preventive approach.[53]

Subsequently, Colin B. Begg, an epidemiologist at Memorial Sloan Kettering Center in New York City, expressed reservations about the Harvard report. He noted that the report echoed countless cohort, case-control, and ecological studies that purported to show that cancer was caused by environmental factors. Critical of the methodology employed by such studies, Begg emphasized, in particular, the omission of any consideration of genetic susceptibility, which could operate independently of environmental risk factors. This criticism was rejected by Graham A. Colditz, one of the editors of the Harvard report. Taking colon cancer as an example, he argued that with "population-wide increases in levels of physical activity and folate intake, and with reductions in alcohol intake, adult weight gain and obesity, red meat consumption, and smoking, up to 70% of colon cancer could be avoided." "It is also time," he added, "to stop chasing after new risk factors."[54]

The effort to link cancer to diet, carcinogens, and behavior—which has been central to the campaign to prevent and control the disease—has been rooted largely in belief and hope rather than fact. Smoking is the one notable exception. Other *proven* carcinogens such as asbestos and high-level radiation hazard other than solar ultraviolet rays affected relatively few individuals. The myriad epidemiological studies of the relationship of diet and behavior to the genesis of cancer—which tended to give results that were constantly changing and usually contradictory—were generally based on questionable epidemiological methodologies. These epidemiological findings, their weaknesses notwithstanding, have caught public attention largely because they seem to confirm the belief that cancer is preventable and that individuals have it within their power to minimize the risk by changing their behavior and lifestyle.

That prevention of cancer in the latter half of the twentieth century remained an elusive goal did not diminish its popularity. Prevention, after all, supported values that placed a premium on individual responsibility for one's own health and well-being. The alternative—that the etiology of cancer was endogenous and not necessarily amenable to individual volition—was hardly an attractive explanation. It is entirely plausible, for example, that cancer is closely related to aging, genetic susceptibility, and genetic mutations, which together impair the ability of the immune system to identify and attack malignant cells and thus permit them to multiply. If there is at present no way to arrest the aging process, then cancer mortality may be inevitable. Moreover, some of the genetic mutations that eventually lead to cancer may occur randomly, and thus cannot be prevented.

Nevertheless, the concept of prevention remains popular. John C. Bailar III, who tracked cancer mortality over several decades, emphasized the failure to find effective therapies. "Age-adjusted mortality rates," he noted in 1986, "have shown a slow and steady increase over several decades, and there is no evidence of a recent downward trend. In this clinical sense we are losing the war against cancer." A decade later he found little improvement even though there had been changes in incidence and mortality rates of specific malignancies. Indeed, the death rate in 1994 was 2.7 percent higher than in 1982, the last year covered in his 1986 paper. In 1986 Bailar wrote that thirty-five years of intensive effort to focus on improving treatment "must be judged a qualified failure." Twelve years later he saw "little reason to change that conclusion." "The best of modern medicine," he concluded, "has much to offer to virtually every patient with cancer, for palliation if not always for cure. . . . The problem is the lack of substantial improvement over what treatment could already accomplish some decades ago. A national commitment to the prevention of cancer, largely replacing reliance on hopes for universal cures, is now the way to go."[55] To be sure, Bailar was overly pessimistic about the efficacy of therapies. In the past decade there have been advances in treating many cancers that extend life even if they do not result in cures. Yet his emphasis on prevention reflected prevailing sentiment.

Aside from behavioral modification to reduce cancer morbidity and mortality, an increasing effort has been underway to urge individuals to take advantage of screening tests to detect cancer. Adults in general have accepted medical claims that finding cancer in its early stages saves lives. One survey found that nearly all women over the age of forty had a PAP test to detect cervical cancer and 89 percent had a mammogram; 71 percent of males aged fifty or over had a PSA (prostate-specific antigen) test to detect prostate cancer; and 46 percent of both sexes had a sigmoidoscopy or colonoscopy. Moreover, most adults were enthusiastic about the prospects of undergoing a total-body CT (computed tomography) scan, a procedure now being aggressively marketed to consumers.[56]

The goal of screening is clear, namely, to detect disease in its earliest stages when it is most treatable and presumably curable. For screening to be successful three requirements must be met. First, the disease must have a recognizable early stage. Second, there must be an accurate way to diagnose the disease. Finally, there must be a therapy that is effective when applied early rather than in later stages when treatments are far less effective.[57]

Yet the evidence that overall cancer mortality has been reduced by screening is not entirely persuasive. The case of prostate cancer is instructive, for it is the most frequently diagnosed cancer in men. During 2007 an estimated 219,000 new cases and 27,000 deaths will occur.[58] Yet most prostate cancers are so slow growing that they are asymptomatic and have little or no effect upon life expectancy. A two-decade-long study of 767 men aged fifty-five to seventy-four years with clinically localized prostate cancer diagnosed between 1971 and 1984 found that there was only a small risk of cancer progression. Their results, the investigators concluded, "do not support aggressive treatment of localized low-grade prostate cancer."[59]

Aside from a digital rectal examination followed by an ultrasound examination and biopsy, the only other screening test is a blood test for prostate-specific antigen. The usefulness of the rectal examination is limited because of the inability to reach all parts of the prostate gland. Ultrasound has a high yield of false positives. Traditionally, a PSA score of 4.0 ng per milliliter or higher was considered suspicious and required further investigation. Aside from a high rate of false positives and false negatives—to say nothing about the fact that normal PSA ranges vary from laboratory to laboratory—recent research has shown that the upper limit of the normal range of the PSA is unknown. As many as 15 percent of men with a "normal" PSA had high-grade cancers. A more recent study led to a finding that variations in five chromosomal regions were associated with a heightened risk of prostate cancer, particularly if there was a family history of the disease.[60]

Nor is there clear evidence that current treatments, including prostatectomy, radiation, and hormone therapy extend life. "Prostate-cancer screening," Edward P. Gelmann has noted, "has resulted in a substantial degree of overdiagnosis of cancers that never would have been presented clinically and that would not have affected morbidity or mortality." Moreover, many treatments have serious side effects, including impotence, incontinence, and a higher risk of death following surgery. Since most prostate cancers grow so slowly that they are harmless, the treatments themselves may pose far greater dangers than watchful waiting. Indeed, Peter C. Albertsen, the principal investigator of the twenty-year outcome study, noted that there was too much prostate screening, resulting in too much treatment. "To me, it is a nightmare," he remarked. "We are just feeding off this cancer *phobia*." A study comparing the impact of screening in the Seattle–Puget Sound area and in Connecticut was revealing. In the Seattle area there was a much higher rate of intensive screening followed by radical prostatectomy and external beam radiotherapy among Medicare beneficiaries aged sixty-five to seventy-nine than in Connecticut. Yet the study, which followed a cohort selected between 1987 and 1990 and followed for eleven years, found no differences in age-adjusted prostate death rates between the two areas. That the benefits of the PSA were shrouded in mystery was reflected in 2008 when the U.S. Preventive Services Task Force (located in the Agency for Healthcare Research and Quality) issued a recommendation statement. It concluded that for men younger than age seventy-five "the benefits of screening for prostate cancer are uncertain and the balance of benefits and harms cannot be determined." It also recommended against screening in men age seventy-five or older, since the harms outweighed the benefits.[61]

Nowhere was the dilemma posed by screening better illustrated than by the introduction of the steroid drug finasteride (Proscar) in the early 1990s to treat enlargement of the prostate (Benign Prostatic Hyperplasia or BPH). In 1993 the Prostate Cancer Prevention Trial was launched to determine if finasteride prevented the disease. The results after seven years showed that prostate cancer was detected in 803 of the 4,368 men taking finasteride (18.4 percent), as contrasted with 1,147 cases out of 4,692 in the placebo group (24.4 percent). This seemed to indicate a 24.8 percent reduction. The finasteride group, however, had a higher rate of more aggressive tumors (6.4 versus 5.1 percent in the placebo group). Thus the same drug that lowered the incidence of prostate cancer was also associated with an increase in the most dangerous form of the disease. A subsequent pathological analysis of the prostate gland of 500 subjects who underwent radical prostatectomies in the original study, however, found that the shrinkage of the prostate by the drug made it easier to detect aggressive tumors. Finasteride decreased the risk by 30 percent of having any tumor without any increase in the aggressive or lethal form.[62]

Yet the use of finasteride to reduce the incidence of prostate cancer posed a series of troubling questions. One authority has pointed out that while 10 percent of men over the age of fifty-five find out that they have the disease, the cancer is lethal in no more than 25 percent of them. If finasteride reduced the incidence by 30 percent, about 7 percent would get a cancer diagnosis, and there would be a reduction in the lethal form of the disease from 2.5 to 1.8 percent. "Finasteride," he concluded, "might make a difference but only in a very small subset of men." Indeed, a new rationale for prescribing the drug emerged, namely, that it would reduce the use of invasive and debilitating treatments that leave men impotent or incontinent for a disease that is generally not lethal. Yet other considerations are involved. What are the risks of taking a drug for years whose long-term side effects are unknown to treat a disease that is often better left undiagnosed? And what costs are involved?[63]

Mammography screening for breast cancer in women presents some of the same problems as screening for prostate cancer. Breast cancer mortality remained fairly stable between 1930 and 1975. Between 1975 and 1990 it increased by 0.4 percent annually, and between 1990 and 2004 it decreased by 2.2 percent annually. Incidence rates followed a slightly different pattern. Between 1980 and 1987 they increased rapidly, followed by smaller increases between 1987 and 2001, and then began to decrease between 2001 and 2004.[64]

What role did mammography play in changing incidence and mortality patterns? The answer to this question is by no means clear. Indeed, controversy has been characteristic. The American Cancer Society, the National Cancer Institute (NCI), and many other organizations and individuals have been adamant in insisting that early detection provides the best opportunity for effective intervention. The Breast Cancer Detection Demonstration Project, begun in 1973 and supported by the American Cancer Society and the NCI, seemed to support the efficacy of mammography. Yet a severe challenge came from John C. Bailar III, the deputy associate director of the NCI. He agreed that annual history, physical examination, and mammography could reduce breast cancer mortality by about a third. Nevertheless, the evidence that mammography alone played a significant role was weak and indirect. Above all, evidence on the long-term effect of associated radiation hazards had not been determined, and he concluded by noting that "promotion of mammography as a general public health measure is premature."[65]

Despite its popularity, mammography remains a controversial screening tool. Some studies of mammography have suggested that claims of efficacy have been somewhat overstated. In reviewing for the Cochrane Collaboration the results of seven trials involving half a million women who had undergone mammograms, two respected Danish figures found severe methodological shortcomings. They noted the absence of large, well-conducted randomized trials with all-cause mortality as the primary outcome. In their eyes it was unclear whether the benefits of the procedure outweighed its risks. They conceded that there was a reduction in mortality. For every two thousand women screened for ten years, one would have her life prolonged. But ten healthy women who would not have been diagnosed if there had not been screening would be diagnosed as breast cancer patients and thus would receive unnecessary treatment that held out potential threats to their health. Many in situ breast cancers that are found by mammography are noninvasive and pose little threat. Over-diagnosis, in other words, is a concomitant of screening that poses its own risk. Moreover, mammography exposes individuals to radiation, which over a lifetime adds to the risk of the procedure. Its enthusiastic proponents notwithstanding, it remains unclear whether the benefits of mammography outweigh the risks.[66]

Conclusion

It seems clear that cherished explanations of the etiology and changing patterns of cancer and heart disease morbidity and mortality lack a solid evidentiary foundation. Indeed, many etiological assertions tend to be based on opinion and hope rather than on clear and unambiguous empirical evidence. This is not in any way to diminish the role of clinical medicine, which has the ability to provide palliative therapies for the various forms of these diseases that improve the quality of life and, to some extent, add to longevity. Yet there is a striking difference between medicine's ability to manage many diseases and its etiological claims. Indeed, etiological claims whose validity is yet to be determined can have a negative impact, if only because they lead to the articulation of proposals for behavioral changes in diet and lifestyle that may or may not be appropriate. Claims to the contrary, our knowledge about disease and basic physiological processes, however impressive, is dwarfed by what remains unknown.

Chapter 5

Transforming Amorphous Stress into Discrete Disorders

The Case of Anxiety

Psychiatry has always helped set many of the most important social boundaries. These include distinctions between abnormality and normality, disease and deviance, symptoms of illness and natural feelings, and states deserving of sympathy or of stigma. During the last half of the nineteenth century, culturally suitable diseases began to require specific diagnoses, sharp boundaries, and particular etiological mechanisms. By the latter decades of the twentieth century, this trend was firmly established and any respected medical specialty had to treat delineated disease entities. Specific diagnoses were necessary for professional authority, legitimate treatments, and monetary reimbursement. Yet the psychiatric profession actually dealt with a huge variety of distressing and impairing psychosocial problems that rarely featured unambiguous boundaries or precise causes. A perennial struggle to carve out explicit diagnoses from an undifferentiated and heterogeneous range of upsetting symptoms has marked the psychiatric profession. More than any other branch of medicine, psychiatry faces tremendous difficulties in separating disease entities from each other and from healthy conditions.[1]

Anxiety provides perhaps the best example of psychiatry's struggle to create explicit diagnostic categories out of ambiguous symptomatic presentations. Signs of anxiety are diffuse and multifaceted. Some are psychic, involving feelings of worry, nervous tension, foreboding, threat, and alarm. Others are somatic, including increased muscular tension, heart palpitations, breathing difficulties, raised blood pressure, and heavy sweating. Many patients with these symptoms also suffer from a variety of psychosocial problems with relationships, finances, and health, among others. The protean mixture of somatic problems, psychic symptoms, and life difficulties in most anxiety states raises difficult boundary questions about distinctions between disease and health and between psychic and physical conditions.

One dilemma diagnosticians confront is how to set boundaries between normal fear and irrational anxiety. Fuzzy and vague boundaries demarcate anxiety disorders from those that are natural responses to external contexts. Symptoms of anxiety can indicate pathology when they occur in the absence of threat or are disproportionately severe or enduring relative to the presence of danger. The same symptoms, however, can be natural and adaptive if they emerge in dangerous, threatening, or uncertain situations.[2] Another diagnostic dilemma is that anxious symptoms characterize numerous physical and mental disorders. Symptoms of anxiety overlap considerably with many common somatic complaints that general physicians typically treat. Likewise, they are ubiquitous in numerous other mental disorders such as depression or schizophrenia. Pure cases of anxiety are rare, especially as conditions unfold over time.

The amorphous qualities of anxiety, its intrinsic overlap with normal worries, and its omnipresence in numerous bodily and psychological conditions render it ill-suited for the categorical and well-bounded diagnostic entities that medically legitimate diseases require. The natural fluidity of anxiety has led the borders between non-disordered and disordered conditions, anxiety and other mental disorders, and different types of anxiety disorders to shift constantly over time depending on prevalent professional, political, economic, and cultural circumstances and interests.

The Evolution of Anxiety Disorders, from Hippocrates to Neurasthenia

Beginning with the earliest Hippocratic writings in the fifth century BC, medical writings have occasionally described cases that would now be recognized as instances of general anxiety, phobic, and obsessive compulsive disorders. Nevertheless, in contrast to conditions such as melancholia, mania, or schizophrenia, psychiatrists and physicians never clearly distinguished anxiety as a distinctive type of disorder until the late nineteenth century. Instead, anxiety was either subsumed as an amorphous type of melancholic disorder that was associated with psychic agitation or was interchangeable with deep feelings of sorrow. The initial formulation of melancholy during the Hippocratic period, for example, explicitly linked anxiety and depression: "When fear and sadness last a long time, this is a melancholic condition."[3]

Admittedly, major psychiatric tracts published before the nineteenth century often noted cases that modern psychiatry would regard as anxiety disorders. Robert Burton's classic seventeenth-century compendium, *The Anatomy of Melancholy,* for example, noted that terrors and frights stemming "from some imminent danger, when a terrible object is at hand" are common causes of melancholic conditions. Burton mentioned a number of particular objects and situations that sometimes are associated with normal fears and sometimes with mental disorders. Yet, he never viewed anxiety as a distinct category but instead included it as one of many causes of more general melancholic conditions. Likewise, the eminent American physician Benjamin Rush insightfully distinguished natural fears from anxiety disorders in a 1798 essay, defining phobia as "a fear of an imaginary evil, or an undue fear of a real one."[4] Psychiatric diagnosticians before the latter part of the nineteenth century, however, did not consider anxiety as a discreet category that was separable from broader mental and somatic states.

Throughout this period anxiety was more commonly connected to philosophical and religious issues than to mental or physical disorders. During the nineteenth century the ideas of the Danish philosopher Soren Kierkegaard became influential. Kierkegaard linked anxiety (Angst) to the normal condition of humanity and not to a somatic illness.[5] He treated anxiety as a pervasive and fundamental state of being that naturally arose because of the perils of life, uncertain existence of a divinity, and inevitability of death.

Institutional circumstances accounted for the ill-defined nature of anxious conditions before the latter decades of the nineteenth century. Until this period psychiatric classifications stemmed from the problems of hospitalized patients. Such patients typically suffered from severe conditions such as schizophrenia, mania, and melancholia. Anxiety was rarely severe or dangerous enough to warrant institutionalization and so was not an important aspect of psychiatric nosologies. Terms, such as "nervous illness," that became widespread during the eighteenth century were non-specific labels used in general medical practice and neurology, not in psychiatry.[6] At the time, diagnoses of nervousness would have allowed people to *avoid* seeing themselves as mentally ill because they allowed them to associate their conditions with somatic problems. Interest in anxiety as a mental disorder in its own right did not emerge until the latter part of the nineteenth century.

Cardiologists developed an interest in anxiety during the middle of the nineteenth century, observing a relationship between anxiety and heart problems, especially among soldiers.[7] They noted that battlefield experiences often stimulated symptoms that included heart palpitations, cardiac pain of various types, rapid pulse, and shortness of breath. Cardiologists subsumed anxiety symptoms as certain types of heart problems, calling them "soldier's heart," "nervous palpitations," or "irritable heart." Nevertheless, there were few points of contact between cardiologists and psychiatrists and these classifications did not penetrate psychiatric conceptions at the time.

The German psychiatrist Carl Westphal developed an early distinct classification of an anxiety disorder in 1872 when he delineated the syndrome of agoraphobia—the "impossibility of walking through certain streets or squares, or possibility of so doing only with resultant dread of anxiety." Nevertheless, most psychiatrists continued to subsume anxiety disorders under the general category of depressive conditions. For example, the most distinguished diagnostician of the nineteenth century, German psychiatrist Emil Kraepelin, devoted considerable attention to Angst—a general state of fear, dread, terror, and apprehension. He also described a condition of Schreckneurose (fright neuroses) that could "be observed after serious accidents and injuries, particularly fires, railway derailments or collisions, etc." Kraepelin, however, generally considered anxious symptoms to have a variety of phobic, obsessional, anxious, depressive, and somatic manifestations that were components of a variety of disorders rather than indicators of a specific disease. Similarly, British psychiatrist Henry Maudsley's influential text, *Pathology of Mind,* classified phobias as a subtype of melancholic disorders. In France, Pierre Janet advocated for a unified family of disorders that encompassed a variety of anxious, depressive, and psychosomatic conditions.[8]

In 1869 the American neurologist George Beard described the indicators of a syndrome that he called "neurasthenia." This condition encompassed a wide variety of physical and psychosocial symptoms including, among others, nervousness, exhaustion, fatigue, dyspepsia, headaches, paralysis, vague pains, sexual dysfunction, and insomnia. This diverse collection of symptoms captured the extremely diffuse conditions of the generally well-off clients of physicians and nerve doctors at the time. Beard insisted that these conditions had somatic bases, which were often inherited, so that people who received labels of neurasthenia would not see themselves as having mental illnesses. The term almost immediately became wildly popular in America, offering a physical-sounding label for many various psychosomatic conditions.[9] Some of the protean symptoms of neurasthenia were related to anxiety conditions but many were not. By the end of the century this condition, which never featured specific manifestations, had become most associated with states of chronic fatigue, exhaustion, and lethargy that more closely resembled depressive or psychosomatic states than anxious conditions.

When psychiatrists and neurologists established community practices independent of inpatient mental hospitals at the end of the nineteenth century, they began to attract non-psychotic clients who suffered from a diffuse collection of psychosomatic, bodily, and nervous complaints variously labeled as "neurasthenia," "hysteria," or "hypochondriasis." Nevertheless, anxiety was rarely recognized as an independent or an important psychiatric condition. Until the turn of that century anxious conditions were seldom considered to be discrete, they lacked sharp boundaries, and they were generally linked to other somatic and mental disturbances. The status of anxiety dramatically changed when the writings of Sigmund Freud gained preeminence.

Freud and the Emergence of the Anxiety Disorders

Before the twentieth century, nearly all psychiatrists practiced in inpatient mental institutions, which very rarely treated patients who primarily suffered from anxiety disorders. Such conditions seldom created enough danger to others, as schizophrenia or manic-depressive might, or danger to self or severe withdrawal from social roles, as melancholia often did. Severely anxious persons consulted general physicians, neurologists, or spa doctors, who avoided applying psychiatric labels and instead treated anxiety as a type of medical condition.[10] Clergy were also a common source of help for general states of anxiety. The emergence of psychoanalytically oriented outpatient therapies dramatically changed conceptions of anxiety disorders.

Far more than any previous thinker, Sigmund Freud made anxiety the central aspect of neurotic disorders. Freud initially posited that anxiety resulted from a transformation of repressed sexual energy. His thinking about anxiety subsequently changed in significant ways, and he came to believe that anxiety was a fundamental cause of repression rather than vice versa: "It was anxiety which produced repression and not, as I formerly believed, repression which produced anxiety." In 1894 he coined the term "anxiety neurosis," separating this condition from the more general state of neurasthenia. In several works, he described the psychic components of threat, irritability, and inability to concentrate and the somatic components of heart palpitations, breathing problems, tremors, sweating, and gastrointestinal disturbances that remain the central components of anxiety disorders.[11] Over the course of his career, Freud also differentiated anxiety disorders from normal fears and from depressive conditions, distinguished several types of anxiety disorders, and developed a causal theory of anxiety. Freud's influence was substantial enough that during the period between roughly 1920 and 1970 psychoanalysts tended to interpret all neurotic symptoms as either manifestations or derivatives of anxiety.

Freud and his followers not only put anxiety at the heart of their theory but also reversed the previous hierarchy of psychiatric classification, relegating depression (or melancholia) to a secondary status. Anxiety, in their view, lay behind most forms of neurotic behavior, including not only such direct manifestations as phobias, obsessions, panic, and general anxiety, but also hysteria, sexual dysfunctions, and psychosomatic problems, among others. "Anxiety," Freud wrote in *Civilization and Its Discontents*, "is always present somewhere or other behind every symptom."[12]

Freud distinguished realistic fears ("realistic anxiety"), which were normal, biologically programmed responses to external or internal dangers, from anxiety neuroses. Fear arose as a reaction to actual dangers, signaling the ego about some threatening situation and so had the "indispensable biological function to fulfill as a reaction to a state of danger." Neurotic anxiety, in contrast, involved a disproportion of internal emotions and external threats. The symptoms of anxiety reactions were not peculiar in themselves; what made them neurotic is that they appeared in contexts that seemed to be either inadequate or inappropriate causes of the response. Even extreme fears were normal when they arose and persisted in contextually appropriate situations. "A person suffering from anxiety," Freud emphasized, "is not for that reason necessarily suffering from anxiety neurosis."[13]

In neurotic disorders fear mechanisms that were constructed to alert people to the presence of actual dangerous situations are transformed to activate in the face of unconscious and, therefore, unknown internal dangers.[14] Freud could not specify what were "realistic" fears or "unrealistic" anxiety disorders, and he stressed the loose boundaries and common mechanisms between normal and abnormal concerns. Although anxiety neuroses, unlike realistic fears, usually arose from internal drives, sometimes anxiety was an appropriate response to internal fears.

Freud grounded normal anxieties in particular stages of the life cycle. As he observed, "The danger of psychical helplessness fits the stage of the ego's early immaturity; the danger of loss of an object (or loss of love) fits the lack of self-sufficiency in the first years of childhood; the danger of being castrated fits the phallic phase; and finally fear of the super-ego, which assumes a special position, fits the period of latency." The fear of castration loomed especially large as a source of normal fear for boys during the oedipal period.

Despite the fact that castration was not a real danger, it was nevertheless realistic for Freud because "what is decisive is that the danger is one that threatens from outside and that the child believes in it." Indeed, for males, the "fear of castration is one of the commonest and strongest motives for repression and thus for the formation of neuroses." Fears of castration that were normal when experienced during the oedipal period could be neurotic when they persisted well beyond this period and became unconscious sources of anxiety symptoms later in life. Most people, however, naturally grew out of their fears as they aged. "The phobias of very young children, fears of being alone or in the dark or with strangers—phobias which can almost be called normal—usually pass off later on; the child 'grows out of them.'"[15]

The appropriateness of the object of anxiety as well as the stage of the life cycle in which a fear arose indicated whether fears were normal or abnormal. Freud used the famous case of Little Hans to illustrate neurotic anxiety. Six-year-old boys normally loved their mothers and feared their fathers. "If 'Little Hans,'" Freud wrote, "being in love with his mother, had shown fear of his father, we should have no right to say that he had a neurosis or a phobia. His emotional reaction would have been entirely comprehensible. What made it a neurosis was one thing alone: the replacement of his father by a horse." Normal oedipal fears became neurotic when they were "directed to a different object and expressed in a distorted form, so that the patient is afraid, not of being castrated by his father, but of being bitten by a horse or devoured by a wolf."[16] The unconscious displacement of the original offensive idea allowed the boy, who simultaneously hated and loved his father, to recognize only his loving feelings while he displaced his hatred of the father onto the bad horse. Fathers were normal sources of fears of castration; horses were not.

Freud emphasized the importance of anxiety as a cause of a variety of psychoneuroses; its frequency among depressives, hysterics, and hypochondriacs; and the difficulties of separating normal fears from neurotic states of anxiety. He also noted the major features of free-floating, phobic, obsessional, and panic anxiety.[17] His conceptions of anxiety strongly influenced subsequent classifications.

Initial Classifications of Anxiety

Psychoanalysis did not use sharply bounded, discrete categories of disorder during the period when it dominated the practice of outpatient psychiatry. Its explanations emphasized unconscious mechanisms, which could manifest themselves through a variety of symptom formations. In addition, analytic therapies were comparable across different conditions because specific diagnoses rarely influenced treatment. Moreover, its clients paid directly for their treatment at the time so that third parties did not require specific diagnoses for payment. No external pressures forced analysts to create sharp boundaries between normal and abnormal conditions or among various types of disorders.

In contrast, public mental hospitals had to account for the diagnoses of their patients. Initial psychiatric classificatory manuals correspondingly emphasized the kinds of conditions found among institutionalized patients. As noted in the introductory chapter, the first such manual in the United States, the *Statistical Manual for the Use of Hospitals for Mental Disorders,* was issued in 1918 and went through ten editions before being superseded by the first *DSM* in 1952.[18] Among its twenty-two principal groups, one dealt with all of the psychoneuroses, including anxiety. Descriptions of the various anxiety disorders in this manual were short and cursory and indicated uncertainty over diagnostic descriptions.

DSM-I, which replaced the *Statistical Manual* in 1952, reflected the movement of psychiatric practice from state mental hospitals to outpatient treatment. It split conditions that were not the result of organic impairments between psychotic disorders that "exhibit gross distortion or falsification of external reality" and psychoneurotic disorders that included a variety of diagnoses including anxiety, phobic, and obsessive compulsive, depressive, dissociative, and conversion conditions. Anxiety was the central conceptual principle behind all the psychoneurotic disorders in the *DSM-I.* The very first sentence of the Psychoneurotic Disorders category stated that the "chief characteristic of these disorders is 'anxiety' which may be directly felt and expressed or which may be unconsciously and automatically controlled by the utilization of various psychological defense mechanisms (depression, conversion, displacement, etc.)."[19] Several psychoneurotic categories—anxiety, phobic, and obsessive compulsive reactions—were explicitly states of anxiety. The manual, following Freud's thinking, viewed the other categories of psychoneuroses—dissociative, conversion, and depressive reactions—as defensive reactions to unconscious anxiety.

Because the *DSM-I* was more concerned with the presumed underlying causal mechanisms than with the resulting symptoms of the neuroses, it provided only cursory definitions of each disorder. As well, it stated that anxiety "is to be differentiated from normal apprehensiveness or fear." While fear stemmed from external threats, neurotic anxiety was the result of some internal threat. The *DSM-II*, published in 1968, made no major changes in the characterization of anxiety. It maintained the central place of anxiety in the psychoneuroses, emphasizing that "anxiety is the chief characteristic of the neuroses."[20]

The *DSM-I* and *DSM-II* were adequate diagnostic schemes during an era when psychodynamic explanations were dominant, the most seriously ill patients were concentrated in inpatient institutions, outpatient clients paid for treatment out of their own pockets, and therapies were nonspecific. By the 1970s this situation had changed considerably.[21] The unfocused nature of analytic categories was no longer acceptable in general medicine, which required well-bounded disorders that had allegedly specific etiological mechanisms. In particular, research-oriented psychiatrists using biological perspectives challenged etiologically based categories that were grounded in unconscious psychological processes, especially unconscious anxiety. The deinstitutionalization of mental institutions and rise of community treatments required psychiatry to place more attention on persons with psychotic forms of disorder, which were rarely amenable to analytic methods of explanation or treatment. The NIMH (National Institute of Mental Health) faced intense political pressures to focus its funding on projects that used narrowly defined types of mental illnesses.[22]

Psychotropic medications, which analysts generally dismissed even though they often employed them, were becoming the treatment of choice for most mental disorders. Psychiatric treatment now required the existence of well-defined, particular diagnoses. Since the early 1960s the FDA required these medications to be effective with specific categories of disorder, not with general psychosocial problems, not to mention Oedipal or castration complexes.[23] Third party payers, as well, insisted that reimbursement would only be forthcoming for the treatment of specific diagnostic entities. A variety of internal and external pressures required psychiatry to develop a classification system with sharp boundaries between mental disorders and normality and with clear distinctions among various types of mental disorders.

DSM-III

Since the late nineteenth century, general medicine had relied on specific disease entities with well-defined etiological mechanisms. "This modern history of diagnosis," according to historian Charles Rosenberg, "is inextricably related to disease specificity, to the notion that diseases can and should be thought of as entities existing outside the unique manifestations of illness in particular men and women: during the past century especially, diagnosis, prognosis, and treatment have been linked ever more tightly to specific, agreed-upon disease categories." By the 1970s culturally legitimate diseases had come to require distinct boundaries and specific, preferably biological, causes. As long as psychiatry relied upon the murky, unconscious-based processes that analysts stressed, it could not be regarded as a legitimate medical specialty. Issues of professional legitimacy dictated that psychiatry adopt a discrete, categorical system.[24] The problem it faced, however, was that little theoretical and empirical knowledge existed about how such a system should be constructed.

It had long been known that, while etiology was the ideal way to classify symptoms, in reality, the causes of mental illnesses were unknown. As far back as 1782, British psychiatrist Thomas Arnold noted, "When the science of causes shall be complete we may then make them the basis of our classification, but till then we ought to content ourselves with an arrangement according to symptoms."[25] In the absence of causal knowledge, manifest symptoms would have to serve as the source of a disease-based classification system.

The publication of the *DSM-III* in 1980 revolutionized psychiatric classification.[26] The central mission of the various task forces on particular categories of disorders was to eliminate the unproven psychoanalytic inferences that underlay the previous *DSM* classifications. The research-oriented psychiatrists, led by the chair of the DSM Task Force, Robert Spitzer, insisted that diagnoses must be based on the presence of manifest symptoms without regard to etiology. Because they would be grounded in observable symptoms these diagnoses would enhance reliability and be more suitable for research purposes. Etiologically agnostic, symptom-based categories not only would be more scientifically useful but also—because they did not favor any particular theory—would be politically valuable in securing the acceptance of the new manual from psychiatrists holding a variety of theoretical persuasions.

To implement their goal of a symptom-based classification system, it was especially important for Spitzer and his allies to get rid of the generalized concept of "neurosis" that underlay and unified the non-psychotic classifications in the *DSM-I* and *DSM-II*. "The predominant American psychiatric theory in 1959," summarized Donald Klein, "was that all psychopathology was secondary to anxiety, which in turn was caused by intrapsychic conflict."[27] This concept was unacceptable to research-oriented psychiatrists not only because it pointed to a specific psychological etiology but also because it was the basis of the loose, overlapping, and vague categorizations that prevented the development of a scientifically based discipline. The bitterest struggles in the creation of the *DSM-III* involved the ultimately successful efforts of Spitzer and his associates to abolish the concept of the neuroses in psychiatric classification and replace it with discrete diagnostic categories. Because anxiety had been the central organizing principle of the neuroses, the defeat of the psychoanalysts inevitably led to a complete reformulation of the nature of anxiety.

Reconstituting such an amorphous condition as anxiety as a categorical disorder presented a challenge to the *DSM-III* task force. The existing psychoneuroses did not just have unproven causal unity but also had huge symptom overlaps with each other and with other disorders, which were especially apparent when conditions were traced over time.

One basis for the new categorical conditions in the *DSM-III* was the Feighner criteria (1972) that stemmed from a group of research psychiatrists at Washington University who were close allies of Spitzer. These criteria split anxiety into three categories: anxiety, obsessive-compulsive, and phobic neuroses. They used hierarchical criteria that provided diagnostic rules for what conditions would take precedence when patients presented more than one disorder. These hierarchies were also useful in the struggle against the analysts because they deemphasized the anxiety disorders: when other conditions were present, diagnoses of anxiety would not be given. Another important stimulus for categorical diagnoses stemmed from the work of psychiatrist Donald Klein, a colleague of Spitzer's at Columbia and an important member of the Anxiety Disorders Task Force. Klein emphasized the intimate relationship of panic attacks and agoraphobia and their distinctiveness from other anxiety states.[28] Based on his finding that the anti-depressant drug imipramine prevented the recurrence of panic attacks and agoraphobia but not chronic anxiety, he claimed that panic and agoraphobia should be split apart from general anxiety conditions.

Using the Feighner criteria and Klein's view as models, the *DSM-III* abandoned the etiological claims that had unified psychoneurotic conditions as defenses against underlying anxiety. Instead, it developed definitions of various anxious states that emphasized how each was a discrete and qualitatively distinct disease.[29] The manual divided the psychoneuroses into separate anxiety, affective, dissociative, and somatoform disorders. Anxiety disorders were now "pure" diagnoses that were independent of depressive, dissociative, and psychosomatic conditions. Each disorder was categorical, requiring a certain number of symptoms for the disorder to be present, rather than continuous in severity.

No single category of anxiety was preeminent. The general category was divided into phobic, anxiety states, PTSD, and ten subtypes. Phobic states were divided into two types of agoraphobia (with and without panic), social phobia, and simple phobia. Anxiety states encompassed panic, generalized anxiety disorder, and obsessive-compulsive disorder. PTSD contained two subtypes of acute and chronic or delayed. Generalized anxiety disorder, which on its face might be viewed as the core anxiety condition, was instead made a residual category; it was only to be diagnosed when symptoms of phobic, panic, or obsessive-compulsive disorders were not present. Finally, the *DSM-III* provided a category of atypical anxiety for "when the individual appears to have an Anxiety Disorder that does not meet the criteria for any of the above specified conditions."[30] To address the problem of multiple diagnoses, the *DSM-III* adopted from the Feighner criteria a hierarchical system of classification that put anxiety on the lowest tier. An anxiety diagnosis was not made if the anxious symptoms resulted from depressive or schizophrenic conditions.

The manuals that followed the *DSM-III*—the *DSM-III-R* (1987), *DSM-IV* (1994), and *DSM-IV-TR* (2000)—altered a number of diagnostic rules. The *DSM-III-R* eliminated many of the diagnostic hierarchies that had minimized diagnostic redundancy. For example, in the *DSM-III* panic disorders that occurred during depressive episodes would not be diagnosed as separate disorders but only as depression. Beginning with the *DSM-III-R*, each disorder was considered a distinct entity regardless of the presence of other disorders. The subsequent versions of the manual also changed the specific symptom criteria of many of the categories. For example, Generalized Anxiety Disorder (GAD) required persistent anxiety with one-month duration in *DSM-III*, unrealistic/excessive anxiety for six months along with at least six of eighteen symptoms in *DSM-III-R*, and only excessive anxiety for six months with at least six symptoms in *DSM-IV*.[31] The basic categorical principles of the diagnostic system, however, have remained unchanged since 1980.

The decision of the DSM-III Task Force to abandon the psychodynamic etiology that infused the first two *DSMs* was grounded in concerns about the scientific status of psychiatry. By the 1970s, it was clear that psychoanalysis could not be the basis for a scientifically oriented psychiatric profession. It was also apparent that, because the etiology of the various mental disorders was unknown, symptoms provided the only possible basis for a new classificatory system. It was far from clear, however, that a categorical system with sharp boundaries between disorders was the best possible way to classify neurotic conditions.

Categorical systems require the construction of sharp boundaries between criteria that are considered to be inside or outside of each category. One especially important boundary was the distinction between each anxiety disorder and normal fears. The *DSM-III* did not use any systematic or consistent criteria to distinguish morbid from natural fears, although it did recognize the importance of this distinction. The disproportion of symptoms to their context was the mark of phobic and obsessive-compulsive disorders, although no operational criteria were provided. Phobic disorders involved "irrational," "unreasonable," or "excessive" symptoms. Obsessive-compulsive disorders were "senseless," "not . . . realistic," and "clearly excessive" relative to appropriate contextual behaviors. Examples of normal panic served to differentiate panic disorders from natural responses to extreme stressors: panic symptoms were not abnormal if they occurred "during marked physical exertion or in a life-threatening situation."[32]

The *DSM-III* made no attempt to distinguish normal from abnormal anxiousness for the other anxiety disorders. Criteria for GAD were purely symptomatic with no indication of whether symptoms were disproportionate to the context in which they arose.[33] However, because GAD was a residual diagnosis that could not be diagnosed in the presence of another mental disorder, this was not a major omission. Likewise, the manual's definition of PTSD was silent about what constituted natural responses to traumatic events. However, because PTSD could only arise in traumatic contexts "that would evoke significant symptoms of distress in almost anyone," contextual qualifiers for this diagnosis were usually redundant.[34] Subsequent *DSMs* have not systematized the haphazard boundaries between anxiety disorders and normal fears. Nevertheless, the diagnostic criteria for the anxiety disorders are far more sensitive to contextual issues than the criteria for the affective disorders.

Another boundary issue regards the standards used to separate one type of disorder from other types of disorders. The categorical nature of the *DSM* diagnoses precluded examining the issue of whether anxiety is more profitably viewed as a dimensional as opposed to a categorical condition.[35] The manual did not allow dimensional diagnoses, not because they are inaccurate but because culturally legitimate medical diagnoses must be categorical disease entities. Dimensions do not fit either the categorical system that has dominated medicine for over a century or the desire of patients for well-defined and bounded conditions. Instead, a central assumption of the *DSMs* since 1980 is that each disorder is independent of the others. This assumption best fits people who present "pure" conditions of a single disorder and where few patients lie on the boundaries of different disorders. Yet, if symptoms highly overlap across disorders, the boundaries will artificially separate conditions that are naturally nonspecific. Individuals can appear to meet criteria for more than one disorder when their symptoms are actually part of the same more general syndrome.

A categorical system not only dictates that possibly overlapping anxiety conditions are distinct but also dictates a separation across different general categories of disorder. A paradox of psychiatric history is that the *DSM-III* is generally viewed as a return to the symptom-based categories that the diagnostician Emil Kraepelin developed.[36] A cornerstone of Kraepelin's thinking was that a great variety of symptomatic presentations in fact represented a single underlying pathology. Although the *DSM-III* followed Kraepelin's emphasis on the need to carefully observe symptoms, it ignored his central contention that distinct psychiatric conditions could only be accurately diagnosed as they unfolded over time.[37] He maintained that cross-sectional snapshots of symptoms were deceptive and could not reveal the nature of a disorder unless their temporal development was tracked. A given manifestation of a condition might actually be an early stage of a disorder that would only become apparent as it developed prospectively. Only the course of an illness, not its symptoms at any particular time, could separate one condition from another.

In sharp contrast to Kraepelin's system, the diagnostic criteria for all of the anxiety disorders were solely based on presenting symptoms at one point in time. This atemporal categorical system disguised any fluctuations in psychological or physical presentations or in anxious or depressive symptoms over time. The categorical system was especially unsuitable for examining whether the unfolding of symptoms of anxiety and depression indicated different stages of a single condition or distinct entities.[38] The categorical system also hindered thinking about various types of anxiety and of anxiety and depression as different manifestations of a common underlying vulnerability that might best be called "neurotic."

The *DSM-III* dealt with the problem of overlapping symptoms by creating a hierarchical system of rules that arbitrarily precluded diagnoses of anxiety when depressive disorders were also present. The *DSM-III-R* and subsequent manuals abandoned most of the hierarchical rules, instead using the concept of "co-morbidity" to give multiple diagnoses to people who meet diagnostic criteria for more than one disorder. The problem, as we will see, is that almost no one has a single anxiety disorder. Instead of recognizing the artificial boundaries across disorders that a categorical system created, the number of people with multiple disorders increased.

Despite its drawbacks, the shift from a fuzzy to a rigid classification system fundamentally altered the nature of psychiatric research. The *DSM-III* initiated a striking move toward the study of specific disorders. Before 1980 most research in psychiatric journals explored general conditions, multiple disorders, and policy questions. Between 1990 and 1992, 83 percent of articles about anxiety disorders concentrated on a single diagnosis. The proportion of articles about specific anxiety disorders published in leading psychiatric journals was just 1.5 percent in 1969 through 1970 and 3.0 percent in 1979 through 1980. By 1989 to 1990, fully16.1 percent of articles in these journals discussed specific types of anxiety, more than a tenfold increase in just two decades.[39] The study of anxiety had become one and the same as the study of specific, categorical, and isolated types of anxiety disorders.

Etiology

The tightly bounded categories of the *DSM-III* were supposed to represent a distinct improvement over the unconscious dynamics that analytic theories had stressed. Freudian categories were inherently unsuitable for the precise identification of distinct diseases. Psychoanalysts viewed overt symptoms as symbolic distortions that represented projections, displacements, introjections, and the like. Ingenious interpretations, rather than direct methods of scientific inquiry, were the methods used to relate manifest symptoms to underlying disorders. Moreover, the central etiological processes were unconscious and so impossible to observe directly. Clinical insight of each individual patient revealed the dynamics of disease. These aspects of analytic theory were not just incommensurate with the norms of scientific medicine, which demanded reliable observation of well-defined disease entities. They were particularly unsuitable for the focus on the biological bases of various mental illnesses, including anxiety, which were becoming ascendant during the 1970s.

The new biological paradigm demanded not only knowledge about genes, neurotransmitters, and neurochemicals, but also a clear idea of what condition was being genetically transmitted. "The part played by heredity in the development of the psychoneuroses is one of the fundamental unsolved problems in psychiatry," noted Felix Brown in 1942, "but the chief difficulty is to define the condition the heredity of which one is attempting to trace."[40] Accurate specifications of phenotypes are essential for the discovery of genotypes connected with various disorders. The specific and well-bounded categories of the *DSM-III* provided sharp definitions that had the promise of defining "the condition the heredity of which one is attempting to trace." The discrete categories of anxiety in the manual implied that the causal mechanisms beneath each category were distinct from the mechanisms that gave rise to the other categories. If the categorical diagnoses of the *DSM* did not correspond to different genotypes, biological psychiatry could be led on a fruitless search for underlying causal processes that do not exist in nature. In particular, the rationale for distinct diagnostic categories would be undermined if the various anxiety disorders shared common causes. Findings from etiological studies do not lend much confidence that the *DSM* categories have discreet, underlying biological causes.

Since 1980, interest in the genetic etiology of the specific anxiety conditions in the *DSM-III* has flourished. The initial studies focused on patterns of familial transmission of these conditions, correlating rates of a condition in a diagnosed individual with rates of various disorders in their blood relations.[41] In general, these studies indicated that afflicted individuals also had family members with histories of mental disorders. However, they rarely showed that family members shared the same specific anxiety disorder as the proband. Instead, what seemed to be inherited was a far more general vulnerability to a variety of disorders.

Many studies found that rates of other disorders—especially depression—could be even higher among family members than rates of anxiety disorders. One major study concluded that depression "in the proband was associated with anxiety disorders, but only slightly with depression or alcoholism, in the relatives; anxiety in the proband was associated with major depression and alcoholism in relatives, but only slightly with anxiety disorders in the relatives."[42] A common underlying etiological factor that might be called "neuroticism" seemed to underlie a variety of anxious and depressive conditions, a finding that in some ways was more similar to the older concept of psychoneurosis than with the bounded categories of the *DSM-III.*

Twin studies, as well, suggested common, rather than specific, genetic influences on anxiety and depression. A number of genetic studies found that no evidence for the inheritance of specific disorders existed, over and above the inheritance of a more general liability to neuroticism or behavioral inhibition.[43] For example, perhaps the most prominent American twin researcher, psychiatrist Kenneth Kendler, concluded that "Genetic influences on (anxiety and depression) were largely nonspecific. That is, while genes may 'set' the vulnerability of an individual to symptoms of psychiatric distress, they do not seem to code specifically for symptoms of depression or anxiety." With the possible exception of panic disorders, there is little evidence that any of the particular anxiety disorders in the *DSM* have distinct patterns of family and genetic transmission.[44] A common biological vulnerability to all of what were formerly characterized as the "psychoneuroses" seems to better account for the results of family and twin studies.

During the 1990s linkage analysis, which examines whether particular types of disorders are likely to have particular locations on chromosomes, became a prominent method for establishing the genetic foundation of mental disorders. To date, these studies have failed to find specific genetic propensities for any particular anxiety disorder. "Searching for genes for categorical diagnoses such as panic disorder," concluded geneticists Jordan Smoller and Ming Tsuang, "may be less fruitful than trying to identify genes influencing an underlying, latent anxiety-proneness such as neuroticism, which may be more directly heritable."[45] These results also seem more congruent with the loosely bounded, indistinct concepts of neurotic disorder than the rigid, tightly bounded categories of the *DSM-III* and subsequent manuals.

Likewise, findings from neuroscientific studies that directly examined brain functioning poorly fit the notion of specific, mechanism-based anxiety disorders. These studies link the detection and response to danger to the amygdala, the oldest part of the brain. Anxiety disorders arise when external or internal learned stimuli that do not signal objective danger serve to trigger anxiety. Unconscious memories stemming from traumatic early learning experiences remain in the amygdala and emerge in contexts when no danger is present. This research suggests that common, rather than distinct, processes explain the emergence of various types of anxiety disorders. One of the most prominent anxiety researchers, Arne Öhman, concludes that "when the symptoms of anxiety characterizing the different anxiety disorders are listed side by side . . . there is a striking overlap among them. . . . The communality among phobic responses, PTSD anxiety, and panic attacks is further underscored by psychophysiological data." Neuroscientist Joseph LeDoux approvingly cites Öhman's conclusion that the major forms of anxiety disorders reflect the "activation of one and the same underlying anxiety response."[46]

To date, familial, genetic, and brain-based studies offer little support for the sharp categorical distinctions in the *DSMs* since 1980. They rarely indicate distinctions among the various particular categories of anxiety or between anxiety and depressive disorders. Their findings also suggest, as has been known since Hippocratic times, that anxiety can reflect the high end of one of a small number of temperamental types that are various aspects of the broader personality construct of neuroticism.[47] Such temperaments, as the French psychiatrist Jean-Etienne Esquirol emphasized in the early nineteenth century, were not themselves pathological but rendered people more vulnerable to develop psychopathology. People who have an underlying susceptibility to develop symptoms of anxiety and depression seem to share a common vulnerability that makes them highly reactive to life stressors. For example, psychologist Robert Krueger examined the symptoms reported by respondents in a large national study without regard to the particular categorical disorders.[48] He found that symptoms of all the anxiety and affective disorders were aspects of a single broad condition, which might best be called "neurotic." As they were in the *DSM-II*, mood and anxiety disorders often seem to be linked types of a common distress-related syndrome.

These findings present a quandary for biological psychiatry. It is possible that distinct genes and/or neural processes for various symptom clusters exist but that the current definitions of these clusters do not map well onto this underlying biological stratum. Alternatively, there might be a shared biological vulnerability to various anxiety and depressive disorders. Genetic and biological factors might trigger more undifferentiated "psychoneurotic" tendencies rather than specific anxiety disorders.[49] The categorical revolution in classification has not helped resolve whether possible biological propensities underlie particular anxiety disorders, any anxiety disorder, or neurotic disorders more generally. Instead, it was a product of efforts to establish professional legitimacy that might disguise the more amorphous natural manifestations of anxious conditions.

Epidemiology

Spurred by the findings of military psychiatry that enormous numbers of soldiers developed psychological disturbances during World War II, psychiatrists and government officials in the postwar period became intensely interested in knowing the extent of psychiatric disturbance in untreated community populations. Interest in community studies exploded during the 1950s and 1960s when psychiatrists joined with social scientists to launch several large studies that examined amount of mental illness and its psychosocial causes in community populations.

Psychiatric epidemiology confronts the major problem that, unlike conditions such as blood pressure or cholesterol, no physical indicators exist to verify measurements of mental disorders. Therefore, it must rely on self-reported symptoms that are subject to many types of uncertainties. The initial studies also faced the dilemma that the psychiatric classifications at the time, the *DSM-I* and *DSM-II,* did not include specific anxiety disorders. Instead, the original research relied on general symptom scales that reflected a nonspecific view of psychic disturbance, although they emphasized symptoms of anxiety. "The prominence of anxiety in psychoanalytic formulations of psychiatric disorders," noted epidemiologist Jane Murphy regarding the symptom scales of the 1950s and 1960s, "meant that depression, at least neurotic depression, was thought of as an epiphenomenon to anxiety."[50]

The Langner scale, developed for use in the Midtown Manhattan Study, illustrates the prominent role of anxiety symptoms in the scales used at the time.[51] Among its twenty-two items, twelve involved symptoms of anxiety: restlessness, nervousness, worries getting you down, being the worrying type, feeling hot all over, heart beating hard, shortness of breath, fainting spells, acid stomach, cold sweats, fullness in the head, and trembling hands. Six others were more related to depression: couldn't get going, low spirits, feeling apart, nothing turns out, nothing seems worthwhile, and feeling weak. The remaining four—poor appetite, trouble sleeping, memory alright, and pains in the head—do not clearly fit either category.

Many of these symptoms were widespread and normal indicators of distress, not necessarily indicators of mental disorder. Not surprisingly, researchers found extraordinarily high rates of what they considered to be mental disturbance. At the extreme, less than 20 percent of members of community populations were classified as "well," that is, they reported no symptoms. Surveys often found that a majority of respondents who had experienced stressful events such as natural disasters, marital separations, or job loss reported serious psychiatric disturbances. The sensitivity of these scales to highly taxing events suggested that they were unable to distinguish between normal worries and anxiety disorders. For researchers, however, the major drawback of these scales was that the general nature of their items was incommensurate with the specific categories of disorders that emerged in the *DSM-III.*[52]

A small number of studies had tried to measure specific anxiety disorders in community populations before the 1980s. They found relatively low rates, ranging from less than 1 to 4.7 percent of the population. For example, one study that measured specific types of anxiety found rates of 2.5 percent for generalized anxiety, 1.4 for phobic disorders, 0.4 for panic disorders, and no cases of obsessive-compulsive disorder in a sample of five hundred persons.

Another study found only a 0.6 percent rate of agoraphobia in the 1960s. These figures led the *DSM-III* to declare in 1980 that it "has been estimated that from 2% to 4% of the general population has at some time had a disorder that this manual would classify as an Anxiety Disorder."[53]

The *DSM-III* provided epidemiologists the tools to specify and to measure symptom-based, distinct disorders in community populations. The initial epidemiological studies that used its criteria did not find strikingly high rates of anxiety disorders. The first such study, the Epidemiologic Catchment Area Study (ECA) conducted in the early 1980s, presented the first nationwide estimates of anxiety disorders from samples generated from five U.S. cities (Baltimore, Durham, Los Angeles, New Haven, and St. Louis). Using six-month prevalence across three of these sites (New Haven, Baltimore, St. Louis), it found rates of 0.8 percent for panic, 3.8 for agoraphobia, and 1.7 for obsessive-compulsive disorder. Comparable to earlier estimates, a summary of epidemiological surveys published in 1986 suggested that the overall annual prevalence of all anxiety disorders approximated 4 to 8 percent. Another summary from the same period estimated a similar range of 2.9 to 8.4 percent.[54]

More recent epidemiological studies of the same disorders present strikingly different figures. The largest and best-known study, the National Comorbidity Study (NCS) found extraordinarily high rates of anxiety disorders. The rates of anxiety disorders reported in the initial NCS, which was conducted in the early 1990s, considerably exceeded those of the ECA although the studies were only conducted ten years apart. Rates of any anxiety disorder in a one-year period rose from 9.9 percent in the ECA to 15.3 percent in the NCS while lifetime rates soared from 14.2 to 22.8 percent, respectively. The NCS restudy (NCS-R) conducted in the early 2000s indicated even higher rates of anxiety disorders: 18.1 percent of the population suffered some anxiety disorder over the past year and 28.8 percent reported one of these disorders over their lifetime. These figures were between seven and fifteen times higher than those presented in the *DSM-III*! Anxiety disorders had become by far the most prevalent class of disorder; simple phobias (12.5 percent) and social phobias (12.1 percent) were the two most widespread particular disorders of any type.[55]

What explains the apparent vast rise in the prevalence of distinct anxiety disorders from studies conducted during the 1960s, 1970s, and 1980s to those of the 1990s and 2000s? No theory of these disorders—whether biological, psychological, or social—posits any factor that could possibly account for such huge leaps in prevalence in such a short period of time. The rise in prevalence rates resulted from the tremendous sensitivity of self-reported symptoms to small changes in the wording of questions used to measure them. These changes, in turn, were products of investigators' decisions that drove prevalence rates in an upward direction.

The measurement of social phobia is illustrative. This condition was not mentioned in the *DSM-I* or *DSM-II*. When it appeared for the first time in the *DSM-III*, the manual noted that the "disorder is apparently relatively rare." The first study that measured the disorder in the early 1980s indicated a lifetime prevalence of 2.5 percent. A standard psychiatric text published in 1988 indicated that "social phobia occurs in from approximately 1.2% to 2.2% of the population."[56]

Subtle changes in the wording used to measure social phobias account for the apparent epidemic of this disorder that began in the early 1990s. The *DSM-III* criteria used in the ECA had required that sufferers have a "persistent, irrational fear of, and compelling desire to avoid, a situation in which the individual is exposed to possible scrutiny by others and fears that he or she may act in a way that will be humiliating or embarrassing." The NCS, however, using slightly revised *DSM-III-R* criteria, stated that the person needed to have only an "unreasonably strong fear" of situations such as meeting new people, talking to people in authority, or speaking up in a meeting or class. Just changing a single question from the ECA wording of having extreme distress when "speaking in front of a group you know" to the NCS inquiry about "speaking in front of a group" increased affirmative responses from 6.5 to 14.6 percent. These seemingly minor changes resulted in an increase of lifetime prevalence from 2.5 percent in the ECA to 13.3 in the NCS, a nearly sixfold increase in prevalence over the course of a decade. In another study, changing cutpoints from "a great deal of interference" to "a great deal of interference or distress" to "moderate interference or distress" resulted in increasing the prevalence of social anxiety disorder from 1.9 to 7.1 to 18.7 percent, respectively.[57]

The fact that small changes in question wording could so greatly enlarge prevalence estimates illustrates how epidemiological studies magnify the problems of symptom-based criteria. Lacking any etiological basis for defining disease, these studies rely on self-reported symptoms to make diagnoses. These symptoms overlap considerably with non-disordered conditions. For example, as much as 90 percent of people self-report feeling shy.[58] Only sophisticated inquiries and clinical judgment can determine whether or not symptoms such as speaking in public or feeling shy at social functions reflect contextually appropriate responses, intense but normal-range worry, or anxiety disorders. Recent epidemiological studies of anxiety disorders fail to distinguish normal fears from anxiety disorders and call both "disorders." The unsurprising result is that they generate extraordinarily high rates of putative anxiety disorders in community populations.

In addition to extremely high prevalence rates, a second major finding of epidemiological studies was the extraordinary amount of "comorbidity" between supposedly distinct disorders. In contrast to most medical diagnoses, where borderline cases that fall in between categories are rare, borderline cases among anxiety disorders outnumber pure cases. "Only a small proportion of individuals," concluded an International Task Force in 1996, "exhibit 'pure' forms of (anxiety) conditions cross-sectionally, and even fewer across the life course." Persons who report experiencing one anxiety disorder also have a high probability of experiencing a different anxiety disorder as well as a mood disorder. All of the anxiety disorders (except obsessive-compulsive disorders) are strongly related to each other and to mood disorders both at a particular point in time and across a lifetime. Over 80 percent of persons who have some other anxiety disorder report a second one; 90 percent of persons who report a generalized anxiety disorder also report another mental disorder at some point in their lives.[59]

Symptoms of anxiety are also ubiquitous in nearly all psychiatric conditions and especially in affective disorders. Scales that measure depression and anxiety typically overlap by about 60 percent. The overlap of anxiety and depressive disorders is comparable in patient populations, where about two-thirds receive both diagnoses over their lifetimes. The overlap among various disorders, especially over time, is far more common than the unique expression of these conditions. One large cross-national study found a strong association of anxiety disorders with major depression across all five sites, with odds ratios ranging between 2.7 to 14.9. Many researchers questioned whether even panic disorders, which had stimulated the categorical system, were actually more serious variants of other anxiety conditions. Comorbidity is more of a rule than an exception: anxious persons generally present concurrent symptoms of depression, and depressed persons show symptoms of anxiety.[60]

Although epidemiologists call the endorsement of enough symptoms of more than one disorder "comorbidity," the co-presence of distinct disorders could result from a system of categorization that creates artificially bounded entities from a more undifferentiated group of symptoms. The enormous amount of comorbidity is consistent with the older idea of a diffuse "psychoneurotic" disposition that makes people vulnerable to a range of epiphenomenal anxious and depressive symptoms depending upon the particular kinds of stresses that are operating when they are examined. The categorical system, however, discourages inquiries about whether the various anxiety disorders are truly distinct conditions or change from one to another over time.[61]

The major thrust of epidemiology since 1980 has been to document putatively high rates of disorders and the overlap of various categories of disorders. It has not made new contributions to the etiology of these disorders. Indeed, its findings regarding the social correlates of anxiety disorders are identical to the stress research of the 1950s and 1960s that showed the link of low social status, negative life events, highly stressful circumstances, low social support, and female gender to the development of anxiety.[62] The fixation on the specific categorical disorders of the *DSM* might hamper, rather than facilitate, the potential contribution of epidemiology to understanding the etiology of anxiety disorders.

The categorical, symptom-based criteria that the *DSM-III* initiated created the possibility to generate such extremely high rates of specific anxiety disorders in community populations. Yet, a number of social forces account for why these estimates are taken seriously. High prevalence estimates, combined with the relatively small, although increasing, proportion of people who seek professional help for their conditions, allow epidemiologists, the NIMH, and mental health policy makers to argue that the conditions they deal with are widespread, undertreated, and in need of substantially increased resources. Robert Spitzer astutely noted that "researchers always give maximal prevalence for the disorders that they have a particular interest in. In other words, if you're really interested in panic disorder, you're going to tend to say it's very common. You never hear an expert say, 'My disorder is very rare.' Never. They always tend to see it as more common."[63] They also serve the ends of mental health advocacy groups such as the National Association for Anxiety Disorders, which justify the need for increased resources because anxiety is such a widespread public health problem.

Pharmaceutical companies are also required to market their products as remedies for specific disorders. The high presumed prevalence of these disorders provides drug companies with huge target audiences for marketing their products. These companies seize on the upper bounds of any range of estimated amounts of pathology, broadcast these figures in ads and brochures, and diffuse them into media stories.[64] While many groups have an interest in expansive definitions of pathology, no organized groups emphasize the normality of fearful emotions. The categorical diagnostic system has created an explosion of pathology, which can best be treated by the ingestion of psychotropic medications.

Treatment

A major justification for delineating specific types of disorders is that each disorder will respond to a different type of treatment. Even while etiology remains unknown, symptom-based diagnoses could be valuable if diverse symptom clusters point to distinct treatments. The *DSM* classifications of anxiety, however, have not yet led to such specificity.

For most of history, no separate treatments existed for mental disorders. Distinct classifications were unnecessary because no discreet treatments were available. Anxious patients would have visited general physicians and received the same nonspecific treatments as others would get. For example, the historian Michael MacDonald showed that a sixteenth-century physician used the same physical remedies to heal mental and physical disorders alike. "Almost every one of Napier's mentally disturbed patients was purged with emetics and laxatives and bled with leeches or by cupping. The clients of other classically trained doctors endured the same treatments." Through the first half of the twentieth century, physicians and psychiatrists used the same drugs, including morphine and opium, across virtually all psychiatric conditions.[65] They were particularly likely to prescribe barbiturates for the range of common symptoms such as "nerves," "tension," or insomnia.

Although Freud distinguished several types of anxiety disorders, analysts tended to treat all anxiety conditions with the same techniques. They used nonspecific methods of psychotherapy to bring unconscious dangers into consciousness so that neurotic anxiety could be handled in the same ways as realistic anxiety. Traumatic neuroses (now called PTSD) were exceptions because they reproduced actual events and so were not subject to the symbolic interpretations of psychoanalysis. Analysts generally discouraged the use of drugs for treating anxiety disorders because they could hinder the search for the causes and meaning of symptoms and reduce valuable processes of vigilance.[66]

A revolution in the treatment of anxiety disorders began in the 1950s. In 1955 the development of meprobamate (Miltown) dramatically changed the nature of treatment for anxiety. "Meprobamate," according to psychopharmacologist David Healy, "opened up the question of the mass treatment of nervous problems found in the community." Miltown became the most popular prescription drug in history; by 1965 physicians and psychiatrists had written 500 million prescriptions for it. By the late 1960s the spectacular success of Librium, which was introduced in 1960, displaced Miltown. Valium, in turn, succeeded Librium by 1970 as the newest blockbuster anti-anxiety drug. In 1981 Valium was the single most prescribed drug of any sort: 20 percent of all women and 8 percent of all men reported using a minor tranquillizer over the past year.[67]

The popularity of these anxiolytics was especially due to their usefulness in treating the diffuse kinds of problems seen in general medical practice: general physicians wrote between 70 and 80 percent of prescriptions for Miltown, Librium, and Valium. In 1968 a prominent anxiety researcher, Karl Rickels, summarized the situation: "An abundance of tensions, fears, worries and anxieties confront mankind today and, in fact, anxiety is seen in the majority of patients visiting the physician's office. Pure anxiety states are relatively rare because such syndromes as depression, hysteria, hypochondriasis, somatization, phobias, and obsessional thinking are often concomitantly present." Drug companies presented the anxiolytics to physicians and psychiatrists as general tranquilizers that treated a variety of nonspecific complaints including anxiety, tension, depression, and mental stress. Advertisements at the time (which were directed to medical professionals, not the general public) typically focused on the interchangeability of symptoms of anxiety and depression.[68]

Studies during the 1950s and 1960s found that only about a third of the minor tranquilizers were prescribed for mental, psychoneurotic, or personality disorders, while the rest were given as a response to more diffuse complaints and psychosocial problems. "Only about 30% of [tranquillizer] use is in identified mental disorders," concluded one review in 1973, "and the remainder covers the rest of medicine." The vocabulary of the era dictated that these drugs would be called "anti-anxiety" or "anxiolytic" drugs, and the problems they treated were considered as problems of generalized "anxiety," although they often involving co-occurring depression. During this period the concept of "depression" barely existed for submelancholic conditions and "anti-depressant" medications were mainly reserved for the serious melancholic conditions found among hospitalized patients.[69] Even after the *DSM-III* sharply split the major categories of mental disorders into affective and anxiety disorders, general physicians continued to treat them non-differentially.

A World Health Organization (WHO) study in 1991–1992 found that benzo-diazipines and anti-depressants were about equally as likely to be given for depressive and anxiety conditions. These classes of drugs were, in practice, prescribed interchangeably.[70]

As noted earlier in this chapter, the notion of specificity of drug treat-ment for anxiety arose in the early 1960s when psychiatrist Donald Klein began experimenting with the anti-depressant drug imipramine on his hos-pitalized patients who had anxiety conditions that were refractory to existing treatments. He found that imipramine effectively prevented the recurrence of panic attacks but did not successfully treat chronic anxiety. He inferred that panic attacks and generalized anxiety states were qualitatively distinct conditions, rather than two forms of the same anxious condition. This was the first suggestion that a psychoactive drug might work with a specific form of anxiety disorder but not with others. It is curious that, while the anxiolytic drugs in general worked nonspecifically across a variety of conditions, the only seemingly effective drug for a specific anxiety disorder was an anti-depressant, not an anxiolytic. Subsequent research, however, showed little support for Klein's notion of drug specificity for panic as opposed to other kinds of anxiety. Moreover, psychological as well as drug treatments success-fully treat panic attacks.[71]

A sharp backlash against the anxiolytics began during the 1970s. Stim-ulated by hostile congressional hearings, the FDA and Bureau of Narcotics began a crusade against this category of medications. The historian Edward Shorter documents how "general hysteria" about the supposedly addicting qualities of the various anti-anxiety drugs swept the United States. This backlash resulted in their classification in 1975 as Schedule 4 drugs, which required physicians to report all prescriptions written for them and limited the number of refills a patient could obtain. As well, press coverage of these medications changed dramatically from their highly positive reception when they were introduced in the mid-1950s to very unfavorable coverage that emphasized their addictive qualities during the 1970s. After twenty years of steadily rising sales since their introduction in the mid-1950s, consumption of the anxiolytics drugs plunged. From a peak of 104.5 million prescriptions in 1973, their use sharply dropped to 71.4 million prescriptions by 1980.[72]

In actual practice the anxiolytics were prescribed nonspecifically. Yet the FDA required that any new medication must have demonstrated efficacy with a specific type of illness; drugs that worked nonspecifically could not be put on the market. As psychopharmacologist David Healy has emphasized, no manufacturer can be interested in drugs that work nonspecifically because they cannot be promoted in this way and thus cannot be profitable.[73] Therefore, drugs had to be marketed for discrete illnesses, regardless of the actual specificity of the condition.

The selective serotonin reuptake inhibitors (SSRIs) now dominate the treatment of non-psychotic mental disorders, including anxiety disorders. When the SSRIs emerged at the end of the 1980s, the anti-anxiety drugs were about twice as likely to be prescribed in outpatient visits to physicians, psychiatrists, and other medical specialists as were anti-depressants. The SSRIs treat depressive and anxious symptoms equally well. Indeed, some psychopharmacologists believe that they treat anxiety disorders more efficaciously than depression.[74] They could just as accurately have been called "anti-anxiety drugs" as "anti-depressants"; had the SSRIs been invented during the 1950s and 1960s, they almost undoubtedly would have been called anxiolytics, not antidepressants. Given the hostile cultural climate toward anti-anxiety drugs in the 1980s, however, it made more sense to market them as anti-depressants rather than as anti-anxiety agents.

Prescribing trends changed sharply after the SSRIs came onto the market. "Individuals treated for anxiety disorders in 1999," summarize psychiatrist Mark Olfson and colleagues, "were 2.7 times more likely to be treated with a psychotropic medication in 1999 than in 1987." This growth was entirely accounted for by the SSRIs: between 1985 and 1993–94 prescriptions for anti-anxiety drugs actually plunged from 52 to 33 percent of all psychopharmacological visits. Conversely, the percentage of visits for anxiety involving an anti-depressant increased from 30 to 45 percent. From 1996 to 2001 the number of users of SSRIs increased even more rapidly, from 7.9 million to 15.4 million. The use of anti-anxiety drugs grew at a much lower rate, increasing from 5.5 million to 6.4 million. The change in prescription patterns among persons in psychotherapy was even more dramatic. In 1997 nearly half (49 percent) received an anti-depressant drug compared to only 14 percent in 1987.[75]

The stagnation or decline of psychosocial treatments for anxiety sharply contrasts with the immense growth of SSRI drug treatments. Rates of psychotherapy, especially long-term psychotherapy, sharply dropped during the 1990s and early 2000s. Despite considerable evidence for the effectiveness of cognitive-behavioral treatments, their use also decreased through the 1990s.[76]

While drug treatments for anxiety have expanded enormously, there is little evidence that the efficacy of the SSRIs has any relationship to the diagnostic categories in the *DSM*. Indeed, the evidence for nonspecificity across diverse conditions is far greater than that for specificity. The way that drugs for anxiety work seems more comparable to the general analgesic effects that aspirin has on arthritis than to the specific effects of insulin on diabetes.[77] The relative responsiveness to drugs might even have more to do with differential temperament or personality as opposed to the nature of the symptoms that individuals display.[78]

The nonspecific nature of the complaints that people bring to their physicians and psychiatrists have not changed over the centuries, although the systems used to classify them have radically altered. When anxious patients list their worries, they speak of the same problems of debt, death, illness, courtship, and marriage that physician Richard Napier's patients had in sixteenth-century England.[79] Their symptoms are still nonspecific, encompassing a wide range of psychic and somatic indicators of anxiety and depression. Especially in primary care, most patients present mixed symptoms of anxiety and depression combined with worries about a variety of psychosocial problems.[80] The current diagnostic system creates the illusion of specificity from a morass of undifferentiated complaints. The categorical diagnoses of the anxiety disorders have little to do with the treatments patients actually receive.

Conclusion

Distressed people have always sought medical or psychiatric help for a protean and diffuse mix of somatic, anxious, and depressive symptoms. The sorts of financial, familial, and health problems that anxious patients bring to treatment differ little over the centuries as do their responses of unfocused apprehension, sleep disturbances, irritability, depression, and tension. A common vulnerability to responding to life stressors with anxiety and depression might best explain these general historical uniformities.

Yet the way in which these problems are classified and treated has varied enormously. Which condition is emphasized depends on prevailing diagnostic fashions. For most of history, specific diagnoses were usually unnecessary and problems involving anxiety were lumped into general categories such as melancholy, nerves, or neurasthenia. During the period of psychoanalytic dominance in the first few decades of the twentieth century anxiety conditions predominated among outpatients, although mixed anxiety-depressive conditions were common.

A major unintended consequence of the *DSM-III* was the reemergence of depression as the central diagnosis of the psychiatric profession. While the manual split anxiety into many distinct conditions in 1980, MDD was clearly the central category of mood disorders. Moreover, the labeling of the SSRIs as "anti-depressants" rather than "anti-anxiety" drugs at the end of the decade led physicians to be more likely to call the conditions they treated "depression" as opposed to "anxiety." While 20 percent of patients in outpatient treatment in 1987 had a diagnosis of some mood disorder, almost all of which were MDD, depressive diagnoses nearly doubled by 1997 to constitute 39 percent of all patients. A decline in diagnoses of general medical conditions, which dropped from 16 to 10 percent of visits, and, especially, a drop from 25 to 12 percent where no condition was specified, accounted for the rise in the proportion of depressive conditions. In contrast, rates of anxiety diagnoses remained stable in this period, only rising from 10.5 in 1987 to 12.5 percent in 1997. During the period from 1996–1997 to 2004–2005 diagnoses of mood disorders were more than three times as common as anxiety diagnoses in office-based psychiatry.[81] What particular condition is predominant at any given time seems more a function of the logic of the classificatory system that is used than of the natural occurrence of these symptoms.

As we move toward the end of the first decade of the twenty-first century, it is possible that anxiety will once again gain diagnostic prominence. The SSRIs are now off-patent for use with depression, and drug companies must search for new, patentable uses for them. The variety of anxiety disorders and the presumed number of people who suffer from them make anxiety an attractive target for pharmaceutical companies. At the beginning of the twenty-first century the drug industry obtained patents to use SSRIs with a variety of anxiety disorders, including GAD, PTSD, and social anxiety, and it is possible that their marketing efforts will shift from depression to anxiety. Which conditions are diagnosed and how they are treated will depend not only on the symptoms that patients display but also on social factors, including professional fashions in diagnoses, the financial rewards from various treatments, cultural images of disorder that are found in advertisements and other media, lobbying efforts by consumer and other advocacy groups, and the focus of government-driven research and funding.

The categorical system of diagnosis has come to influence all aspects of the anxiety disorders. Simple phobias, social phobias, agoraphobia, panic disorder, obsessive-compulsive conditions, generalized anxiety disorders, and post-traumatic stress disorder have become discrete conditions with specialists who treat and study each diagnosis. Research focuses on these particular diagnoses, conferences are organized to discuss them, publications derive from them, curricula are developed to study them, and careers revolve around them. But research has not yet demonstrated that these various disorders have different clinical courses, family and genetic clustering, or responses to treatment. Convenience and convention should not be confused with knowledge.[82] Extant studies actually seem more congruent with the notion of a general neurotic syndrome that prevailed before the development of the *DSM-III.*

While the *DSM* categories of anxiety are now firmly entrenched in the psychiatric canon, the extent to which they have improved the diagnosis, treatment, or causal understanding of anxiety disorders is not clear. What is unquestionable is that the psychiatric and other mental health professions have successfully expanded their control over the protean condition of "stress." Until psychiatry develops sound etiologically based classifications of the disorders it studies and distinguishes anxiety disorders from normal states of fear, however, its classifications will be of limited help in furthering the understanding of and successful response to these conditions.

Chapter 6

Depression

Creating Consensus from Diagnostic Confusion

Major Depressive Disorder (MDD) has become firmly entrenched in psychiatric research, treatment, and teaching; the mental health and health care systems; media reports about the condition; pharmaceutical advertisements for anti-depressants; and patient self-conceptions. It is so taken-for-granted and widely institutionalized that it is difficult to realize that it only emerged in its current form in 1980. Although depressive conditions have been recognized since the earliest known medical writings, the diagnostic criteria for MDD in the *DSM-III* were a major departure from previous conceptions of depression. Indeed, as late as 1979 numerous controversies raged on how to measure depression, the number of forms the disorder took, and its relationship to normal emotions of sadness and to other mental conditions, among many others. The seeming naturalness of the current MDD criteria disguises a number of arbitrary aspects of the classification of depressive mental disorder.

The current definition of depression, called Major Depressive Disorder (MDD), is found in the *Diagnostic and Statistical Manual* of the American Psychiatric Association (*DSM-IV-TR*).[1] A diagnosis of MDD requires that five symptoms out of the following nine be present during a two-week period, one of which must be either depressed mood or diminished interest or pleasure: (1) depressed mood;(2) diminished interest or pleasure in activities; (3) weight gain or loss or change in appetite; (4) insomnia or excessive sleep; (5) psychomotor agitation or retardation; (6) fatigue or loss of energy; (7) feelings of worthlessness or excessive or inappropriate guilt; (8) diminished ability to think or concentrate or indecisiveness; (9) recurrent thoughts of death or suicidal ideation or suicide attempt. With one major exception, anyone who meets these symptom criteria for a two-week period should be given a diagnosis of MDD. The exception is that patients are exempt from an MDD diagnosis if their symptoms are due to bereavement after the death of a loved one that lasts no more than two months and is not of extreme severity. The explicitness, clarity, and measurability of these criteria perhaps accounts for the nearly universal adoption of the definition of MDD since its first appearance in the *DSM-III* in 1980.[2]

Depression in many ways is now the most important condition in the contemporary psychiatric canon. Far more people receive a diagnosis of depression than of any other mental disorder: by the end of the twentieth century fully 40 percent of psychiatric outpatients received this diagnosis. Since about 1990, anti-depressant medications, in particular, the selective serotonin reuptake inhibitors (SSRIs), have been by far the most widely prescribed drugs for mental disorders. More published research articles concern depression than any other psychiatric condition. By 2020, the WHO estimates that depression will become the second leading cause of worldwide disability, behind only heart disease.[3] Depression seems to be a ubiquitous disease that causes a tremendous amount of suffering, impairment, and social cost. Yet its recent history illustrates how a seemingly natural and consensual condition is in many ways a thoroughly social creation.

Historical Conceptions of Depression in Early Writings

As long as emotions have been recorded, sadness has been viewed as one of a small number of core human feelings. Likewise, depressive mental disorder is one of a limited number of psychiatric conditions whose symptoms have remained relatively constant over millennia. Diagnosticians have always distinguished normal states of sadness from pathological depressive conditions. Hippocrates provided the first known description of depressive symptoms (which he called "melancholia") in the fifth century BC. The symptoms Hippocrates noted as characteristic of depression—"aversion to food, despondency, sleeplessness, irritability, restlessness"—are remarkably similar to those found in the *DSM* definition noted above. Hippocrates' definition of melancholia—"When fear or sadness last a long time, this is a melancholic condition"—indicated that the chronicity of melancholic disorders separated them from natural emotions of sadness and fear that are grounded in situations of loss or threat.[4]

The Hippocratic corpus and the ancient commentators who followed it noted a number of conditions that discriminated depressive mental disorders from symptomatically similar—yet distinct—conditions. One major distinction in early thought was between depressive symptoms that were "without" or "with" cause. Aristotle (or one of his students) noted that an excess of black bile could produce "groundless despondency." "Groundless" serves to differentiate despondency that is an appropriate response to life circumstances from comparable conditions that are not grounded in realistic external situations. Symptoms that were "without cause" either arose in the absence of situations that would normally produce sadness or were of disproportionate magnitude or duration to their provoking causes.[5] They were thus "groundless" because they were not related to external conditions that might expectably produce sadness or to a melancholic, but not disordered, temperament.

In contrast, the same symptoms might be "with cause," that is, natural, proportionate responses to serious losses such as deaths of intimates, economic reversals, disappointments in attaining valued life goals, and the like. Because both types of melancholia shared the same symptoms, the essential difference between conditions that were "with" or "without" cause lay in the fact that the social environment evoked and maintained the first type while factors internal to the individual produced the second type.[6] Melancholic disorders were limited to conditions that were "without cause."

A second distinction embedded in traditional thought was between mental disorders and melancholic personality dispositions. Ancient commentators recognized that some people were prone to melancholic temperaments, which they explained as a result of a preponderance of the humor of black bile, and thus to an inherent inclination to sadness. An abundance of black bile, however, was not necessarily a sign of a disorder but could indicate a personality disposition, which in some cases could even be beneficial. Aristotle, for example, linked melancholic temperaments to outstanding artistic, philosophical, and political achievements.[7] Melancholic disorders had to be distinguished from natural proneness to melancholic reflection.

Historically, most commentators also recognized that the boundaries between melancholic and other types of disorders were loose and amorphous. Although the core symptoms of melancholia consisted of despondence and anxiety, the manifestations of these states varied considerably. Consequently, melancholic states were often difficult to isolate and shared many symptoms with other conditions, most prominently, with anxiety. Sadness and fear, as in Hippocrates' definition, were commonly linked; anxious concerns and worries often accompanied melancholic conditions.

The major distinctions that arose with the Hippocratic corpus persisted for thousands of years, until the eighteenth century, when theories regarding the central nervous system replaced humoral conceptions as key explanations for the emergence of mental disorders.[8] For most of the eighteenth, nineteenth, and twentieth centuries, melancholic conditions no longer dominated conceptions of mental illnesses. Nevertheless, descriptions of these conditions retained the core distinction between melancholic disorders and ordinary sadness that was "with cause," on the one hand, and melancholic personality dispositions, on the other. Likewise, the boundaries between melancholia and other mental disorders were often fluid and unstructured. Specific diagnoses did not become important aspects of psychiatric practice until the nineteenth century.

Pre-*DSM* Developments

The German psychiatrist Emil Kraepelin is justly considered to be the originator of modern psychiatric diagnostic systems.[9] General paresis provided the underlying conception for Kraepelin's diagnoses of mental disorders. The isolation of this disease showed that mental disorders, like physical disorders, could stem from specific brain-based physical pathologies. Careful observation of the symptoms of general paresis also showed how they changed dramatically over time and differed markedly at different stages of the disease. These different manifestations, however, represented the unfolding of the same underlying disorder. A mild symptom of syphilis, for example, might indicate the early stages of what would sometimes progress to become a very severe disorder at a later time. Thus, for Kraepelin, not symptoms at any particular time but only symptoms over the entire course of an illness served to identify a disease.[10]

Using paresis as a model, Kraepelin outlined distinct categories of manic-depression and schizophrenia that were based on careful observation of symptoms, traced the varying courses of the disorders over time, and grounded these categories in brain pathologies. Manic depressive insanity included mania, which involved irrational ideas, exaltation, and overactivity, and depression, which incorporated inhibited thought, depressed mood, and psychomotor retardation. Kraepelin did not think that that all mild states of sadness would develop into depressive disorders; instead, he asserted that full-blown disordered conditions often started as mild states. Nineteenth-century psychiatry generally followed Kraepelin's contention that melancholic disorders were brain diseases that often had a strong hereditary causal factor.

The emergence of psychoanalysis at the end of the nineteenth century provided a thoroughly distinct perspective from the Kraepelinian approach to depression. Sigmund Freud and his followers concentrated on the psychological etiology of depression. They understood pathological symptoms in terms of unconscious mental processes, not of brain pathologies. Unlike Kraepelin, the Freudians did not emphasize depression but subsumed this condition under the more general processes of the psychoneuroses that arose from unconscious feelings of anxiety.

Freud stressed the differences between natural processes of mourning and pathological melancholia, which were analogous to previous distinctions between depressions that were with and without cause. Both types of conditions shared common symptoms, including profound dejection, loss of interest in the external world, inhibited activity, and an inability to feel pleasure, which resembled the symptoms in the current *DSM*. However, despite their common appearance, Freud explained that "although grief involves grave departures from the normal attitude to life, it never occurs to us to regard it as a morbid condition and hand the mourner over to medical treatment. We rest assured that after a lapse of time it will be overcome, and we look upon any interference with it as inadvisable or even harmful."[11] Grief, or mourning, was a natural process that was self-healing; it was not a mental disorder. Melancholia, in contrast, was a pathological redirection of internalized hostility toward earlier love objects onto one's self. Their common appearances notwithstanding, grief was a normal reaction to loss that should not be subject to medical treatment while melancholia stemmed from unconscious losses that the sufferer could not understand without the aid of a therapist.

In the United States Adolf Meyer's view of depression as a reaction type was especially influential during the middle third of the twentieth century. Meyer emphasized a contextual approach to depression, stressing how the nature of depressive illnesses was too heterogeneous to be encompassed within a single disease condition. Unlike Kraepelin, he did not privilege biological processes. Instead, he stressed that most depressive states were reactions to environmental demands that arose from a variety of personality and biological characteristics, life circumstances, and general experiences. While depressive symptoms were universal, depressive disorders were pathological conditions that were out of proportion to their precipitating environmental contexts.

Freud's and Meyer's views were the major influences on the first diagnostic manuals in the United States that were developed for use in a broad range of treatment settings, the *DSM-I* and *DSM-II*. Following Meyer, the *DSM-I* called depression "depressive reaction."[12] The *DSM-II* emphasized psychodynamic formulations, especially the distinction between depressive neurosis and depressive psychosis. Following Freud, the *DSM-II* conceived of depression as stemming from unconscious attempts to deal with anxiety and guilt stemming from some loss. It changed the label of depression from "depressive reaction" to "depressive neurosis," defining this condition as follows: "This disorder is manifested by an excessive reaction of depression due to an internal conflict or to an identifiable event such as the loss of a love object or cherished possession."[13] This definition stressed the differences between "excessive," disproportionate responses to conflicts and losses, which are disorders, and non-excessive, proportionate responses to the same situations. The latter, which are "with cause," are not disorders. The manual did not list any symptoms of the disorder but implied that the distinction between disorders and normal sadness lies in the context in which symptoms arise, not in the nature of the symptoms themselves.

During the period between roughly 1920 and 1980 numerous controversies surrounded the study of depression. One issue involved whether depression was a single disorder, as Kraepelin argued, or more than one distinct disorder. British psychiatrist Aubrey Lewis was the most influential supporter of the unitary view. He emphasized that depressive conditions lay on a single continuum running from mild to severe disorders and encompassing both endogenous conditions with no apparent environmental cause and exogenous conditions that arose in response to external stressors.[14]

In contrast to Kraepelin and Lewis, most researchers argued that melancholic depression—a particularly serious state marked by vegetative symptoms, delusions, and hallucinations—was not an extreme point on a continuum but a distinct type of disorder.[15] They believed in a distinction between endogenous disorders that emerged "out of the blue" and exogenous disorders that were provoked by distinct losses. Endogenous conditions gradually came to be associated with the extreme symptoms they featured rather than with the lack of a precipitating, external cause. The term "psychotic" more accurately characterized the nature of these conditions. They were believed to be discrete conditions that had distinct responses to medication. Unlike reactive (or exogenous) depressions, they were thought to be highly responsive to anti-depressant medications but not reactive to placebos.[16] Despite their many disagreements, psychiatric researchers generally felt that depression was not a homogeneous illness category but included a psychotic type as well as a variety of less distinct and difficult to classify non-psychotic conditions.

While most researchers agreed on the existence of a separable, psychotic form of depression, they did not reach consensus on the nature of non-psychotic types of depression. The question of whether depressive illnesses were best regarded as a continuum or characterized by discrete types was unresolved. Similarly, those who argued for discrete types couldn't agree on how many types existed. Some concluded that depression had a single neurotic type as well as a melancholic, psychotic type. Others argued for the existence of three or more distinct, neurotic states of depression. Various classifications of depression embraced from a single to as many as nine or more separate categories. Still others conceived of neurotic depression as more closely resembling a personality or temperament type rather than a disease condition.[17]

The only thing that was clear about the state of depression research at the end of the 1970s was the extraordinarily broad range of unresolved opinions on how best to diagnose the condition. In 1976 the prominent British psychiatric diagnostician R. E. Kendell published an article whose title accurately conveyed the classificatory situation at the time: "The Classification of Depressions: A Review of Contemporary Confusion." In his summary of the state of research about the classification of depression he noted that "there is no consensus of opinion about how depressions should be classified, or any body of agreed findings capable of providing the framework of a consensus."[18] Kendell outlined twelve major systems of classification, most of which had little to do with the others. Different researchers emphasized distinctions between psychotic and neurotic, endogenous and reactive, and bipolar and unipolar conditions. While almost everyone agreed that psychotic (or endogenous) depressions were distinct from neurotic states, no accord existed on the nature of non-psychotic conditions.[19] Researchers did not agree on whether non-psychotic depressions were continuous or discontinuous with psychotic forms, on the one hand, or with normality, on the other.

None of the issues about depression that initially emerged in the works of the ancient Greeks had been decided. Researchers and clinicians disputed how many forms neurotic conditions took and sometimes even if they had any discreet forms at all. Debates continued about whether depression was better seen as a neurotic personality type than as a disease. It is hard to imagine that anyone would have thought that the development of the *DSM-III* in 1980 would seem to resolve all of these controversies in a single stroke.

The Foundation of the *DSM-III*

During the period that psychoanalysis dominated American psychiatry, the major outpost of medically minded psychiatry was at Washington University in St. Louis. Led by psychiatrists Eli Robins and Samuel Guze, the mission of the Washington University group was to develop easily measurable, symptom-based criteria that would serve as the basis for empirical research. The Washington University group scorned the definitions of the *DSM-II,* which were based on the assumption that unconscious anxiety was at the root of the various psychoneuroses. Realizing that the causes of the various mental disorders were unknown, this group's first priority was to purge unwarranted etiological elements from definitions of each disorder. They developed criteria for a small number of disorders, fifteen in all, that were solely based on the symptoms each disorder displayed. These diagnostic criteria were called the "Feighner criteria" after the name of the psychiatric resident in the Washington University department who was the first author of the published version of the descriptions.[20]

Given the extant lack of agreement about the nature of depression, however, there was little consensual basis on which to build empirical criteria to replace the existing vague and etiologically based definition of depression in the *DSM-II.* The Feighner criteria split the Affective Disorders category into primary affective disorders that were not preceded by any other mental or physical illness and secondary affective disorders that were preceded by another psychiatric illness or were accompanied by a life-threatening physical illness. They subdivided the primary and secondary types into two categories, depression and mania. Depression required the presence of dysphoric mood and at least five of the following symptoms: poor appetite, sleep difficulty, loss of energy, agitation, loss of interest in usual activities, guilt, lack of concentration, and recurrent thoughts of death. The Mania category was not related to depression but instead to a psychotic state marked by exuberance and hyperactivity. The criteria, in effect, contained one form of depressive illness (that could be independent of or preceded by other mental and physical conditions).

The Feighner criteria took little note of previous research on the topic and in many respects had little resemblance to it. "No evidence," noted Kendell in regard to the Feighner approach, "has been offered to suggest that it is anything more than a convenient strategy."[21] Although they did allow for a diagnosis of "probable" depression when four instead of five symptoms were present, the criteria were categorical, assuming that depression was a discrete rather than dimensional disorder. The criteria abandoned the classical distinction between symptoms that were "with" or "without" cause, so they considered both symptoms that were related or unrelated to precipitating causes to be disorders. They were thus purely symptom-based, so that anyone who met the symptom criteria received a diagnosis of depression. Even bereaved people who satisfied the symptom criteria were viewed as having a depressive disorder.

Perhaps the most striking aspect of the Feighner criteria is that they considered all depressive conditions to fall under a single category. Most previous researchers, if they did not take a dimensional view of depression, considered psychotic (or endogenous) depression to be distinct from less serious forms of the condition. Psychotic unipolar depression simply disappeared in the Feighner criteria, which only recognized the manic form of affective psychosis. The criteria also did not take note of the controversies regarding how many forms of non-psychotic depression existed. Finally, although the criteria followed Kraepelin in asserting the primacy of careful observation of symptoms in making diagnoses, they discarded the basic Kraepelinian dictum that accurate diagnoses required observations over long periods of time. They were cross-sectional, requiring one-month duration of symptoms. Depressive conditions stemming from dysfunctional psychological mechanisms that led people to be unable to experience pleasure, those that featured chronic pessimism, and those that arose from situations of loss were treated as comparable, as long as they satisfied the symptomatic criteria.

In 1979, just a year before the publication of the *DSM-III*, psychiatrists Nancy Andreasen and George Winokur noted the presence in research about depression of "a hodgepodge of competing and overlapping systems."[22] Likewise, Kendell's review gave no special primacy to the Washington University classification, treating it as one of twelve ways to classify depression. Despite their uncertain grounding in the extant research literature, the Feighner criteria quickly generated a consensus among empirically minded psychiatric researchers. By 1989, the article in which the Feighner criteria appeared was the single most cited article in the history of psychiatry.[23] The criteria clearly met the need of research psychiatrists for easily measurable diagnostic entities. Most importantly, they became the basis for the new classification of depression that appeared in the *DSM-III* in 1980.

DSM-III

The *DSM-III* is justifiably viewed as a revolution in psychiatric classification.[24] It presented explicit definitions of several hundred diagnostic entities (including depressive disorders), which remain the standard of what counts as a mental disorder. They are used in all settings that require diagnoses, including general medical practice, private mental health practice, and hospital clinics. They are also the central measures used in epidemiologic investigations, research studies, and treatment outcomes. In effect, the definition of depression that the *DSM-III* initiated and that has remained basically intact through the subsequent *DSM-III-R, DSM-IV,* and *DSM-IV-TR* manuals is the arbiter of what is currently considered to be a depressive disorder.[25]

The *DSM* definitions of depressive disorders were primarily grounded in the Feighner criteria. However, unlike the Washington University measures that were developed for use in research studies, the *DSM* was a manual intended for clinical use as well as for research. No single paradigm dominated the practice of psychiatry by 1980, so the manual had to be useful for clinicians of all theoretical persuasions, not just for empirically minded researchers such as Robert L. Spitzer and the Washington University group. Because it would have been politically unacceptable for the *DSM-III* explicitly to favor any particular theoretical group, the symptom-based Feighner criteria had the advantage of not relying on any specific theory of mental illness, whether biological, psychological, or social.

The *DSM-III* diagnosis of MDD, outlined above, was very similar to the Feighner criteria. It retained the primary distinction between bipolar disorders and major depressive disorders, so that all unipolar depressive conditions were part of one illness. It also maintained virtually intact the particular symptoms from the earlier diagnosis, requiring the presence of dysphoric mood or loss of pleasure in activities along with at least four from the same list of eight additional symptoms of poor appetite, insomnia, psychomotor agitation, fatigue, loss of interest, feelings of worthlessness, lack of concentration, and recurrent thoughts of death.[26]

What led research psychiatrists to rally around the Feighner criteria, which were no more empirically supported than many other possible schemas? One reason was that they were perfectly posed to solve the reliability problems that bedeviled the psychiatric profession. Because the criteria considered all symptoms, regardless of the context in which they arose, as potential signs of depressive disorder, they did not need to rely on tricky judgments of whether or not a given collection of symptoms was a natural response to a given contextual situation. This quality made it easier to generate agreement on whether a given patient had a depressive condition. In addition, the Feighner criteria made no assumptions about etiology. Diagnostic judgments did not depend on the causes of symptoms, which were often hard to determine. The purely symptom-based nature of the criteria also made them potentially useful to psychiatrists of all theoretical persuasions. These attractive qualities, however, would not be sufficient in themselves for the Feighner criteria to overcome the decades of disagreement about appropriate ways to classify depressive disorder. Political considerations, in particular, the allegiances of the key actors responsible for constructing the MDD criteria for the *DSM-III*, were a crucial factor in leading to the adoption of the Washington University definition of depression.

Spitzer and his colleagues, who were either based at Washington University or were close collaborators of the Washington University group, controlled the development of the new edition of the *DSM*. The five members of the Advisory Committee on Schizophrenic, Paranoid, and Affective Disorders whose work primarily concerned depression were Spitzer himself, his two close collaborators from Columbia, Jean Endicott and Janet Williams (Spitzer's wife), and two psychiatrists from Washington University, Paula Clayton and Robert Woodruff. Every member of the depression subgroup was therefore part of the research network centered on the Washington University group and their allies at Columbia.[27] The close personal affiliations among this group insured that the in-house instruments of the Feighner criteria and the Research Diagnostic Criteria that were developed from the Feighner measures would serve as the basis for the new depression diagnosis in the *DSM-III*.[28]

The *DSM-III* did make several changes in the Feighner criteria. The distinction between primary and secondary affective disorders, which commentators had called the "most important feature of this classification," disappeared in the *DSM-III* definition.[29] The *DSM* also lowered the duration of required symptoms from one month to two weeks. Although, the MDD criteria maintained the purely symptom-based focus of the Washington University group, they added an exclusion for bereavement so that non-psychotic symptoms due to bereavement that didn't last longer than three months (later changed to two months) would not receive a MDD diagnosis. The addition of this exclusion was likely due to work of Paula Clayton, a prominent member of the Washington University group and of the *DSM-III* Advisory Group on Affective Disorders. Her work showed that, although high proportions of bereaved people could satisfy one-month duration criteria for depression, their symptoms were typically self-healing and remitted shortly after this period.[30] The *DSM-III*, however, did not apply the same logic to any other serious loss: it made no comparable exclusions for depressions arising in response to events such as natural disasters, divorce, unemployment, or the diagnosis of a serious physical illness. Aside from the bereavement exclusion, the diagnostic criteria did not recognize the ages-old separation of depressive conditions that were "with" or "without" cause.

Major Depressive Disorder was the primary category of depression in the Affective Disorders category of the *DSM-III* (and subsequent manuals). The larger Affective Disorders category also included the psychotic state of bipolar disorder. The *DSM-III* also added a subtype of Major Depressive Disorder with Melancholia, which was a subclassification of MDD. People could only qualify for a diagnosis of Melancholic MDD if they already met the criteria for MDD. It required symptoms of greater severity in the morning, early-morning awakening, marked psychomotor retardation, weight loss, and excessive guilt. This category corresponded to a considerable amount of earlier research that had delimited a distinct category of psychotic, but non-manic, depression, but its submersion into the broader MDD category ensured its fall into obscurity.[31] Melancholic depression, as defined in the *DSM-III*, lost the primacy it had maintained through thousands of years of psychiatric history. Psychotic types of mood disorders became identified with bipolar disorder; unipolar states of psychotic depression were virtually indistinguishable from major depression.

The group that constructed the Affective Disorders category also had to find some way of dealing with the traditional category of neurotic depression that, although ignored by the Washington University diagnosticians, was an important diagnosis for the psychoanalytic component of the psychiatric profession. Spitzer and his research-oriented allies were firmly opposed to including a term such as "neurosis," which implied a distinct etiology of symptoms rooted in unconscious psychological conflicts.[32] Psychoanalysts, however, bitterly contested attempts to abolish a concept that had been part of the core of the discipline for the past half-century. As a compromise, Spitzer introduced a new category of "dysthymic disorder" with the term "neurotic depression" following in parentheses. The final wording in the *DSM-III* was "Dysthymic Disorder (or Neurotic Depression)."[33]

Dysthymia was an attempt to capture the central features of what psychoanalysts had considered to be neurotic depression. In the past, neurotic depressions would have been contrasted to psychotic depressions and differentiated by their lesser severity. In the *DSM-III*, however, the symptom requirements for dysthymia had little resemblance to any previous use of this term. Diagnoses of dysthymia, like those of MDD, required the presence of either depressed mood or loss of interest in most activities but only three additional symptoms (changed to two additional symptoms in the *DSM-IV*) from a list of thirteen possible symptoms.[34] However, the symptoms had to endure for a two-year period (one year for children and adolescents), in contrast to the two-week period required for an episode of MDD. Dysthymia was thus a curious amalgam of low-grade but long-lasting symptoms that seems more similar to a melancholic personality disposition than to a psychiatric disorder. The extreme duration requirement for dysthymic states ensured that they were not analogous to transient, mild states of depression. In any case, it was MDD, not dysthymia, that became the core diagnoses of the Affective Disorders category.[35]

The *DSM-III* was initially intended to be a provisional document that would be subject to revision based on new empirical evidence.[36] In fact, its success in seeming to resolve the problems of psychiatric legitimacy, reliability, and theoretical confusion ensured that it quickly became reified and its diagnostic entities taken for granted. The developers of the *DSM-III* did not envision that depression, as embodied in the MDD criteria, would soon become the most central diagnosis of the psychiatric profession.

Post-*DSM-III* Developments

Depression is one of a small number of diagnoses that has been continuously described throughout psychiatric history. For the first part of the twentieth century, however, it was not an especially important or widespread condition.[37] Since the latter part of the nineteenth century "nerves," "tension," and "stress" were the core features of psychological problems seen in general medical as well as psychiatric practice. Their accompanying psychological and somatic features had much more resemblance to anxiety than to depression. Anxiety, not depression, dominated characterizations of the psychoneuroses before the *DSM-III*.

As the preceding chapter noted, during the 1990s depression replaced anxiety as the core condition experienced by typical clients of outpatient psychiatry and general medical practice. While diagnoses of anxiety remained stable throughout the decade, the proportion of patients receiving diagnoses of depression in outpatient psychiatric therapy about doubled from 20 percent in 1987 to 39 percent in 1997.[38] The medications used to treat neurotic conditions changed from being labeled "anxiolytics" or "tranquillizers" to being called "anti-depressants." Images of depressed people were also transformed. During the 1960s portrayals of depression typically contained older women who were often formerly hospitalized patients.[39] By the end of the 1990s advertisements featured attractive, younger and middle-aged women who were restored to exceptional health after treatment with anti-depressant medication. What factors led to the sudden emergence of depression at the top of the hierarchy of outpatient psychiatric diagnoses during the 1980s?

One of these factors was the inadvertent result of the *DSM* classifications themselves. MDD was unquestionably the core diagnosis within the Affective Disorders category. What was formerly called "endogenous depression" became a subcategory within the MDD diagnosis and by now has virtually disappeared as an independent entity. Dysthymia never gained traction as a diagnostic entity and is rarely found in research, treatment, or clinical practice. In contrast, major depression, which did not even appear as a diagnostic label until 1979, was by 1984 the most cited term used in research articles. By 2000 it was used far more frequently than all other diagnostic terms for depression put together.[40]

In contrast to the unity of the depressive disorders, the category of Anxiety Disorders subdivided into many entities, none of which was dominant.[41] Panic, Agoraphobia, Specific Phobia, Social Phobia, Obsessive-Compulsive Disorder, PTSD, and GAD all developed into viable diagnostic categories with their own researchers, treatments, and clinics. GAD, which might seem to be the central category of anxiety, became a residual category that was not diagnosed when some other psychiatric condition was present. The *DSM* cleared a path for major depression to dominate the labeling of the amorphous group of conditions that before 1980 were considered to be "neurotic," "nerves," or "anxious" conditions.

A second critical development was the emergence of a new category of drugs, the SSRIs, at the end of the 1980s. As chapter 5 outlines, the tranquilizing drugs, which were called "anti-anxiety" or "anxiolytic" medications, dominated the treatment of non-psychotic conditions during the 1950s and 1960s. Correspondingly, the conditions they treated were seen as problems of nerves or anxiousness that were sometimes combined with depression. Beginning in 1962 the FDA required that medications could only be approved, marketed, and advertised for the treatment of specific disease conditions, not for general psychosocial problems.[42] The dominance of the anxiety conditions at the time ensured that these medications would be promoted as treatments for anxiety rather than for depression.

The specificity requirement led to a search for specific diseases that existing medications could treat. The major research question was whether a specific disease state could be linked to the sites in the brain where the drugs were biologically active. The SSRIs act very generally to raise levels of serotonin in the brain. Serotonergic drugs treat a wide variety of depressive and anxious conditions, among others; they are not specific to any single disorder. They could just as easily have been marketed as anti-anxiety as anti-depressant medications when they first appeared in the late 1980s. By the 1980s, however, anti-anxiety medications were linked to dependency and many negative side effects.[43] The media had turned sharply against their use and broadcast many stories featuring their potential for addiction, use in suicide attempts, and other destructive consequences. Patients, with backing by organized groups of advocates, filed many lawsuits against the drug companies that manufactured the tranquillizers. Government agencies attempted to restrict their use and adopted an openly adversarial stance toward the pharmaceutical industry. Sales of anti-anxiety drugs plunged from their peak usage in 1975 and continued to plummet throughout the 1980s. Pharmaceutical companies faced a tough situation in marketing anti-anxiety drugs. "By the mid-1980's," writes psychopharmacologist David Healy, "it had become impossible to write good news stories about the benzodiazepines."[44]

Before the late 1980s, anti-depressant medications were mainly associated with the treatment of severe depression, not with common psychosocial problems treated in general medical practice or outpatient psychiatry. In contrast to the anti-anxiety drugs, anti-depressants were not connected to problems of dependency.[45] When the SSRIs came onto the market in the late 1980s it made much more marketing sense to promote them as anti-depressants, not as anti-anxiety agents. The publication of Peter Kramer's wildly popular *Listening to Prozac: A Psychiatrist Explores Antidepressant Drugs and the Remaking of the Self* in 1993 cemented the coupling of the SSRIs with the treatment of major depression.[46] Network television shows, national newsmagazines, and best-selling books widely featured anti-depressant medications. Depression had become the disease that the new drugs would treat.

SSRI use increased spectacularly over the 1990s, growing by 1,300 percent. Between 1996 and 2001 alone, overall spending on anti-depressants rose from $3.4 billion to $7.9 billion. By 2000, three SSRIs—Prozac, Zoloft, and Paxil—were among the eight most prescribed drugs of any sort; the anti-depressants were the best-selling category of drugs in the United States.[47]

As had so often happened in psychiatric history, the development of a treatment shaped the nature of the illness for which it was supposedly a response. Because a drug was called an "anti-depressant," depression must be the condition that was being treated. Between 1987 and 1997, the proportion of the population receiving outpatient treatment for conditions that were called "depression" increased by more than 300 percent. While 0.73 persons per 100 received outpatient treatment for depression in 1987, ten years later the rate had leaped to 2.33 per 100. Depression became by far the single most common diagnosis in outpatient treatment. At the same time, the proportion of individuals treated for depression receiving a psychotropic medication nearly doubled over this period from 44.6 percent to 79.4 percent.[48] After controlling for socio-demographic characteristics, treatment for depression was 4.5 times as likely to involve medication in 1997 compared to 1987.

The FDA approval of direct-to-consumer (DTC) drug advertisements in the late 1990s both enhanced the popularity of the SSRIs and reinforced their link to depressive illness. "Such advertising," explains sociologist Nikolas Rose, "seeks not just to market a drug, but to reshape the potential patient's understanding and presentation of their condition to their doctor in the form of a particular *DSM* disorder for which a specific drug has been licensed and marketed."[49] These ads typically linked the most common symptoms of depression from the *DSM* diagnosis—sadness, fatigue, sleeplessness, and the like—with very common psychosocial situations involving problems with interpersonal relationships, employment, and achieving valued goals. For example, a widely broadcast ad for Paxil featured a woman on one side and her husband and son on the other side, with a list of symptoms drawn from the MDD diagnosis separating the two sides. The ad implied that the symptoms of depression are the cause, rather than the result, of the family's problems.[50] SSRI consumption was presented as the solution to the kinds of widespread family, work, and motivational problems the ads depicted, which were called "major depression."

The DTC ads had the additional consequence of changing the conditions that the general medical sector treated from anxiety to depression. Since the middle of the nineteenth century, general physicians had called the amorphous collection of psychological, somatic, and psychosocial problems they treated as "nervous" or "stress" conditions. DTC ads urged potential patients to "consult your doctor" about receiving SSRI medications for problems of depression. The result of these successful advertising campaigns was to increase the proportion of people obtaining treatment for a psychological condition in the general medical sector as opposed to the specifically mental health sector. During the period from 1990–1992 to 2001–2002, the percentage of emotional disorders treated in the general medical sector grew from about one-third to about one-half, an increase of about 150 percent.[51] These conditions were now considered to be problems of depression instead of anxiety.

The findings of epidemiological studies also helped to boost the status of major depression as a central problem of the modern age. Rates of depression in the community were rarely studied before 1980. Community studies instead examined generalized conditions using scales where symptoms of anxiety predominated. The ECA Study was the first study to use the *DSM-III* category of MDD. Conducted in the early 1980s, it found rates of one-year prevalence of MDD that varied from 1.7 percent to 3.4 percent across the five different sites in the survey. Lifetime rates of MDD varied from 2.9 to 5.8 across these sites. Other community studies from a variety of countries indicated comparable rates.[52]

The NCS, conducted during the early 1990s, found sharply higher rates of MDD than earlier surveys had, although it used similar *DSM-III-R* criteria. In the NCS, 10.3 percent of respondents reported MDD over the past year; 17.1 percent reported this condition over their lifetime. Its rates were between three to six times higher than those reported in earlier studies. These differences were explained as the product of methodological changes regarding question placement and memory probes.[53] Although there is no compelling reason to believe that the NCS rates are more accurate than those found in earlier studies, they became the standard for claims that about a tenth of the population suffers from depression at any particular time and that nearly a fifth will have this disorder at some point in their life. Pharmaceutical ads, public health campaigns, Internet Web sites, and media stories all widely trumpeted the tremendous amount of depressive disorder in the population. While as recently as the late 1970s depression was a relatively uncommon disorder, just fifteen years later it had become a widespread public health problem.

The widely disseminated findings of the WHO about the burdens that depressive illness creates also helped to raise the profile of this condition. One of the major concerns of the WHO was to raise worldwide public awareness of the seemingly immense costs of depression. It used ratings of severity that combined prevalence estimates based on epidemiological findings about the number of people who suffer from depression with expert ratings of the severity of depression, which considered it comparable in disability to the conditions of paraplegia and blindness and more severe than conditions such as Down syndrome, deafness, and angina. Based on these figures, the WHO projected that by 2020 depression would become the second leading cause of worldwide disability, behind only heart disease, and that depression is already the single leading cause of disability for people in midlife and for women of all ages.[54] "The response from psychiatry to this news," David Healy drolly comments, "appeared to be satisfaction that the discipline was now the second most important in medicine after cardiology." Healy goes on to note that the "emergence of a comparable epidemic of any other serious illness on this scale would have led to serious questioning as to what had happened. There appeared to be no such questioning in the case of depression."[55] The WHO figures helped solidify the appearance of the dire social and economic impacts from depressive illness.

Since the 1980s, the NIMH has promoted depression as a central form of mental disorder. The perception of its widespread prevalence combined with its terrible consequences made it the most promotable threat to public health that any mental illness posed. The NIMH not only became the major sponsor of research about depression but also developed widespread public education campaigns with the aim of raising public consciousness about this condition and promoting professional help-seeking among untreated people with depression. It also became heavily invested in promoting the benefits of pharmaceutical treatments for the disorder.

The NIMH is the most credible, respectable, and prestigious source of information about mental disorder. Because of its enormous cultural capital, it has been a leading force in changing public discourse about the nature of mental illnesses. The symptom-based criteria of the *DSM* generated very large estimates of depressive illnesses. These estimates, in turn, allowed the NIMH to expand its mandate, make claims that mental illness is rampant in the population, and protect and expand its budget. The creation of ubiquitous depressive disease states also depoliticized the NIMH's previous concern with the problematic social consequences of poverty, racism, and discrimination. Political support is far more likely to accrue to an agency that is devoted to preventing and curing a widespread disease than to one that confronts controversial social problems. The consequences of chronic states of social deprivation as well as of stressful life situations are now viewed as diseases that fall within the mandate of mental health professionals. A variety of intraprofessional, economic, political, and cultural reasons coalesced to make depression the central diagnosis to emerge from the *DSM-III* revolution.

The Expansion of Depression

One of the major controversies surrounding the nature of depression before 1980 was whether depression was categorical or continuous in nature. The

DSM arbitrarily resolved this controversy, requiring that a diagnosis of MDD required at least five symptoms. Persons who otherwise met requirements for an MDD diagnosis but who only had four or fewer symptoms would not receive the diagnosis. This requirement was not based on empirical research that showed any sharp breaking point at the five-symptom cutoff but was adopted from the Feighner criteria as an approximation to the point where a reasonable break might lie between a disordered and non-disordered state.

Clinicians need to use some cutting point in order to generate a diagnosis and to receive reimbursement. Yet even the proponents of the *DSM-III* diagnosis recognized that the particular number of symptoms required for delineating patients who meet or do not meet the MDD requirements is somewhat arbitrary and a matter of convention.[56] Research subsequent to the *DSM-III* showed that potential symptoms of MDD were not discontinuous between four and five symptoms or between any other adjacent points. Instead, depressive symptoms fell on a linear continuum of varying severity and duration with no sharp breaks at any point. "Our current *DSM-IV* diagnostic conventions," geneticists Kenneth Kendler and Charles Gardner summarize, "may be arbitrary and not reflective of a natural discontinuity in depressive symptoms as experienced in the general population."[57] The seeming continuous nature of depression gave rise to a movement that aimed to establish considerably lower cut points than those of the MDD diagnosis, with a resulting tremendous expansion of depressive disorder.

One of the reasons for establishing the categorical system of the *DSM-III* was the extremely high, and widely ridiculed, estimates of community studies of the 1950s and 1960s, which indicated only a small proportion of the population did not show some sign of a mental disorder. Indeed, the best-known community study of this time found that only 20 percent of the population of Midtown Manhattan was "well," that is, symptom-free.[58] These findings arose because symptoms among community members lie on a continuum that ranges from a small to a large number of symptoms. Although the five-symptom requirement of the MDD diagnosis generates very high amounts of mental disorder in the population, lowering the criteria produces even greater estimates. The number of people who report a small number of symptoms far exceeds those reporting many symptoms. For example, in the ECA study 8.7 percent of respondents had just one depressive symptom in the past month compared with 2.3 percent who met the full criteria for MDD.[59]

The continuous distribution of symptoms in the general population posed a challenge for the categorical distinction of MDD in the *DSM*. This distribution does not suggest any natural cutoff point for a diagnostic decision. Likewise, the social impairments and physical disabilities that accompany depressive symptoms increase as the number of symptoms rises.[60] When symptoms are used as the basis for defining depressive disorder, a small number of symptoms can seem to indicate a milder form of disorder rather than a non-disordered condition.

The arbitrary nature of the MDD diagnosis led to a flood of studies about "minor" or "subthreshold" conditions that have fewer than five symptoms of depression. The most common definition of this condition stipulates that two to four symptoms of depression (including sad mood or loss of pleasure in activities) during the same two-week period indicate minor or subthreshold depression.[61] Such studies produce extremely high calculations of depression. For example, in a one-month period nearly a quarter (22.6 percent) of the respondents in the ECA study reported one or more symptoms of depression. When "mild depression" is defined as the presence of two to four symptoms, the lifetime prevalence of depression increases from 15.8 to 25.8 percent.[62]

Because the *DSM* definition of depression is symptom-based, the subthreshold movement has the potential to pathologize an extreme amount of ordinary behavior. For example, the most common depressive symptoms in the ECA study are "trouble falling asleep, staying asleep, or waking up early" (33.7 percent), being "tired out all the time" (22.8 percent), and "thought a lot about death" (22.6 percent).[63] People who worry about an important event, those who must work overtime, or those taking the survey around the death of a famous person would all expectably, but naturally, experience such symptoms. The lack of context in the *DSM* diagnosis makes the problem of mistaking normal symptoms for signs of depressive disorder progressively worse as fewer symptoms are required for a diagnosis.

Advocates of the subthreshold movement justifiably argue that depression is a continuous disorder. In addition, they rightly note (as Kraepelin did) that the presence of a small number of symptoms can indicate the early stages in the development of a more serious disorder. Moreover, research into genetic, biological, and personality susceptibilities shows that the same vulnerabilities are likely to be present in both mild and severe forms of depression.[64]

The problem is that the subthreshold movement's lowered criteria were not accompanied by a contextual definition that separated natural sadness from depressive disorder. The existence of a small number of symptoms is often the natural product of transitory, distressing situations as opposed to a mental disorder. Moreover, the fewer the symptoms that are required for a depressive diagnosis, the more likely they are to indicate natural sadness rather than depressive disorder. Even more than the MDD diagnosis, the subthreshold criteria confounds ordinary distress with pathological depression.

The subthreshold movement repeats the major themes of the post–World War II community studies: depression is continuous; all points along the continuum are disorders; even a low point on the continuum is worrisome because it is associated with some impairment; and a low score at one point in time can predict a full-blown future case of depression. For example, one of the major proponents of the subthreshold depression movement, psychiatrist and former NIMH director Lewis Judd, argues that this condition is "a truly hidden, unrecognized public health problem that has an enormous 1-year prevalence in the society" and that it should be a major focus of research and preventive efforts.[65] These arguments echo the attempts in the 1960s to pathologize and treat common sources of human unhappiness. When the continuous notion was applied in the 1960s, the result was the pathologization of a large proportion of the population, the extension of mental health services to many non-disordered people who had problems of living, and the failure to direct treatment resources to people with serious mental disorders.[66] If successful, the movement to pathologize minor depression threatens to lead to the same mistakes that the community mental health movement made during an earlier decade.

Conclusion

The *DSM* category of Major Depressive Disorder has generated a remarkable amount of consensus in the mental health field and has become firmly institutionalized in mental health practice.[67] Its explicitness, clarity, and ease of measurement have led the definition to become the standard for diagnoses, research, and treatment. Moreover, it has become the common language for discussions of depression not only in the United States but also worldwide.[68] It might appear as if the *DSM* definition has solved the perennial problems of defining and classifying depression. The appearance that the MDD criteria resolved the problems of measuring depression is deceptive. Under the surface of definitional consensus lies a host of unanswered questions.

For millennia, diagnosticians separated depressive disorders from ordinary sadness. The *DSM-III* blurred this distinction; its symptom-based criteria considered all depressive emotions except for uncomplicated bereavement as signs of mental disorder. The trend toward using fewer symptoms of "subthreshold" depression as indicators of disorder greatly expanded the range of

conditions that were treated as pathological. The consequences were vast estimates of the amount of depressive disorder, reaching nearly half of the population in some community studies. Such figures have led to the questioning
of the criteria that lead to such results.[69] While the *DSM* definition excludes
conditions that result from normal bereavement, it does not make exclusions
for conditions that arise from other forms of loss. Comparable exclusions
to the bereavement criteria for further types of losses lead to a considerable
drop in rates of MDD.[70] Ultimately, the unrealistic estimates of rates of depressive disorder that result from a definition that does not distinguish natural
unhappiness from mental disorder could lead to a fundamental rethinking of
the conception of mental disorder that underlies the *DSM* criteria.

Another unresolved issue involves the status of melancholic depression,
which had been at the core of conceptions of depression for thousands of
years but which all but disappeared in the diagnostic manuals since 1980.
Before this date it seemed apparent that melancholia was the best delimited
type of depression that also had the most distinctive response to medication
treatment. The perceived need for a new, separate melancholic category led a
major psychiatric journal to devote an entire issue to this topic in 2007. Others, however, dismiss the need for such a category, arguing that melancholia
is simply the most severe type of major depression.[71] The issue of whether
melancholy has any special standing as a core form of depressive disorder
remains unresolved.

The controversy over whether depression is actually a dimensional, as
opposed to a categorical, disorder is also unsettled. Just before the publication of the *DSM-III*, British diagnostician R. E. Kendell concluded that the
pros and cons of categories and dimensions were "fairly evenly balanced."
This topic, of great concern before 1980, was resolved by fiat with the categorical diagnosis of MDD that appeared in the *DSM-III*. Most empirical analyses,
however, indicate that no discrete breaks occur at five, or any other number
of particular symptoms, so that depression is by its nature more dimensional
than categorical.[72] A dimensional system, however, is not conducive to clinical practice, which requires decisions about whether an illness is present
or not. A number of prominent researchers have called for a new diagnostic
system that would feature dimensional as well as categorical measures of
depression.[73] The calls for dimensional measurement echo the debates that
were very active in the half-century preceding the *DSM-III*.

The question of how depressive disorders relate to depressive temperaments, which has concerned diagnosticians since Hippocrates, also remains

uncertain. The dysthymic category that emerged in the *DSM-III* as a political compromise with the psychoanalysts does nothing to resolve this issue. It provides no guidance regarding how to distinguish long-term but low-grade depressive disorders from comparable symptoms that reflect a melancholic but natural personality disposition. Accordingly, Aristotle's contribution to the distinction between depressive disorders and personality dimensions seems more accurate than the portrayal of dysthymia in the current *DSM*.

The *DSM* has generated a consensus about the operational definition of depressive disorder. It has not, however, resolved any of the issues about classification that have continuously surrounded this condition since the earliest times. Whether depression is continuous or categorical, how many categories it has, what its relationship to melancholic personality is, and how it can be distinguished from normal sadness are no closer to resolution now than they were when the *DSM-III* arose.

"Are we still confused?" asks an article written in 2008. It responds, "The answer to this question is surely 'yes.' Our current nosologies remain as 'working hypotheses' and have no greater validity than the definitions of depression that existed when Kendell wrote in 1976. Consequently, the 'true' classification of depression remains as elusive as it was 30 years ago."[74] Despite strenuous efforts, depressive disorders—as defined in the *DSM*—have none of the characteristics of diseases: they remain without well-defined phenotypes, any identifiable etiologic factors, predictable courses, or distinct responses to treatment. No biological marker or gene has yet been found that is helpful for making a diagnosis of major depression or that predicts a response to any specific treatment.[75] It is hardly surprising that a diagnosis that emerged because of the social and political pressures facing psychiatry during the 1970s has been unable to achieve the fundamental goals of accurate classification systems. It is unlikely that this situation will change in the absence of better diagnostic criteria that distinguish depressive disorder from normal sadness and from melancholic personality types as well as from other forms of mental disorder.

Chapter 7

Post-Traumatic Stress Disorder

The Result of Abnormal Environments or Abnormal Individuals?

Post-traumatic stress disorder and its historical antecedents have always been problematic diagnoses for psychiatry. Their basic tenet—that some traumatic event in the external environment can lead to lasting psychopathological consequences in previously normal people—does not easily fit the psychiatric profession's traditional focus on the biological and/or psychological roots of mental illness. While psychiatric explanations have periodically emphasized how a heterogeneous range of social, moral, and lifestyle factors influence who becomes mentally ill, they generally regarded these environmental forces as precipitants of mental disorder in already predisposed individuals. The view of trauma found in the PTSD diagnosis, in contrast, considers some external event as a necessary and sometimes sufficient cause of disorder. It thus focuses attention on how exposure to traumatic situations can itself cause mental disorder, threatening one of the profession's core assumptions that some internal vulnerability underlies pathology. Likewise, the environmental emphasis of the PTSD diagnosis challenges psychiatry's usual therapeutic focus on changing disordered brains and minds. Psychiatry has faced great difficulties with integrating PTSD into the paradigms that have guided the profession since its inception in the nineteenth century.

PTSD also reveals in their most manifest form the political and moral conflicts that are latent in many psychiatric diagnoses. Because of its intrinsic tie to traumatic events, PTSD is rooted in social and political contexts to an unusually great extent. These contexts often involve intense clashes between, on the one hand, victims who seek to hold liable and gain restitution from the party they believe is responsible for their trauma and, on the other hand, potential wrongdoers who reject these accusations. Successful PTSD judgments often lead to secondary gains for people who have suffered the traumatic event. Indeed, PTSD is one of the few psychiatric diagnoses that are valued rather than stigmatized. "It is rare," notes psychiatrist Nancy Andreasen, "to find a psychiatric diagnosis that anyone likes to have, but PTSD seems to be one of them."[1] Diagnoses can become part of moral crusades that involve sufferers' demands for redress, on one side, and claims of deception, malingering, and exploitation of the sick role, on the other. It is difficult for medical personnel to remain neutral in these controversies, which are often related to the benefits of disease status and its accompanying sick role.

While PTSD-like diagnoses originated during the latter decades of the nineteenth century, the proximate roots of the current diagnosis are found in the *DSM-III*, which was published in 1980. Since that time, the diagnosis has exploded in popularity. "At the beginning of the twenty-first century," write historians Paul Lerner and Mark Micale, "PTSD is perhaps the fastest growing and most influential diagnosis in American psychiatry."[2] Although Lerner and Micale probably exaggerate the role of PTSD within the psychiatric profession, they are certainly correct to emphasize its mounting importance within the mental health professions more generally.

A number of indicators show the rising impact of the PTSD diagnosis. A large trauma industry has developed that encompasses medical and mental health professionals, grief counselors, lawyers, and claimants. An active subculture that responds to traumatic events peddles proprietary workshops, trade magazines, and books to public safety, military, school, and hospital organizations. The expanding rate of publications about PTSD between 1980 and 2005 exceeds any other anxiety diagnosis.[3] Traumas and their psychological consequences are also major stock-in-trade of daytime talk shows, television documentaries, and news programs. Laypersons routinely use the term "PTSD" to describe their reactions to traumas. While the extent of this "culture of trauma" is new, the controversies it involves have a long history in medicine and psychiatry.

Origins of PTSD

Wars, natural disasters, violence, accidents, and plagues have been regular aspects of the human experience. Victims of these traumas have undoubtedly always suffered from intense psychic disturbances. "Shell shock had not yet been heard of," notes a historian of the American Civil War, "but families recognized that after cannonade and bayonet charge a man might come home and seem queer for a while. The warp of battle might remain in him a long time."[4] Until the latter decades of the nineteenth century, however, conceptions of mental illnesses were limited to conditions resembling insanity. Before this time, no psychiatric diagnostic category existed that defined, organized, and classified the psychological consequences of traumatic experiences. PTSD did not become a culturally recognized condition until expanding forces of industrialization created the potential for massive man-made catastrophes.

The emergence of psychological trauma as a psychiatric diagnosis was connected to the spread of mechanized technologies during the nineteenth century and to the resulting changes in conceptions of liability when their malfunctioning caused injury. While accidents themselves were nothing new, the scope and violence of train wrecks were unprecedented and they captivated the public imagination. Most importantly, railroad companies could be held liable for injuries resulting from the shock and trauma of these crashes. "Railway spine" was the first diagnosis that captured the psychic consequences of disasters, emerging during the 1860s and 1870s when railroad accidents became increasingly widespread.[5] It was characterized by patient reports of intense pain, the loss of muscular control, paralysis, neurological problems, and general health impairments without any discoverable physical pathology. Sufferers demanded monetary compensation because their conditions rendered them unable to resume their normal occupational, familial, and social activities.

During the period when railway spine first became an issue, most psychiatrists accepted the centrality of hereditarian explanations. Their views emphasized how psychiatric disorders only emerged in individuals who already had inherited predispositions for them. "After 1870," explains historian George Makari, "biologic inheritance was widely accepted as the cause of psychic functions and the central precondition that led to a mind breaking during accidental events."[6] Persons without pre-existing susceptibilities who developed psychogenic problems did not fit established psychiatric theories; they were likely to be regarded as malingerers who stood to gain from consciously simulating symptoms. No conception existed that would explain why previously normal persons who were not already predisposed could develop psychogenic conditions after a severe environmental shock.

The initial debates over railway spine centered on whether physical traumas such as train wrecks could lead a malfunctioning nervous system in the absence of any predisposition that was present before the traumatic event. In 1866 the eminent British surgeon John Erichsen wrote the first text on railway spine and related conditions, *On Railway and Other Injuries of the Nervous System.*[7] While Erichsen could not specify the mechanisms through which powerful shocks damaged the nervous system, his work led to a lively debate on the nature of nervous shocks. Like Erichsen, a number of neurologists and physicians claimed that nervous shocks were common results of physical traumas and were as deserving of compensation as more precisely demonstrable physical symptoms.

Yet almost as soon as neurologists developed theories that emphasized how physical shocks could produce nervous conditions, they were countered by other physicians who claimed that personal vulnerabilities and desires for monetary compensation lay behind claims of railway spine. Whenever individuals stood to gain from a diagnosis, their motives became suspect. These controversies showed the keen awareness of physicians and psychiatrists about the advantages and disadvantages of granting victims of psychic trauma the benefits of the sick role. Many commentators stressed how injuries would remain chronic as long as they were reinforced by the reception of compensation. One skeptical reviewer of Erichsen's text noted that "the only differences which . . . are to be found between railway and other injuries are purely incidental and relate to their legal aspects. A man, whose spine is concussed on a railway, brings an action against the company, and does or does not get heavy damages. A man, who falls from an apple-tree and concussed his spine, has—worse luck for him—no railway to bring an action against." Others claimed that the distinctiveness of diagnoses of railway spine was "due, not to the specific peculiarities of train accidents, but to the annoying litigation and exorbitant claims for pecuniary damage that are constantly the grave result of their existence."[8] The distinctive aspect of railway spine for skeptics was that unlike other diagnoses it led to monetary rewards. The secondary gains accruing from acknowledging and rewarding victims have remained a constant theme of the response to trauma-related diagnoses.

The notion that psychic injuries stemmed from desires for compensation rather than actual damage was linked to a corresponding argument that personal vulnerabilities and not traumatic events were responsible for mental symptoms. By 1890 the prominent American neurologist Morton Prince could divide trauma medicine into two sharply contrasting schools.[9] The first emphasized the grounding of railway spine in actual traumatic events leading to damaged nervous systems; the second located injury in psychological susceptibilities to conditions such as hysteria or neurasthenia. These two contrasting traditions and variants upon them have dominated discussions of traumatic injuries up to the present.

The work of French neurologist John-Martin Charcot during the 1870s and 1880s and his students Pierre Janet and Sigmund Freud in the 1890s also strongly influenced explanations of psychological trauma. Charcot's work had made hysteria the defining diagnosis of the psychiatric profession at the time.[10] This condition featured physical symptoms such as paralysis, fainting, fatigue, headache, and pain in the absence of any discernable organic cause. Charcot noted that many people who were exposed to severe traumas did not become symptomatic while minor stressors could lead predisposed individuals to develop hysterical symptoms. Consequently, he grounded the psychic consequences of trauma in underlying flaws of the nervous system that stemmed from hereditary weaknesses. Although traumas could cause hysteria and other neuroses, they simply triggered a more basic vulnerability in their victims. By linking the psychological symptoms stemming from trauma to hysteria, Charcot greatly raised the profile of such symptoms.[11]

While Charcot's writings focused on men who had often experienced railway accidents, Janet's work primarily explored trauma among female victims of rape, incest, and sexual seduction.[12] He focused on the impact of trauma on memory, emphasizing how the original trauma created psychic dissociation that precluded later recollections of the event. These traumas generally occurred far earlier in life than their resulting symptoms, which were repressed until brought to light many years later by therapeutic means. Like Charcot, Janet emphasized that heredity played a dominant role in determining which individuals would succumb to traumatic experiences and develop hysteria and other neuroses.

Unlike Charcot and Janet, Freud rejected hereditarian explanations and insisted that repressed mental conflicts explained the development of the psychoneuroses. His initial theories focused on how traumatic events in childhood had profound psychic consequences in later life when they were the preeminent cause of hysteria and other neurotic conditions. By 1897, however, Freud had already begun to doubt that repressed childhood traumas were the source of later neurotic symptoms. Freud's later theories emphasized the *differences* between traumatic and hysterical neuroses. In contrast to hysterical neuroses that originated in childhood experiences, traumatic neuroses arose from unexpected contemporaneous external events and would generally abate when the conditions surrounding the trauma dissipated. Freud wrote, regarding war neuroses, that "when war conditions ceased to operate, the greater number of the neurotic disturbances brought about by the war simultaneously vanished." His confrontation with the psychic effects of war neuroses led him to revise his theories in major ways. In addition to sexual instincts, he came to emphasize aggressiveness, cruelty, and violence as inherent aspects of the unconscious. In addition, in contrast to the general analytic principle that dreams represented the fulfillment of wishes, he stressed that efforts to cope with wartime traumas through dreams involved the compulsion to repeat, and therefore to master, the traumatic experience.[13] Freud never successfully resolved the tension between the psychic consequences of overt traumas and the symbolic and unconscious nature of the neuroses.

Because traumas were not products of unconscious memories, they were also not amenable to traditional methods of psychoanalysis. "Traumatic neurosis," according to psychoanalyst Charles Rycroft, "is the one form of psychological illness for which interpretative psychotherapy is not indicated."[14] Moreover, many analysts believed that repetition of the traumatic memory was not neurotic but manifested healing processes that helped the sufferer anticipate, react to, and get over the distressing experience. Traumatic neuroses, therefore, largely remained outside of the mainstream of analytic thought because they mirrored a real event, did not reflect symbolic distortions, and were not subject to typical analytic techniques. Psychoanalysts faced great difficulties with integrating the psychic impacts of realistic traumas into their core conceptions about the sources of mental distress.

Shellshock and Malingering in the World Wars

World War I created an especially intense opposition between those who focused on traumatic occurrences and others who stressed personal vulnerabilities to traumas. This war produced a sudden, unexpected, and huge number of soldiers with psychic rather than physical wounds. British medical units alone treated tens of thousands of psychic cases.[15] Initial conceptions of the etiology of psychic symptoms recapitulated arguments from railway spine and focused on how the shock from exploding shells damaged the nervous system with resulting "shell shock." The term stuck, despite the fact that the vast majority of affected soldiers had not been near exploding shells but suffered from debilitating fatigue, fear, and horror. The problem became so overwhelming, however, that some sort of medical response was necessary.

Most military officers and politicians felt that psychological damage was a product of cowardice and malingering, which could only be overcome through harsh discipline. Likewise, most military psychiatrists deemphasized the triggering events and wartime experiences themselves and focused on psychic and hereditary predispositions that led some but not other soldiers to develop hysterical symptoms. They stressed that psychic weakness and desire to escape from combat, on the one hand, and the allure of a comfortable bed and cushy pension, on the other, created and perpetuated symptoms of shell shock.[16] While normal individuals would naturally recover from traumas without long-term effects, the minority of men who developed chronic disorders likely had constitutional predispositions to become mentally ill. After the war ended, most physicians continued to resist the idea that external traumas were the primary causes of chronic psychic traumas, instead emphasizing the subjective and material rewards that flowed from diagnoses of shell shock.[17] Many questioned whether neurotic soldiers were using their premorbid weaknesses to exploit the availability of public pensions.

A few medical thinkers, however, concluded that the war experience showed the importance of environmental stressors in causing psychic disturbances among otherwise healthy individuals. Most notably, military psychiatrist (and anthropologist) W.H.R. Rivers found no evidence of pre-existing personal weaknesses and attributed breakdowns to war experiences themselves. This minority maintained that the severity of wartime trauma led normal men to become shell-shocked. "The war," stated anatomist Grafton Smith and psychologist Tom Pear in 1917, "has shown us one inescapable fact, that a psychoneurosis may be produced in almost anyone if only his environment be made 'difficult' enough for him." In the early 1920s the prominent psychiatrist Thomas Salmon joined with the American Legion to lobby successfully for the establishment of a network of veteran's hospitals that provided services for psychically disabled veterans in the United States.[18] The American Legion promoted the view that these veterans were normal, patriotic men who had succumbed to the intense stress of wartime combat.

The debate over shell shock during and after World War I reproduced the debate among neurologists and physicians about railway spine. It pitted those who emphasized how "nature" produced personal susceptibilities to traumatic events against those who stressed "nurture," so that "every man has his limit" in dealing with powerful environmental stressors. Because it occurred in the highly charged context of what military actions constituted bravery and cowardice and what sorts of wartime injuries entailed soldiers to receive compensation, it aroused deep moral passions.

When the United States began to prepare for war in 1940, the initial involvement of psychiatrists was with the Selective Service System. Even before the nation entered the war, prominent psychiatrists became involved in a massive screening program whose goal was to identify individuals with neuropsychiatric problems (which at that time included homosexuality) from entering the army in the first place. These programs combined a few standardized questions about mental health with brief psychiatric interviews. The results of screening led to a huge number of deferments on psychiatric grounds, amounting to more than 1.75 million men or about a quarter of all draftees. Despite these screening efforts, the war produced an enormous psychic toll. By the end of 1942 psychiatric disorders accounted for more than a quarter of hospital admissions among soldiers. After the war nearly two-thirds of patients in Veterans Hospitals were psychiatric casualties and nearly half a million veterans received pensions for psychiatric disabilities.[19]

The well-established patterns of debates over the nature of railway spine and shell shock continued in discussions of what were now called "war neuroses." Some influential psychiatrists accentuated factors that led soldiers to regress to childhood vulnerabilities. They emphasized how constitutional factors such as psychopathy, mental instability, and individual defects determined which soldiers would succumb to the stress of combat. Yet, in contrast to World War I, most psychiatrists found that predisposition was not a significant factor leading to psychological breakdowns. The bulk of American psychiatrists "underwent a marked change of view, switching from their initial belief that 'a clear cut distinction (could) be made among men as between the 'weak' and the 'strong,' to the view that 'every man has his breaking point.'"[20]

Military psychiatrists generally believed that they were not dealing with abnormal men but with normal men in abnormal conditions. Psychiatrist John Appel's research showed that the longer that men remained in battle the greater were their chances of becoming victims of psychic trauma. In the North African campaign, for example, combat veterans were more likely to breakdown than inexperienced soldiers. Appel emphasized how factors related to the stressful situation and military organization, such as the degree of combat exposure, loss of comrades, weak unit cohesion, and ineffective leadership, accounted for rates of psychiatric casualties. A generation of psychiatrists who served in the military during World War II and took positions of professional leadership in the postwar era assumed that environmental factors played a major role in the etiology of mental disorders. The most influential psychiatrist during this period, William C. Menninger, concluded that the "history or the personality make-up or the internal psychodynamic stresses" were less important than "the force of factors in the environment which supported or disrupted the individual."[21]

Wartime experiences also showed that most men who became psychological casualties were not permanently damaged. Indeed, brief periods of support and reassurance accompanied by adequate food, rest, and sleep successfully dealt with the symptoms of the majority. Temporarily relieving soldiers of their duties and assuring them that distress was natural led to rapid recovery while long-term hospitalization was ineffective and served to prolong healing. Likewise, after the war, "a job and a girl" were the most effective routes to successful reintegration. Most former soldiers proved to be resilient and coped with the impact of traumatic events on their own or with the help of family, friends, religion, and community. While most psychiatrists agreed that combat exposure was the best predictor of acute psychological breakdowns, some emphasized how constitutional susceptibilities could account for which soldiers would not recover and would become chronic patients after they were removed from dangerous situations.[22]

Overall, World War II reinforced the association of highly stressful conditions with massive numbers of mental casualties and prepared the way for the social emphasis that came to dominate American psychiatry during the 1950s and 1960s. The dramatic social and cultural changes that the New Deal had already brought to American life and thought paved the way for a new environmental emphasis in psychiatry as well as in the culture at large. The ideological climate of the postwar period was conducive to sympathetic attitudes toward psychological injuries and the idea that traumatic environments could produce disturbances in otherwise normal individuals. It also legitimated the concept of the welfare state, enlarged the scope of federal intervention in making social reforms, and strengthened the role of psychiatrists in formulating mental health policies. More than anything else, this war helped to unify the beliefs that environmental stress contributed to mental maladjustment and that purposeful human interventions could alter psychological outcomes. Issues of predisposition and malingering receded into the background of mainstream psychiatric thinking during and after World War II.

DSM-I and DSM-II

The epidemic of war neuroses that arose during World War II demonstrated the inadequacies of extant psychiatric manuals, which had been developed for institutionalized patients. The existing diagnostic system embodied in the *Statistical Manual for the Use of Hospitals for Mental Disorder* could not ade-quately classify the vast majority of symptoms that psychically impaired sol-diers displayed. In particular, it could not classify chronic but non-psychotic conditions that stemmed from exposure to traumatic events. The insufficien-cies of the *Statistical Manual* led the Veterans Administration to develop its own diagnostic system, which in turn spurred the American Psychiatric Association to create its first classification manual, the *Diagnostic and Statis-tical Manual of Mental Disorders* (or *DSM-I*), in 1952.[23]

None of the major functional categories in the *DSM-I*—brain disorders, mental deficiency, psychotic disorders, psychoneurotic disorders, or per-sonality pattern disturbance—could encompass long-lasting symptoms that arose after an environmental trauma among people with no previous histo-ries of psychological problems. The *DSM-I* created a category called Transient Situational Personality Disorders for people with normal personalities who developed acute symptoms as a way of adjusting to an overwhelming situa-tion. These disorders were distinguished from psychoneuroses, which were assumed to arise from unconscious conflicts stemming from childhood expe-riences, and from personality disorders, which were developmental defects that had minimal anxiety. Among these transient situational reactions was "Gross Stress Reaction." This diagnosis followed the environmental tradition and was only to be applied for "previously more or less 'normal' persons who have experienced intolerable stress." The *DSM-I* specified wartime combat and catastrophic events in civilian life as the two traumatic conditions lead-ing to this reaction. Because gross stress reactions arose in normal individu-als who had undergone unusually stressful experiences, the manual stated that they would "clear rapidly" once the individual was removed from the stressful situation.[24] If symptoms persisted, a different diagnosis, usually some psychoneuroses, was indicated. The manual, therefore, could not ade-quately deal with chronic symptoms that resulted from some environmental trauma among people without some pre-existing vulnerability.

By the time that the *DSM-II* appeared in 1968, the influence of military psychiatrists had receded; no organized group had an interest in trauma-related diagnoses. This manual dropped the category of Gross Stress Reaction. It did include a general diagnosis of "Transient Situational Disturbances" that stated that if "the patient has good adaptive capacity his symptoms usually recede as the stress diminishes. If, however, the symptoms persist after the stress is removed, the diagnosis of another mental disorder is indicated." In other words, persistent conditions would not be classified in this category but must be psychoneuroses, personality disorders, or psychoses. Chronic symptoms, therefore, must be due to individual predispositions rather than to experiences of a traumatic stressor. Within the general category of Transient Situational Disturbances was a diagnosis of "adjustment reaction of adult life." Among its brief descriptions was the example of "fear associated with military combat and manifested by trembling, running and hiding."[25] The absence of a suitable diagnostic category for chronic combat-related stress in the *DSM-II* was highly significant when the psychic casualties from Vietnam returned from the war.

The Vietnam Experience and the *DSM-III*

Psychiatric casualty rates during the Vietnam War itself were remarkably low compared to previous conflicts. For example, psychological reasons accounted for fewer than 5 percent of evacuations of soldiers out of Vietnam from 1965 to 1967, the period of most intense combat. Overall rates of breakdowns during the war were only about 5 per 1,000 troops. This favorably compared to previous conflicts: 37 per 1,000 soldiers experienced psychological breakdowns in the Korean War, and 70 per 1,000 during World War II. Although the reasons for this low rate are not clear, a number of factors could have been responsible, including improved treatment in combat zones, expectations of quick recovery, the ready availability of alcohol and illegal drugs as ways of coping with the stresses of war, or the underreporting of psychiatric casualties.[26]

Veterans entered a highly turbulent environment when they returned to the United States. Although most felt that they received a warm welcome and few felt rejected by their peers, the cultural climate had significantly changed.[27] Distrust of authority, rejection of the war, and a highly politicized anti-war atmosphere pervaded much of the country. A strong, vocal, and well-organized subculture of anti-war veterans emerged, most notably the Vietnam Veterans Against the War (VVAW).

Within the VVAW, a subgroup developed that consisted of anti-war psychiatrists (most prominently, Robert Jay Lifton and Chaim Shatan), disillusioned Veteran's Administration therapists, and psychologically disturbed veterans. They created a network of therapeutic "rap groups" where veterans could discuss their problems in the company of sympathetic peers. Based on their experiences in dealing with these groups, Lifton, Shatan, and others became convinced that massive numbers of veterans were experiencing a "post-Vietnam syndrome" marked by survivor guilt, flashbacks, rage, psychic numbing, alienation, and feelings of being scapegoated.[28] They emphasized both that symptoms could have a delayed onset that began well after their wartime experiences had ended and that veterans who did not receive appropriate treatment for this syndrome would become chronically disabled.

The anti-war psychiatrists openly advocated veterans' interests, making no claims to be dispassionate scientists. Shrewdly using the national media, they successfully projected images of Vietnam veterans as "ticking time bombs" whose psyches had been badly wounded by their wartime experiences. A powerful stereotype of a "crazy Vietnam vet" who was "angry, violent and emotionally unstable" dominated many media presentations of veterans.[29] The diagnostic categories of the *DSM-II,* however, could not encompass veterans who displayed chronic pathology where traumatic memories compulsively intruded into their present lives.

Coincidentally, at the same time as the veteran's group was mobilizing against the psychiatric establishment, the APA created a task force in 1974 to revise the *DSM-II.* It consisted of a number of subgroups that were charged with evaluating existing data and developing specific criteria for each of the disorders that would appear in the *DSM-III.* The overriding goal of the new manual was to replace the psychoanalytically based system of the *DSM-II* with ideologically free, scientific classifications. A cardinal principle of the new diagnostic system was to use manifest symptoms that carefully described each syndrome and delineated it from other syndromes without reference to the cause of symptoms. The *DSM-III* eschewed etiological diagnoses because there was not enough evidence for particular causes of psychiatric conditions. The Task Force on Nomenclature and Statistics declared that it "was the unanimous opinion of the Committee that etiology should be a classificatory principle only when it is clearly known."[30] Etiological discoveries would only follow from accurate descriptions so that the new manual, unlike the previous *DSMs,* would not be based on causal assumptions.

PTSD is a stark exception to the data-driven, causally agnostic descriptions of the other diagnoses in the *DSM-III.* Empirical studies had not examined how traumas produced specific symptoms that some pre-existing diagnostic category did not capture. The most prominent researchers of post–Vietnam War psychopathology—sociologist Lee Robins and psychiatrist John Helzer—believed that the categories of mood, anxiety, and substance abuse disorders adequately reflected the psychic consequences of combat.[31] They argued not only that existing diagnoses could sufficiently account for veterans' symptoms but also that the creation of a new diagnosis grounded in etiology would reproduce exactly the sort of unproven causal assumptions of previous manuals that the *DSM-III* was supposed to eliminate. Moreover, Helzer and Robins were close allies of Robert Spitzer and members of the group of Washington University researchers who dominated the deliberations of most of the particular task forces.

Despite their presumably weak political position relative to the research-oriented psychiatrists, the anti-war psychiatrists took advantage of the revision process of the manual to aggressively promote veterans' interests and remedy the absence of a diagnostic category that covered the conditions of disordered combatants. Lifton and Shatan modeled their efforts after the activist groups that had recently succeeded in eliminating the diagnosis of homosexuality from the *DSM-II*. In addition, they operated within an ideological climate that was still hostile to the war effort and sympathetic to veterans' claims. Lifton and Shatan were able to persuade Spitzer, the head of the *DSM* revision process, to appoint them and a Vietnam veteran (Jack Smith, the sole member of the roughly 150 persons on the various *DSM* task forces to have no graduate degree), to the six-member advisory committee working on the Reactive Disorders section of the new manual. They realized that they would have to convince at least one additional member (the others were psychiatrists Nancy Andreasen, Lyman Wynne, and Spitzer himself) to be able to secure a diagnosis that they thought would displace blame from the soldier onto the war itself.[32]

The creation of the new diagnosis of PTSD in the *DSM-III* had none of the trappings of other diagnoses, such as field trials of criteria, tests of reliability, and statistical analyses of data. Instead, the veterans' advocates relied on anecdotes from clinical experience as well as the moral argument that failing to include a PTSD diagnosis in the new manual would be tantamount to blaming victims for their misfortunes. In an ideological climate that was still highly charged from the aftermath of the war, their moral position was able to transcend the data-driven arguments that prevailed in the creation of other diagnoses. They were able to persuade Nancy Andreasen, who specialized in the treatment of burn victims, that the diagnosis was not limited to war veterans but could be applied to "an enormous number of stressful situations," including the experiences of victims of sexual violence, civilian disasters, accidents, or concentration camp survivors. "They were," reports sociologist Wilbur Scott, "well organized and politically active, and their opposition in St. Louis was neither of these."[33] The result was that the *DSM-III* incorporated a diagnosis of "post-traumatic stress disorder" that almost completely mirrored the recommendations of the anti-war psychiatric group.

The event criterion of the diagnosis required the "existence of a recognizable stressor that would evoke significant distress in almost everyone."[34] It was based on the environmental model of trauma, which assumed traumatic events produced chronic symptoms in otherwise normal individuals. The horrific quality of events themselves, not pre-existing vulnerabilities, were responsible for resulting symptoms. The clear causality in the diagnosis moved from a traumatic event to the denoted symptoms and left little room for factors connected to individual vulnerabilities. The rationale for the diagnosis was grounded in the fact that traumatic events were linked to a *particular* set of resulting symptoms. If, for example, traumas produced depression, anxiety, substance abuse, and other well-recognized diagnoses, there would be no need for a specific diagnosis intrinsically connected to the results of the traumatic experience.

Nancy Andreasen takes credit for writing the text of the syndrome, stemming from her experience with burn victims and the research literature. "I wrote the entire text description of the syndrome," she stated, "which was based on my experience caring for burn patients and the substantial literature available at the time." The large literature on psychological traumas of disaster victims that existed at the time, however, had little in common with the symptomatic criteria of the PTSD diagnosis. It emphasized psychological outcomes such as depression, anxiety, and delusions as well as social outcomes such as family, work, and social readjustment. Each of these outcomes could also occur in the absence of traumas and none required any new diagnostic category.[35] This literature was quite dissimilar to the distinctive pathology of Vietnam veterans, whose memories compulsively intruded into their lives many years after their traumas had occurred.

The symptom criteria required three sorts of characteristic symptoms, all tied to the patient's active memory of the event.[36] The first involved re-experiencing the trauma through intrusive recollections, dreams, or feelings of reoccurrence. The second stemmed from numbed responsiveness to the external world that began some time after the trauma as indicated by diminished interest, detachment, or restricted affect. Finally, the criteria required two symptoms that followed the trauma from among hyperalertness, sleep disturbance, survivor guilt, trouble concentrating, avoidance of activities that arouse recollection, or intensification of symptoms when exposed to similar traumatic events.

These criteria were not commonly found in the extant literature and were quite distinct from, for example, the depressive and anxious symptoms and social disabilities that burn victims reported in Andreasen's studies. They were also quite distinct from the paralyses, seizures, daze, and trembling that marked the symptoms of shell shock during the First World War and those of restlessness, fatigue, sleep difficulty, and anxiety that characterized the war neuroses of the Second World War. It is the case that some of the symptoms, such as recurrent dreams of the event, had been widely noted as aspects of reactions to traumas. Others, however, seemed more related to the experiences of small rap groups of Vietnam veterans. The prominence given to flashbacks to the traumatic event as responses to environmental cues raised particular questions. Some historians have not been able to find any corresponding experiences in victims of past wars. Others claim that the flashback criteria actually arose from cinematic portrayals of disturbed veterans in movies such as *Taxi Driver*.[37] Whatever their actual genesis might have been, the symptom criteria were virtually unique among *DSM-III* diagnoses in lacking grounding in the research literature.

To overcome the absence of any stressor-related diagnosis for chronic symptoms in previous manuals, the *DSM-III* criteria allowed for not only conditions that had acute onset and limited duration but also those that lasted for six months or more and those that had delayed onset of at least six months after the trauma. Symptoms could emerge at any time subsequent to the experience of the trauma and did not need to coincide with the traumatic event. This allowed the diagnosis to encompass both stressors that usually produced almost immediate symptoms and the conditions of combat veterans who became symptomatic well after the time of the stressor itself.

The task force had to place the PTSD diagnoses within one of the broader sixteen diagnostic categories of the manual. The category of Adjustment Disorders was not suitable because it only included short-term conditions that both arose at the time of a stressor or shortly thereafter and remitted when the stressor ended.[38] Although few of the symptoms of PTSD were comparable to those of any anxiety disorder and some, such as diminished interest, detachment, and restricted affect, would be unusual among anxious persons, the diagnosis was placed in the category of the Anxiety Disorders. In addition, other types of anxiety disorders relate to future threats; PTSD, in contrast, focuses on past traumas. Nevertheless, the veterans' advocates had successfully convinced the other members of the task force to support the new diagnosis. From its delineated origin in the conditions of Vietnam veterans, PTSD was to become one of the most influential psychiatric diagnoses in history.

The initial studies of how much PTSD existed in the community, using *DSM-III* criteria, found relatively low lifetime rates of between 1 to 3 percent of the population. The first large population study, the ECA, using data from the St. Louis site, found that only 5 men and 13 women per 1,000 met PTSD criteria at any time during their lives. This study found that only Vietnam War veterans who had suffered wounds had substantial rates of PTSD, with 20 percent of this group meeting full criteria for the disorder and 60 percent suffering from at least one PTSD symptom. Only fifteen members of this population sample, however, were wounded Vietnam veterans. Another study based on the North Carolina site of the same broader study found a similarly low lifetime prevalence of 1.30 percent and a six-month prevalence of 0.44 percent.[39]

PTSD seemed to be confined to a small proportion of people who had experienced seriously traumatic events, especially wounded combat veterans. This assumption did not endure for long. Indeed, almost as soon as the figures from the ECA were published, they were rejected on moral grounds. "We believe," asserted two Veterans Administration psychologists, "that post-traumatic stress disorder is not a de novo diagnosis whose entrance into the *DSM-III* was politically motivated, but rather that it is a serious psychiatric condition affecting many men and women who have survived life-threatening events, including combat, rape, political torture, and other disasters that often occur in the course of world events. Its effects should not be minimized."[40] A new era of contention had begun.

PTSD after *DSM-III*

Given its highly politicized genesis, it is not surprising that the PTSD criteria have undergone more changes in subsequent editions of the *DSM* than any other diagnosis. The first revision of the *DSM-III*, the *DSM-III-R* (1987), made minor changes in the stressor criterion to require "an event that is outside the range of normal human experience and that would be markedly distressing to almost anyone" and added a list of examples of such events.[41] The revisions to the symptom criteria were more substantial.

During the 1980s a prominent social movement had developed that emphasized the widespread prevalence of repressed and then recovered memories of childhood sexual abuse. The basic tenet of this group, echoing Pierre Janet's theories and Freud's early views that he quickly repudiated, was that early traumas in childhood were forgotten but stored as unconscious memories. Traumatic impacts not only stemmed from the distant past but also were not accessible to normal processes of recollection. "The ordinary response to atrocities," according to a leader of the recovered memory movement, psychiatrist Judith Herman, "is to banish them from consciousness." The repression of traumatic experiences had little connection to the intense memories of veterans who were all too able to recall their symptoms. A large cadre of therapists had developed who were committed to using techniques that would bring memories into consciousness after many years of repression.[42] This group required symptom criteria that recognized traumatic experiences could be repressed as well as intrusive.

Primarily in response to the recovered memory movement, the revised criteria changed the category of numbed responsiveness to the external world to include the "inability to recall an important aspect of the trauma." Traumatic symptoms now encompassed recurrent and intrusive memories as well as the inability to remember some trauma. The *DSM-III-R* also significantly lowered the duration requirement of symptoms from six months to one month so that long-lasting symptoms were no longer necessary for a diagnosis of PTSD.[43]

The altered symptom and duration requirements substantially increased the number of persons who met criteria for PTSD diagnoses. Community studies that used the *DSM-III-R* criteria, which only required one-month instead of six-month duration, yielded far higher rates than the initial studies that had used *DSM-III* criteria. The National Comorbidity Survey found that 61 percent of men and 51 percent of women reported experiencing at least one traumatic event according to the revised criteria. This study found PTSD rates of 10.4 percent of women and 5.0 percent of men, with an overall 7.8 percent rate. One study of residents of the Detroit area comparably found that 11.3 percent of women and 6.0 percent of men reported PTSD, with an overall prevalence rate of 9.2 percent. Lifetime prevalence for women in the Detroit study was nine times higher than the ECA study that used *DSM-III* criteria; that for men was thirty-five times higher![44] Subsequent changes in the diagnostic criteria expand the pool of people who potentially qualified for PTSD diagnoses to an even greater extent.

PTSD in *DSM-IV*

The *DSM-III* and *DSM-III-R* criteria had limited traumatic events to those that would lead to significant distress in "almost everyone," leaving little room for the importance of individual biological and psychological susceptibilities. These criteria were largely products of, first, veterans groups and, later, women's groups, who focused on traumatic experiences and felt that an emphasis on internal susceptibilities amounted to blaming the victims of such experiences. The next revision of the *DSM* in 1994, the *DSM-IV*, greatly enlarged the scope of the stressor criterion of the diagnosis and thus provided an opportunity to enhance the causal status of vulnerability factors.[45]

The *DSM-IV* was supposed to be conservative, making only minimal changes to existing diagnostic criteria.[46] Once again, the PTSD diagnosis was an exception. Among the major diagnoses in the *DSM*, only PTSD uses etiology rather than descriptive phenomenology to define a disorder. It is a unique diagnosis because someone who has the defining symptoms without having experienced the stressor cannot have the disorder. Therefore, it is the sole condition where broadening the criteria of exposure can also increase the number of people who qualify for the diagnosis.

Although the *DSM-IV* made minimal changes to the symptom and duration criteria of PTSD, it substantially revised the exposure criteria in two different ways. The new criteria dropped the requirement that events must "cause distress in almost everyone" and be "outside the range of normal human experience." It replaced them with the requirement that "the person experienced, witnessed, or was confronted with events that involved actual or threatened death or serious injury, or a threat to the physical integrity of self or others" and that "the person's response involved intense fear, helplessness, or horror." Although the intention of the revision was to overcome the "vague, inaccurate, and unreliable" aspect of the earlier criteria, in fact, the altered definition both expanded the class of people who were considered to be exposed to traumatic stressors and increased the ambiguity regarding just what constituted a traumatic experience.[47]

The revised definition included all cases that the earlier definitions had captured but added many other experiences that the previous diagnosis did not encompass. The "confronted with" criterion extended the notion of exposure so that persons who were not even present at a traumatic event could potentially meet diagnostic criteria for PTSD. The stressor criteria was now heterogeneous enough to encompass not just persons who were directly involved in traumas but also those who only witnessed or were confronted with them. For example, someone who learns of the sudden and unexpected death of a close relative or friend who has died from natural causes would meet the new stressor criterion. Even people who watched a disaster unfolding thousands of miles away on television could be seen as being exposed to a traumatic stressor.

The *DSM-IV* criteria changed the nature of traumatic exposure in a second way. The requirement that the person's response involve "fear, helplessness, or horror" shifted the definitional criteria from the nature of the stressor itself to the subjective experience of the victim.[48] Individual temperament, personality, and reactivity now entered into what defined an event as "traumatic." This introduced a subjective element into the nature of the stressor itself because only people who have a certain emotional reaction to the stressor are considered to have experienced a traumatic event in the first place. The *DSM-IV* radically changed definitions of trauma both to include a great heterogeneity of experiences and to partially locate the nature of trauma within the individual rather than the environment.

These changes in the criteria of who was considered to be exposed to a trauma had major consequences. First, the boundaries of pathology expanded to encompass ever-widening groups of claimants. The PTSD criteria came to be applied to a broad range of events including sexual and workplace harassment, exposure to hazardous materials, automobile accidents, crime victimization, child abuse, the discovery that a spouse is having an affair, or hearing news about the death of intimates who were far removed from their original application to combat experiences. Advocates for victims of sexual harassment, for example, argued that up to a third of such victims suffered from PTSD symptoms, which should be "reflected in judicial decisions regarding the appropriate monetary compensations for victims of sexual harassment."[49] A new legal specialty of trauma law developed that provides assessment and diagnoses for people seeking compensation for the psychological damage from traumatic injuries.

Second, the revised criteria in the *DSM-IV* meant that virtually everyone had experienced some traumatic event. Community surveys using the *DSM-IV* criteria showed that about 90 percent of the population reported traumatic events that met the stressor criterion of the definition. This was about a 60 percent increase in the number of people who had been exposed to traumatic events according to the previous criteria.[50] The most common traumatic event, reported by 60 percent of the population, was the sudden, unexpected death of a close relative or friend. While hearing about deaths of loved ones is surely a distressing experience, in many cases it is of a different order of magnitude than participating in combat or being the victim of a sexual assault.

Third, under certain circumstances, the broadened criteria could mean that not just individuals but entire populations could be exposed to traumatic events. The plethora of research about PTSD in the wake of the terrorist attacks of September 11, 2001, demonstrated how new understandings of the condition could encompass a vast and heterogeneous group of "exposed" persons. Mental health researchers launched a number of studies immediately after the attack that measured the psychological impact of this event. These studies did not focus on people who were actually in the World Trade Center and so would be most directly traumatized. Instead, relying on the expansive *DSM* definition of PTSD, research encompassed the entire population of the country, almost all of whom had presumably "witnessed" or "were confronted with" the terrorist attacks and so met the exposure criteria for PTSD.[51]

Surveys taken during the first week after 9/11 could not practically use full-scale diagnostic interviews. Instead, they took affirmative responses to such ordinary emotions as "fears of future terrorism," "fear of future harm to family as a result of terrorism," or reporting "quite a bit" of anger at Osama bin Laden as indicators of PTSD. Such studies indicated that nearly half of the U.S. population experienced some "symptom" of PTSD. Over half of respondents said that at least one child was upset by the attacks. One to two months following the attacks, more than 10 percent of New York metropolitan area residents had "clinically significant" levels of distress.[52]

These studies raise the issue of what the meaning of being "exposed to 9/11" is. The *DSM-IV* criteria encompassed both the actual experience of being in the World Trade Center at the time of the attacks and watching these events on television as potential triggers of PTSD. In a society where terrorist attacks, school shootings, natural disasters, and other horrors are widely and continuously broadcast on television, virtually everyone is "confronted with" traumatic events on a regular basis. Indeed, the "exposure" indicator of the extent of television watching of the events of 9/11 was the best predictor of resulting symptoms of PTSD. Despite dire predictions that 9/11 would result in an enormous amount of psychological disorder, especially PTSD, in fact, symptom levels dropped precipitously soon after the attacks. While about 7.5 percent of New York City residents reported rates of full-blown PTSD a month after the attacks, three months later rates had declined to 1.7 percent. By six months after the attack a negligible 0.6 percent had PTSD.[53] The almost immediate "recovery" of most people who were not directly affected by the attacks calls into question whether they were ever exposed to a genuine trauma in the first place.

At the same time as the *DSM-IV* criteria expanded the class of people exposed to a traumatic event, it also provided new opportunities for the study of individual vulnerabilities to traumas. When the *DSM-III* was published in 1980, biological psychiatrists were just beginning to establish their dominance in the profession.[54] By 1994, however, the nature of psychiatric explanation had vastly changed. PTSD, like its predecessor diagnoses, has a distinct etiology originating in an external stressor. It inherently directs attention to the environment as a primary cause of distress that follows the event. This focus was in considerable tension with the basic assumptions of the psychiatric profession that had become firmly entrenched by the early 1990s, when biological approaches were clearly ascendant. Biological psychiatry located the origins of disorders in damaged brains and genes, emphasizing individual vulnerabilities and predispositions. This foundational assumption would be called into question if stressors themselves could lead to pathology in otherwise normal persons. Biological approaches would have little to contribute to the study of PTSD if events triggered symptoms in previously unimpaired individuals.

The growing heterogeneity of the sorts of events that were encompassed in the *DSM-IV* criteria for what constitutes a "trauma" ensured that factors having to do with individual responses to events would have a more powerful impact than when traumas were limited to events that "would be markedly distressing to almost everyone." Traumatic exposure in itself inevitably recedes in importance while individual susceptibilities become of greater explanatory importance. In addition, the logic of the PTSD diagnosis in the *DSM-IV* leaves a wide opening for those who wish to emphasize the importance of individual vulnerability. Comparing rates of pathology in groups that are exposed or unexposed to traumas would show the massive role of traumatic exposure in causing PTSD. Yet, as epidemiologist Naomi Breslau pointed out, unexposed groups *cannot logically* develop the disorder.[55] Traumatic exposure itself is a constant, not a variable; the sole possible comparisons lie *within* a group that has been exposed to trauma. Only factors that vary across exposed individuals can explain who develops PTSD and who does not. PTSD researchers were quick to exploit this aspect of the diagnosis.

For example, numerous studies of levels of PTSD after natural disasters or catastrophes caused by humans showed that about 10 to 30 percent of persons who experienced traumas met criteria for PTSD. If a much high proportion of people experienced traumatic events than actually developed PTSD, the reasoning went, individual factors must account for why some exposed people but not others developed the disorder. The fact that PTSD emerged in only a minority of persons exposed to traumatic events was then used to show how risk factors other than trauma must be invoked in explanations of the disorder.[56] This allowed PTSD researchers to ask not only the question of "what is the extent of pathology following a traumatic event" but also "what leads some people but not others to develop PTSD after a traumatic event"?

The gap between the great number of people reporting traumas and the smaller number reporting PTSD symptoms was a fortuitous finding for the by now dominant style of psychiatric explanation that focused on individual vulnerabilities. Many studies began to examine biological differences between people exposed to traumatic events that meet or do not meet PTSD criteria. For example, some researchers reported an association between stress exposure and smaller-sized hippocampi and postulated that small hippocampus volume is a pre-traumatic risk factor for the emergence of PTSD. Others compared the responses of fraternal and identical twins to traumatic events in order to access the extent that heritable genetic tendencies such as neurocognitive abilities influenced psychological vulnerability to PTSD among people who are exposed to traumas. Research using functional magnetic resonance imaging and positron emission tomography indicated that people with PTSD had distinctive patterns of brain activation in response to trauma-related stimuli. Others stressed the existence of biological markers of susceptibility to PTSD such as the hypersuppression of cortisol in respond to environmental stimuli.[57]

Another strand of research emphasized the importance of individual characteristics and psychological traits to explain why only a minority of persons who were exposed to traumatic events develop PTSD. Female gender, poor coping ability, high levels of neuroticism, and personal and family histories of psychiatric disorders predicted who was likely to develop PTSD.[58] These factors are identical to virtually every other anxiety and mood disorder, calling into question the uniqueness or even the need for a PTSD diagnosis. Moreover, the causal link that stimulated the initial diagnosis—that some stressor leads to a distinct set of stressors—is reversed. Vulnerabilities that predated the occurrence of the stressor led some people but not others to develop PTSD.

"Overall," psychologists Marilyn Bowman and Rachel Yehuda summarized, "research demonstrates that PTSD is best understood as the periodic expression of long-standing dispositions that often are risk factors for both threatening exposures and subsequent dysfunctions." Echoing earlier neurologists and psychiatrists who studied sufferers of railway spine, shellshock, and combat neuroses, traumatic experiences resulted from personal dispositions rather than from horrific events. Research in the wake of 9/11, for example, showed that poor individual coping styles, pre-existing anxiety and mood disorders, and family histories of mental illness predicted who developed PTSD after the attacks.[59] Just as in the previous eras, arguments emphasizing predisposing qualities replaced the prominence given to the traumatic qualities of events themselves. "Individual differences," claimed Bowman, "are significantly more powerful than event characteristics in predicting PTSD." By the beginning of the twenty-first century, psychiatry was able to claim both that traumatic events produced huge levels of pathology and that biological and psychological weaknesses accounted for which individuals exposed to traumas would actually develop PTSD.[60]

Despite the re-emergence of a research tradition that concentrated on individual vulnerabilities, the major focus of research about PTSD remained on the large number of people who developed and required treatment for this condition after disasters. PTSD remains an exception to the otherwise overwhelming dominance of biological and psychological approaches. By the 1990s and early 2000s the core assumption of the trauma community that tragic events could provoke PTSD in large proportions of the population was too well entrenched to be displaced by a concentration on internal susceptibilities. A largely autonomous profession that studied and treated trauma had emerged with its own ideology, journals, conferences, and training capacity. Grief and trauma counselors who placed more emphases on exposure than vulnerability were firmly institutionalized in schools, hospitals, disaster relief organizations, and other establishments. A focus on the vulnerability of a minority of exposed people contradicted a basic principle of the trauma community: responses to catastrophes must be immediate and encompass entire populations that are at risk of developing severe symptoms.

The Response to PTSD

The expansion of the criteria defining what situations counted as "traumatic" meant that virtually the entire population could be viewed as vulnerable to developing PTSD and other mental disorders in the wake of disasters. A deeply established PTSD community now attempts to implement massive mental health interventions for as widespread a group as possible.[61] It believes that large proportions of people will develop PTSD unless mental health interventions are implemented immediately after catastrophes occur.

In particular, techniques of psychological debriefing became popular and often mandatory after any sort of disaster in the English-speaking world.[62] Toward this end a large industry of grief counselors emerged that sends therapists to scenes of natural disasters, schools, and workplaces whenever a highly stressful event has occurred. Because everyone who has experienced the disaster is presumed to be at risk, its goal is to treat as many people as quickly as possible.

The research literature regarding the effectiveness of such interventions shows that debriefing neither relieves distress nor prevents the emergence of subsequent PTSD. The sorts of single-debriefing sessions that trauma and grief counselors provide have no efficacy and occasionally produce detrimental effects compared to no intervention. Debriefing by mental health professionals can interfere with the natural processing of traumatic events, suggest that people are not capable of handling tragedies on their own, and imply that they are at risk if they do not participate in interventions. Other research shows that prevention efforts can backfire. In one study, schoolchildren given prevention training for a possible earthquake that never occurred showed higher levels of distress two months later. A Cochrane Review Report concluded that "compulsory debriefing of victims of trauma should cease."[63]

In spite of the evidence that widespread debriefing efforts do not have positive results, they continue to flourish. For example, emergency personnel in New York City were required to participate in mental health treatment after 9/11. Likewise, after the collapse of the investment bank Bear Stearns in 2008, the company called in grief counselors to help its employees deal with their feelings about impending layoffs and losses of life savings. The trauma industry has become so embedded in schools, work organizations, hospitals, police and fire departments, and the military that it is impervious to efforts to limit its interventions. Indeed, the industry has spread worldwide to dispense Western-style therapy to victims of natural disasters.[64]

The military has also undergone a vast change in its assumptions about the extent of PTSD that will emerge as a result of combat experiences. Unlike military psychiatry in previous conflicts, which assumed that the vast majority of soldiers were resilient, the Veterans Administration expected that PTSD would commonly arise as a result of the Iraq and Afghanistan wars.[65] Like the broader mental health culture at the time, it embraced a view that PTSD was a widespread consequence of combat, that all soldiers could be potential victims, that short screening tools could indicate what soldiers would suffer from it, and that as many affected soldiers as possible should be treated for it. In contrast to the screening tools developed for World War II, which were used to identify vulnerable persons before they entered the armed services, the military now uses very short instruments that try to discover which veterans are likely to contract PTSD and other mental disorders after their service is completed.

The most common instrument, the Primary Care PTSD screen (PC-PTSD), uses just four items that ask about intrusive thoughts, avoidance, being easily startled, and feeling detached and so is fast, efficient, and can be administered to large numbers of soldiers.[66] Respondents are considered to be at mental health risk if they give positive responses to two PTSD questions or to one question about the presence of depression, interpersonal conflict, aggressive ideation, or suicidal ideation. One widely reported study that used these criteria reported that 27.0 percent of active soldiers and 35.5 percent of National Guard and reserve soldiers were "mental health risks." Other studies indicated about 20 percent of soldiers had some mental disorder prior to deployment to Iraq and about 30 percent after deployment. Notably, 10 percent had PTSD *before* deployment to Iraq.[67]

Results of this research also showed that half of the soldiers who reported three or more PTSD symptoms had improved six months later. Strikingly, "an inverse relationship existed between receiving mental health services and improvement in symptoms by the time of the [reassessment]." In other words, recovery was related to *not* receiving mental health treatment. Moreover, among those soldiers who were referred for treatment, recovery rates were highest among those who did not follow up and make an appointment for therapy.[68]

The expectations that high proportions of veterans will suffer from PTSD and other psychiatric disabilities reflect a profound cultural change. Before the popularization of the PTSD diagnosis after the Vietnam War, the assumption was that most soldiers who faced traumas were resilient and would be strengthened by their battlefield experiences.[69] While soldiers who have suffered from the emotional consequences of trauma deserve the best possible treatment if they desire it, an over-emphasis on the emotional impact of wartime experiences can turn attention away from other salient aspects of postwar adjustment. Perhaps, as in the past, a "job and a girl (or boy)" are the surest sources of successful reintegration into the community after military service for most returning veterans.[70] By the early twenty-first century, however, PTSD was seen as omnipresent, and professional therapy as the best way to overcome its impact.

PTSD seems to be one of the most resistant disorders to the therapeutic armamentarium of psychiatry. Some techniques, particularly those that attempt to recover repressed memories of childhood sexual abuse, seem to have been iatrogenic in many cases. Other, more traditional psychotherapeutic or medication therapies are not harmful but they do not have high success rates. A major review conducted by the Institute of Medicine at the request of the Veterans Administration concluded that "the scientific evidence on treatment modalities for PTSD does not reach the level of certainty that would be desired for such a common and serious condition among veterans."[71] This review found that the evidence base was so weak that they could not issue recommendations on issues such as the timing and types of interventions and the efficacy and length of either psychotherapeutic or medication treatments. While catastrophic events undoubtedly cause much psychic devastation, therapeutic techniques that focus on the intra-psychic consequences of traumas might have inherent limitations. Psychotherapy and medications can help some people cope with traumatic symptoms, but they cannot deal with the root causes of the disorder, which lie outside of individuals.

Given the failure of traditional mental health therapies to respond to PTSD, what can be done to help people who suffer from this devastating disorder? Participation in supportive communities of victims of similar traumas provides a promising mode of response. Programs that deal with overcoming actual adversities in the wake of traumas might also have better outcomes than those that provide therapy to individuals. For example, a major study conducted in the wake of Hurricane Katrina estimated that about a third of residents of the New Orleans metropolitan area suffered from PTSD five to seven months after the hurricane.[72] Yet the persistence of disaster-related stressors such as property devastation, geographic relocation, and job loss, rather than a mental disorder, could account for the endurance of thoughts and memories of the event. Victims of natural disasters might benefit more from economic and social assistance that helps them overcome the genuine devastation in their circumstances than from individual therapy. Likewise, widespread efforts to screen and then treat as much combat-related PTSD among soldiers as possible can not only misidentify many soldiers as disordered but also waste substantial amounts of mental health resources that could be used in more effective ways for economic and social reintegration.[73] A focus on intra-psychic processes can redirect attention from social circumstances to interior conditions that are among the most highly resistant to successful therapeutic interventions.

Conclusion

The history of trauma-related diagnoses shows an uneasy co-existence between emphases on the traumatic event itself and emphases on individual responses to the event. On the one hand, the importance of train wrecks, combat, or terrorist attacks in creating traumatic symptoms seems unquestionable. Yet, on the other hand, such claims do not easily fit the fundamental strand of psychiatric explanation that accounts for symptoms in terms of individual vulnerabilities and susceptibilities. Social and cultural factors influence the degree of prominence given to exposure and vulnerability in various historical eras. Ideologies emphasizing personal responsibility and individual agency mark some historical eras. Explanations that focus on internal vulnerabilities are most congruent with such periods. In contrast, environmental considerations dominate explanatory styles at other times. Such concerns are more compatible with accounts that accentuate the power of intense stressors to bring about traumatic experiences.

When trauma-related diagnoses first emerged, the psychiatric profession relied on hereditarian explanations. The initial claims that train wrecks could cause psychological symptoms in the absence of some individual predisposition were immediately countered by the view that only people with weak constitutions could develop nervous conditions after traumas. The latter emphasis, which was more congruent with broader individualistic cultural trends, dominated psychiatric explanations of trauma until the onset of World War II. Even psychoanalysts, who rejected hereditarian views, could not successfully integrate traumatic neuroses into their theories about the causes and treatments for the neuroses. By the time World War II ended, environmental considerations were leading aspects of theories of human behavior, and explanations that emphasized the power of exposure to traumatic events prevailed over those that focused on individual susceptibilities. The *DSM-III* clearly embraced the view that traumatic events in themselves brought about PTSD.

By 1994, when the *DSM-IV* was published, the vulnerability view had regained a prominent role in both psychiatry and the culture at large. Yet the major impact of the *DSM-IV* has been to expand the range of events that are considered to be traumatic rather than to bring PTSD in line with the dominant focus in psychiatry on biological susceptibilities to developing mental disorders. In large part, the existence of a large and well-entrenched trauma profession outside of psychiatry accounts for the failure of vulnerability to gain much traction as an explanation of PTSD. As it has been throughout its history, PTSD remains a difficult diagnosis to integrate into mainstream psychiatric explanations.

The connection between external causes, individual responses, and resulting symptoms raises fundamental issues that cannot be conclusively resolved about the relative importance of environmental and internal forces in provoking mental disorder. From the earliest inception of traumatic diagnoses through major world wars, sexual politics, and terrorist attacks, psychiatry has never satisfactorily been able to define and treat the psychic consequences of traumatic events. Yet despite the problems it entails, PTSD cannot be eliminated from the psychiatric canon because of the tremendous suffering that follows in the wake of all individual and collective traumas.

Where Do We Go from Here?

The "lessons" of history are far less clear and often obscure and contradictory. Indeed, history suggests that there is a price to be paid for implementing ideology ungrounded in empirical reality and for making exaggerated rhetorical claims. In this volume we have employed both historical and contemporary materials to deal with some fundamental problems within the American medical care system. Our goal has not been to denigrate the theory and practice of the American medical care system. Nevertheless, there are numerous elements that raise important doubts about the validity of many medical explanations, diagnostic categories, therapeutic interventions, and claims. It is of vital importance that we address issues too frequently subordinated to exaggerated rhetorical claims that have little basis in fact.

One general problem is that the enthusiasm for new diagnostic categories and the consequent deployment of drugs often occurs in a partial vacuum of knowledge. There is a tendency, for example, to smile at diagnostic categories of the past, such as the more than one hundred fevers listed in mid-nineteenth-century classifications that have, with some exceptions, disappeared from the medical lexicon. Yet there is relatively little awareness of the contingent nature of contemporary categories. Hence we take seriously RLS, CFS, fibromyalgia, and the current diagnosis of depression as exemplified in the *DSM*. We fail to understand, however, that they differ but little from many earlier diagnostic categories in their underlying characteristics. This failure is not simply a play on words, for they have consequences. Nor are many contemporary diagnoses that lack an empirical foundation neutral, for sometimes they lead to therapies that are at best questionable and at worst harmful.

Another general problem is that evidence to support many etiological claims rests on dubious grounds. The insistence that CHD was related to behavioral risk factors, for example, ignored data that demonstrated that a rise in mortality from this disease occurred in the absence of those risk factors and that the mortality decline took place when the operation of risk factors was at their maximum. Nor have the claims that cancer etiology was somehow related to diet or other behavioral attributes been substantiated by evidence other than conclusions based on correlational studies. While conceding that correlation is not causation, proponents tend to ignore this caveat and nevertheless proceed to make causal claims. The result has been to bombard the public with behavioral advice that not only has undergone continuous change, but has frequently been contradictory.

Likewise, highly differentiated, specific categories of mental illnesses have been foundational for psychiatry since the publication of the *DSM-III* in 1980. Although flourishing research communities have developed that center around the study of each specific diagnosis, progress in discovering the causes of any mental disorder remains limited. In particular, the widely trumpeted claims that "mental illnesses are brain diseases" and that "mental illnesses result from chemical deficiencies" remain more slogans than firmly grounded evidentiary claims. Much the same has been true of many widely deployed therapies. That medicine has the capacity to develop effective therapies is clear. It is equally clear, however, that many therapies have come into use and persist in spite of lack of evidence demonstrating efficacy. Drugs that were introduced with considerable fanfare were subsequently withdrawn because of adverse reactions or labeled with a "black box" indicating special hazards.

The increase in the number of practitioners trained as specialists and the consequent decline in the number of general practitioners and internists is also a matter of concern. Most specialties tended to be oriented toward surgery and the use of technology, and often their dramatic interventions are based more on logic than on evidence. Spinal fusion surgery for lower back pain is an example of an intervention of dubious efficacy. The studies of Richard Deyo and his colleagues found that such surgery "had few scientifically validated indications and was associated with higher costs and complications rates than other types of back surgery." He and others participated in a panel sponsored by the federal Agency for Health Care Policy and Research to develop evidence-based guidelines for managing acute back problems of recent onset. The panel recommended nonsurgical approaches in most instances. The North American Spine Society then launched a lobbying campaign against the recommendations, partly because the guidelines (as well as subsequent research) suggested that the use of pedicle screws had severe shortcomings. The results of lobbying by spine surgeons and Medtronic (the manufacturer of the screws) resulted in a 25 percent cut in the agency's budget and the abandonment of its congressional mandate to develop clinical guidelines. Despite the lack of evidence of efficacy, spinal fusion operations increased 77 percent between 1996 and 2001.[1]

The efficacy of therapies for most mental illnesses also remains uncertain. Since 1990, rates of drug treatment have soared while those of psychotherapy have declined.[2] Yet there is no evidence that this class of medication is any more effective than various forms of interpersonal and cognitive psychotherapies. Changes in the organization and financing of mental health care rather than the success of drug treatments have dictated these changes. Indeed, apart from the most serious types of mental illnesses, the value of medication does not greatly exceed that of placebos.[3]

Nevertheless, new classes of psychotropic drugs are typically introduced with assertions that they are superior to older classes. For example, second-generation anti-psychotic drugs were heralded as having greater effectiveness and fewer adverse side effects than first-generation drugs. Careful studies, however, show that as a group the newer class of drugs is neither more efficacious nor more benign than the category it replaced, although it is far less cost effective.[4] Similar questions are being raised about whether the SSRIs have any advantages over the tranquillizers and older anti-depressants that they superseded.[5] The ability of a medication to generate profits seems more related to how frequently it is used than to its therapeutic benefits.

The lack of safe and effective treatments has not deterred the mental health field from implementing new screening programs that strive to identify and then treat vast numbers of people who have not spontaneously sought treatment on their own. In 2003, for example, the President's New Freedom Commission recommended that every teenager in America should be screened for signs of mental illness and suicidal tendencies; such screening programs have been widely implemented in schools across the country.[6] Its rationale was that early detection of mental illnesses such as depression and anxiety can prevent not just impairments such as poor school performance, teenage pregnancy, and substance abuse that arise during adolescence, but also the development of mental illnesses later in life. Yet no evidence exists that screening and subsequent treatment actually fulfill these preventive objectives. In fact, screening programs generate far more false positives than actual cases of mental disorder and have the potential to lead to a vast amount of pathologizing of natural distress.[7] The enthusiasm for widespread screening programs considerably exceeds the ability of current detection and treatment technologies to provide more benefits than risks for people identified as having a mental illness. Likewise, the wisdom of screening for some other conditions such as prostate cancer is beginning to be questioned because such a high proportion of detected tumors would have benign outcomes even when they are not discovered.[8]

The etiological claims of medicine and the proliferation of therapies of dubious efficacy conceal an even more significant problem, namely, the medicalization of everyday life. Aging, for example, was in the past considered a normal stage of the life course. In the last half century, however, there is a growing tendency to define aging not as a normal phase, but rather as a disease. The example of osteoporosis is instructive. Human bones grow during early years. When bones cease growing after puberty, they continue to strengthen through a process of mineralization. During the fifth decade of life a gradual process of demineralization begins and lasts until death. The process is a normal accompaniment of life, and relatively few people demineralize to the extent that fractures are unavoidable. Nevertheless, osteoporosis and osteopenia (or scant bone) have acquired the status of a disease. The result has been a proliferation of therapies, including dietary supplements, hormone replacement therapy, and such drugs as Fosamax (Merck) and Actonel (Procter & Gamble). The claims of efficacy of these interventions, however, are largely exaggerated. In a placebo controlled trial (funded by Merck) women free from fracture but with bone mineral density measurements 1.6 standard deviations below the mean for normal young adult white women took alendronate (Fosamax) for four years. In the placebo group the incidence of radiographic vertebral fractures was 3.8 percent as compared with 2.1 percent in the treated group. To be sure, there was a 44 percent reduction in risk. The absolute reduction, a much more meaningful statistic, was only 1.7 percent. Nor did this modest reduction take into account the adverse side effects of the drug. Some years after its introduction it was associated with osteonecrosis (death of the bone) of the jaw. "Osteopenia," concludes Nortin M. Hadler (an authority on musculoskeletal disorders), "is an example of a New Age social construction, propelled to its status in a decade by aggressive marketing and vested interests."[9]

The emergence of genetic technologies has also created new opportunities for a vast growth in the medicalization of emotional life. For example, an extensive body of research on the 5-HTT gene, which controls the way that serotonin passes messages through brain cells, has emerged in the study of depression. The results of a large study in New Zealand that indicated that the short allele of the 5-HTT gene interacts with highly stressful environments to produce depression has been especially influential. This study found that among people who have experienced four or more stressful life events, 43 percent with two short alleles and 33 percent with one short allele developed major depression compared to only 17 percent of those with two long alleles who did.[10]

The identification of the 5-HTT gene as a risk factor for depression created the possibility that genetic tests could identify a new type of condition—being "at risk" for developing depression even when a person showed no actual depressive symptoms—that long-term regimens of drug therapy might prevent from ever actually arising. The market for such therapies is potentially huge. In the New Zealand study, for example, 17 percent of the sample had genotypes with two copies of the short allele of the 5-HTT gene and an additional 51 percent had one copy of the short allele. In theory, then, two-thirds of the population has a genotype that is associated with a susceptibility to becoming depressed. Biotechnology companies are making large investments in techniques for uncovering possible genes for depression and other mental illnesses. Correspondingly, pharmaceutical companies are striving to develop new classes of more refined, genetically tailored medications that might be prescribed to presumably at-risk populations.[11]

The proliferation of diagnoses, the use of numerical scales that tend to expand and thus to include ever larger numbers of persons, and the medicalization of hitherto normal phenomena have created vast entrepreneurial opportunities. The pharmaceutical industry sponsors diseases and promotes drugs for diagnoses that are at best questionable and at worst nonexistent. Its efforts to promote medical education are often synonymous with its marketing strategy. Its close ties to the medical profession lead physicians to prescribe drugs to a willing public eager to believe claims of efficacy that rest on a shaky empirical foundation or whose benefits are far outweighed by the risks. The problem, however, is even more serious. Academic medical centers hold equity interests in companies that also sponsor research within the same institution. Many articles in medical journals are prepared by drug company employees or medical publishing companies hired by them. Prominent researchers are then paid substantial sums and are listed as authors even though they had little to do with the study. Faculty investigators have ties to companies that support their research. They receive compensation for consulting and speaking and often have equity interests in the company. This problem is especially acute in psychiatry, where several prominent researchers did not disclose millions of dollars in payments from the pharmaceutical industry.[12] It is "absurd," according to Marcia Angell (a former editor of the *New England Journal of Medicine*), "to look to investor-owned companies for unbiased evaluations of their own products. Yet many academic investigators and their institutions pretend otherwise, and it is convenient and profitable for them to do so."[13]

Much attention has been focused on Americans who are either uninsured or underinsured. That this is a serious problem is indisputable; access to medical care can assuage or alleviate many disorders that detract from or are dangerous to the quality, if not the length, of life. Yet relatively little attention has been paid to the extraordinarily high costs of drugs and medical procedures, many of which have not been shown to be efficacious. Equally significant, their risks sometimes outweigh any possible benefits. All too often Americans have been urged to undergo testing and imaging for reasons that are unclear, to take drugs for conditions that hardly merit a medical diagnosis or have little evidence that the benefits outweigh the risks, to submit to surgical procedures for which efficacy has not been established, to say nothing about the large costs of what goes under the name of alternative or holistic therapies. All of these, in addition to the very large administrative costs of a decentralized system that relies on private-for-profit insurance firms, have combined to make the health care system the most expensive in the world even though the health indicators in the United States compare unfavorably with those of other industrialized nations.[14]

That the United States faces serious problems in its health care system is clear. As we have tried to demonstrate, many of these problems are related not only to the high costs of a decentralized medical care system and the fact that millions cannot afford health insurance, but to the inner dynamics of the system and exaggerated claims of physicians and biotechnology and pharmaceutical firms. Until some of these problems are addressed, the claims of the American health care system will continue to exceed its actual achievements.

Notes

Chapter 1 – Rhetoric and Reality in Modern American Medicine

1. For a discussion of this development see Gerald N. Grob, *The Deadly Truth: A History of Disease in America* (Cambridge: Harvard University Press, 2002).
2. See Mark Schlesinger, "A Loss of Faith: The Sources of Reduced Political Legitimacy for the American Medical Profession," *Milbank Quarterly* 80 (2002): 185–235.
3. Aaron Catlin et al., "National Health Spending in 2006: A Year of Change for Prescription Drugs," *Health Affairs* 27 (2008): 14–29.
4. Cathy Schoen et al., "In Chronic Condition: Experiences of Patients with Complex Health Care Needs, in Eight Countries, 2008," *Health Affairs* 28 (2009): W1–W16.
5. WHO World Mental Health Survey Consortium, "Prevalence, Severity, and Unmet Need for Treatment of Mental Disorders in the World Mental Health Surveys," *JAMA* 291 (2004): 2581–2590.
6. Ellen Nolte and C. Martin McKee, "Measuring the Health of Nations: Updating an Earlier Analysis," *Health Affairs* 27 (2008): 58–71; Cathy Schoen et al., "U.S. Health System Performance: A National Scorecard," *Health Affairs* 25 (2006): W457–W475; Cathy Schoen et al., "Toward Higher-Performance Health Systems: Adults' Health Care Experiences in Seven Countries, 2007," *Health Affairs* 26 (2007): W717–W734; Steven A. Schroeder, "We Can Do Better—Improving the Health of the American People," *New England Journal of Medicine* 357 (2007): 1221–1228.
7. Kenneth E. Thorpe, David H. Howard, and Katya Galactionova, "Differences in Disease Prevalence as a Source of the U.S.–European Health Care Spending Gap," *Health Affairs* 26 (2007): W678–W686.
8. Schroeder, "We Can Do Better," 1224–1225; David Mechanic, "Population Health: Challenges for Science and Society," *Milbank Quarterly* 85 (2007): 533–559; Karen Davis et al., "Mirror, Mirror on the Wall: An International Update on the Comparative Performance of American Health Care," *The Commonwealth Fund*, vol. 59 (May 16, 2007); Majid Ezzati et al., "The Reversal of Fortunes: Trends in County Mortality and Cross-County Mortality Disparities in the United States," *PloSMedicine* 5 (2008): e66 doi:10.1371; John Komlos and Benjamin E. Lauderdale, "Underperformance in Affluence: The Remarkable Relative Decline in U.S. Heights in the Second Half of the 20th Century," *Social Science Quarterly* 88 (2007): 283–305; John Komlos, "Stagnation of Heights among Second-Generation U.S.-Born Army Personnel," *Social Science Quarterly* 89 (2008): 445–455.
9. Elizabeth A. McGlynn et al., "The Quality of Health Care Delivered to Adults in the U.S.," *New England Journal of Medicine* 348 (2003): 2635–2645 (quote from 2643–2644); Mark A. Schuster, Elizabeth A. McGlynn, and Robert H. Brook, "How Good Is the Quality of Health Care in the U.S.?" *Milbank Quarterly* 76 (1998): 517–563.
10. Seth W. Glickman et al., "Pay for Performance, Quality of Care, and Outcomes in Acute Myocardial Infarction," *JAMA* 297 (2007): 2373–2380.

11. Julie Appleby, "The Case of CT Angiography: How Americans View and Embrace New Technology," *Health Affairs* 27 (2008): 1515–1521; Laurence C. Baker, Scott W. Atlas, and Christopher C. Afendulis, "Expanded Use of Imaging Technology and the Challenge of Measuring Value," *Health Affairs* 27 (2008): 1467–1478; Rita F. Redberg and Judith Walsh, " Pay Now, Benefits May Follow—The Case of Cardiac Computed Tomographic Angiography," *New England Journal of Medicine* 359 (2008): 2309–2311; Julie M. Miller et al., "Diagnostic Performance of Coronary Angiography by 64-Row CT," *New England Journal of Medicine* 359 (2008): 2324–2336; Alex Berenson and Reed Abelson, "Weighing the Costs of a CT Scan's Look Inside the Heart," *New York Times*, June 29, 2008; Alexandra Kirkley et al., "A Randomized Trial of Arthroscopic Surgery for Osteoarthritis of the Knee," *New England Journal of Medicine* 359 (2008): 1097–1107; Martin Englund et al., "Incidental Meniscal Findings on Knee MRI in Middle-Aged and Elderly Persons," *New England Journal of Medicine* 359 (2008): 1108–1115. For a provocative critique of many medical therapies see Norton M. Hadler, *Worried Sick: A Prescription for Health in an Overtreated America* (Chapel Hill: University of North Carolina Press, 2008).

12. Stephanie Saul, "Need a Knee Replaced? Check Your Zip Code," *New York Times*, June 11, 2007; Elliott S. Fisher et al., "The Implications of Regional Variations in Medicare Spending. Part 1: The Content, Quality, and Accessibility of Care, Part 2: Health Outcomes and Satisfactions with Care," *Annals of Internal Medicine* 138 (2003): 273–299.

13. Fisher et al., "Implications of Regional Variations," 273–299; John E. Wennberg et al., "Extending the P4P Agenda, Part 1: How Medicare Can Improve Patient Decision Making and Reduce Unnecessary Care, Part 2: How Medicare Can Reduce Waste and Improve the Care of the Chronically Ill," *Health Affairs* 26 (2007): 1564–1585.

14. James N. Weinstein et al., "Trends in Geographic Variations in Major Surgery for Degenerative Diseases of the Hip, Knee, and Spine," *Health Affairs–Web Exclusive,* October 7, 2007, VAR-81–89; Richard A. Deyo et al., "United States Trends in Lumbar Fusion Surgery for Degenerative Conditions," *Spine* 30 (2005): 1441–1445; Brook I. Martin et al., "Expenditures and Health Status among Adults with Back and Neck Problems," *JAMA* 299 (2008): 656–664.

15. Katherine Baicker, Kasey S. Buckles, and Amitabh Chandra, "Geographic Variation in the Appropriate Use of Cesarean Delivery," *Health Affairs* 25 (2006): W355–W365.

16. For an illuminating discussion, see John C. Burnham, *Bad Habits: Drinking, Smoking, Taking Drugs, Gambling, Sexual Misbehavior, and Swearing in American History* (New York: New York University Press, 1993).

17. See especially Sheila M. Rothman and David J. Rothman, *The Pursuit of Perfection: The Promise and Perils of Medical Enhancement* (New York: Pantheon Books, 2003).

18. William B. Schwartz, *Life Without Disease: The Pursuit of Medical Utopia* (Berkeley: University of California Press, 1998), 3, 149.

19. Susan Sontag, *Illness as Metaphor* (New York: Farrar, Straus and Giroux, 1978), 64–66.

20. Ronald C. Kessler and Ellen E. Walters, "The National Comorbidity Survey," in *Textbook in Psychiatric Epidemiology*, 2nd ed., ed. Ming T. Tsuang and Mauricio Toheh (New York: Wiley-Liss, 2002), 343–362.

21. Allan V. Horwitz and Jerome C. Wakefield, *The Loss of Sadness: How Psychiatry Transformed Normal Sorrow into Depressive Disorder* (New York: Oxford University Press, 2007).

22. Rene Dubos, *The Dream of Reason: Science and Utopias* (New York: Columbia University Press, 1961), 84–85. See also his classic *Mirage of Health: Utopias, Progress, and Biological Change* (New York: Harper & Brothers, 1959) and *Man Adapting* (New Haven: Yale University Press, 1965).

23. David J. Weatherall, *Science and the Quiet Art: The Role of Medical Research in Health Care* (New York: W. W. Norton, 1995), 223–224.

24. Robert B. Belshe, "The Origins of Pandemic Influenza—Lessons from the 1918 Virus," *New England Journal of Medicine* 353 (2005): 2209–2211.

25. Linda T. Kohn, Janet M. Corrigan, and Molla S. Donaldson, eds., *To Err Is Human: Building a Safer Health System* (Washington, DC: National Academy Press, 2000), 26–48; John P. Burke, "Infection Control—A Problem for Patient Safety," *New England Journal of Medicine* 348 (2003): 651–656; Mary Ann Baily, "Harming Through Protection?" *New England Journal of Medicine* 358 (2008): 768–769; Guy M. McKann, "Cognitive Outcome after Coronary Artery Bypass: A One-Year Prospective Study," *Annals of Thoracic Surgery* 63 (1997): 510–515; Dean Fergusson et al., "Association between Suicide Attempts and Selective Serotonin Reuptake Inhibitors: Systematic Review of Randomised Controlled Trials," *British Medical Journal* 330 (2005): 396–399; Mark Olfson, Steven C. Marcus, and David Shaffer, "Antidepressant Drug Therapy and Suicide in Severely Depressed Children and Adults," *Archives of General Psychiatry* 63 (2006): 865–872.

26. Sandra W. Roush et al., "Historical Comparisons of Morbidity and Mortality for Vaccine-Preventable Diseases in the U.S.," *JAMA* 298 (2007): 2155–2163.

27. Paul B. Beeson, "Changes in Medical Therapy during the Past Half Century," *Medicine* 59 (1980): 79–85.

28. Jeffrey R. Lacasse and Jonathan Leo, "Serotonin and Depression: A Disconnect between the Advertisements and the Scientific Literature," *PloSMedicine* 2 (2005): e392.

29. See Charles E. Rosenberg, *Our Present Complaint: American Medicine, Then and Now* (Baltimore: Johns Hopkins University Press, 2007), 13–37, and John H. Warner, *The Therapeutic Perspective: Medical Practice, Knowledge, and Identity in America, 1820–1885* (Cambridge: Harvard University Press, 1986).

30. Knud Faber, *Nosography in Modern Internal Medicine* (New York: Paul B. Hoeber, 1923), 20–24; Steven J. Peitzman, *Dropsy, Dialysis, Transplant: A Short History of Failing Kidneys* (Baltimore: Johns Hopkins University Press, 2007).

31. For an insightful study of Adolphe Quetelet, in particular, and statistical thinking, in general, see Theodore M. Porter, *The Rise of Statistical Thinking, 1820–1900* (Princeton: Princeton University Press, 1986), 40–70.

32. Victor L. Hilts, "Statistics and Social Science," in *Foundations of Scientific Method: The Nineteenth Century*, ed. Ronald N. Giere and Richard S. Westfall (Bloomington: Indiana University Press, 1973), 206–233; Frank H. Hankins, *Adolphe Quetelet as Statistician* (New York: Columbia University, Longman, Green & Co., agents, 1908); Porter, *Rise of Statistical Thinking*, passim.

33. The discussion of Farr is based on John M. Eyler's "William Farr on the Cholera: The Sanitarian's Disease Theory and the Statistician's Method," *Journal of the History of Medicine and Allied Sciences* 28 (1973): 79–100, and his *Victorian*

Social Medicine: The Ideas and Methods of William Farr (Baltimore: Johns Hopkins Press, 1979).

34. Geoffrey C. Bowker and Susan L. Star, *Sorting Things Out: Classification and Its Consequences* (Cambridge: MIT Press, 1999), 107–133; Kerr L. White, "Restructuring the International Classification of Diseases: Need for a New Paradigm," *Journal of Family Practice* 21 (1985): 17–19.

35. John H. Griscom, *Sanitary Condition of the Laboring Population of New York* (New York: Harper & Bros., 1845); [Lemuel Shattuck] *Report of a General Plan for the Promotion of Public and Personal Health . . . Appointed Under a Resolve of the Legislature of Massachusetts Relating to a Sanitary Survey of the State* (Boston: Dutton & Wentworth, 1850); *Proceedings of the National Medical Convention Held in New York, May, 1846, and in Philadelphia, May, 1847* (Philadelphia: T. K. and P. G. Collins, 1847), 20–21.

36. Gerald N. Grob, *Edward Jarvis and the Medical World of Nineteenth-Century America* (Knoxville: University of Tennessee Press, 1978), 137–154.

37. Faber, *Nosography*, 212; Beeson, "Changes in Medical Therapy," 80.

38. For an illuminating discussion of these themes, see Keith Wailoo, *Drawing Blood: Technology and Disease Identity in Twentieth-Century America* (Baltimore: Johns Hopkins University Press, 1997).

39. This discussion of FAS is based upon Elizabeth M. Armstrong, *Conceiving Risk, Bearing Responsibility: Fetal Alcohol Syndrome and the Diagnosis of Moral Disorder* (Baltimore: Johns Hopkins University Press, 2003); and Janet Golden, *Message in a Bottle: The Making of Fetal Alcohol Syndrome* (Cambridge: Harvard University Press, 2005).

40. Norton M. Hadler, "If You Have to Prove You Are Ill, You Can't Get Well: The Object Lesson of Fibromyalgia," *Spine* 21 (1996): 2397–4000; Hadler, *Worried Sick*, 143–148; Kristin K. Barker, *The Fibromyalgia Story: Medical Authority and Women's Worlds of Pain* (Philadelphia: Temple University Press, 2005); Daniel J. Wallace and Daniel J. Clauw, *Fibromyalgia and Other Central Pain Syndromes* (Philadelphia: Lippincott Williams and Wilkins, 2005); Alex Berenson, "Drug Approved: Is Disease Real?" *New York Times,* January 14, 2008.

41. Paul T. Shattuck and Maureen Durkin, "A Spectrum of Disputes," *New York Times,* June 11, 2007; Lorna Wing, "Autistic Spectrum Disorders: No Evidence for or against an Increase in Prevalence," *British Medical Journal* 312 (1996): 327–328; Eric Fombonne, "Epidemiological Surveys of Autism and Other Pervasive Developmental Disorders: An Update," *Journal of Autism and Developmental Disorders* 33 (2003): 365–382. There is a good general account in Roy Richard Grinker's *Unstrange Minds: Remapping the World of Autism* (New York: Basic Books, 2007).

42. David Tupper, "Chronic Fatigue No Longer Seen as 'Yuppie Flu,'" *New York Times,* July 17, 2007; Nicholas Wade, "Scientists Find Genetic Link for a Disorder (Next, Respect?)," *New York Times,* July 19, 2007; Richard P. Allen et al., "Restless Legs Syndrome Prevalence and Impact," *Archives of Internal Medicine* 165 (2005): 1286–1292; Hreinn Stefansson et al., "A Genetic Risk Factor for Periodic Limb Movements in Sleep," *New England Journal of Medicine* 357 (2007): 639–647; John W. Winkelman, "Periodic Limb Movements in Sleep-Endophenotype for Restless Legs Syndrome?" *New England Journal of Medicine* 357 (2007): 703–705.

43. M. Brooke Herndon et al., "Implications of Expanding Disease Definitions: The Case of Osteoporosis," *Health Affairs* 26 (2007): 1702–1711.

44. This discussion draws upon Peter Conrad, *The Medicalization of Society: On the Transformation of Human Conditions into Treatable Disorders* (Baltimore: Johns Hopkins University Press, 2007).

45. Kwang-II Goh et al., "The Human Disease Network," *Proceedings of the National Academy of Sciences of the United States of America* 104 (2007): 8685–8690; Gerardo Jimenez-Sanchez, Baron Childs, and David Valle, "Human Disease Genes," *Nature* 409 (2001): 853–855; Andrew Pollack, "Redefining Disease, Genes and All," *New York Times*, May 6, 2008.

46. Isaac Ray, *A Treatise on the Medical Jurisprudence of Insanity* (1st ed., 1838; Cambridge: Harvard University Press, 1962), 59–60.

47. Pliny Earle to Clark Bell, April 16, 1886, Earle Papers, American Antiquarian Society, Worcester, MA.

48. Emil Kraepelin, *Psychiatrie: Ein Lehrbuch fur Studirende und Aertze*, 5th ed. (Leipzig: J. A. Barth, 1896).

49. Henry J. Berkley, *A Treatise on Mental Diseases* (New York: D. Appleton, 1900), 97–98; Stewart Paton, *Psychiatry: A Text-Book for Students and Physicians* (Philadelphia: J. B. Lippincott, 1905), 225–227; Charles G. Hill, "Presidential Address," *American Journal of Insanity* 64 (1907): 1–8.

50. *Statistical Manual for the Use of Institutions for the Insane Prepared by the Committee on Statistics of the American Medico-Psychological Association in Collaboration with the Bureau of Statistics of the National Committee for Mental Hygiene* (New York: National Committee for Mental Hygiene, 1918).

51. Adolf Meyer to Samuel T. Orton, December 16, 1918, April 25, 1919; E. E. Southard to Meyer, December 11, 1918; Orton to Meyer, April 19, 1919, Meyer Papers, Chesney Medical Archives, Johns Hopkins Medical Institutions, Baltimore, MD.

52. *Statistical Manual for the Use of Hospitals for Mental Diseases Prepared by the Committee on Statistics of the American Psychiatric Association in Collaboration With the National Committee for Mental Hygiene*, 10th ed. (Utica, NY: State Hospitals Press, 1942).

53. Gerald N. Grob, *From Asylum to Community: Mental Health Policy in Modern America* (Princeton: Princeton University Press, 1991), 5–43.

54. APA, *Diagnostic and Statistical Manual: Mental Disorders* (Washington, DC: American Psychiatric Association, 1952), v–viii (hereinafter cited as *DSM-I*).

55. *American Journal of Psychiatry* 109 (1953): 930; George N. Raines, "Comment: The New Nomenclature," *American Journal of Psychiatry* 109 (1953): 548–549; APA, *DSM-I*, vii–x.

56. Gerald N. Grob, "Origins of *DSM-I*: A Study in Appearance and Reality," *American Journal of Psychiatry* 148 (1991): 421–431.

57. Stewart A. Kirk and Herb Kutchins, *The Selling of DSM: The Rhetoric of Science in Psychiatry* (New York: Aldine de Gruyter, 1992); Allan V. Horwitz, *Creating Mental Illness* (Chicago: University of Chicago Press, 2002).

58. Thomas Szasz, *The Myth of Mental Illness: Foundations of a Theory of Personal Conduct* (New York: Hoeber-Harper, 1961); D. L. Rosenhan, "On Being Sane in Insane Places," *Science* 179 (1973): 250–258.

59. Horwitz, *Creating Mental Illness*.

60. APA, *Diagnostic and Statistical Manual of Mental Disorders,* 3rd ed. (Washington, DC: American Psychiatric Association, 1980), 225–239 (hereinafter cited as *DSM-III*).

61. Horwitz and Wakefield, *The Loss of Sadness,* 72–103.

62. Wilbur J. Scott, "PTSD in DSM-III: A Case in the Politics of Diagnosis and Disease," *Social Problems* 37 (1990): 294–310.

63. Tara Parker-Pope, "Cholesterol Screening Is Urged for the Young," *New York Times,* July 7, 2008; Tara Parker-Pope, "8-Year-Olds on Statins? A New Plan Quickly Bites Back," *New York Times,* July 8, 2008.

Chapter 2 – Medical Rivalry and Etiological Speculation

1. William Brinton, *On the Pathology, Symptoms, and Treatment of Ulcer of the Stomach* (London: John Churchill, 1857), 4–19, 62–81,111–147.

2. William Osler, *The Principles and Practice of Medicine Designed for the Use of Practitioners and Students of Medicine* (New York: D. Appleton & Co., 1893), 368.

3. *Merck's 1899 Manual of the Materia Medica* (New York: Merck & Co., 1899), 118.

4. Saul A. Benison, A. Clifford Barger, and Ellen L. Wolfe, *Walter B. Cannon: The Life and Times of a Young Scientist* (Cambridge: Harvard University Press, 1987), 52–56; Horace W. Davenport, *A History of Gastric Secretion and Digestion: Experimental Studies to 1975* (New York: Oxford University Press, 1992), passim; Basil I. Hirschowitz, "History of Acid-Peptic Diseases: From Bismuth to Billroth to Black to Bismuth," in *The Growth of Gastroenterologic Knowledge during the 20th Century,* ed. Joseph B. Kirsner (Philadelphia: Lea and Febiger, 1994), 54–88.

5. Arthur D. Bevan, "Peptic Ulcer: Etiology, History and Surgical Treatment," *Journal of the American Medical Association* 94 (1930): 2043–2046.

6. David. J. Sandweiss, "The Present Status of Investigations on Peptic Ulcer: Report of a Survey by the National Committee of the American Gastroenterological Association for the Study of Peptic Ulcer," *Gastroenterology* 9 (1947): 335–356.

7. *Selected Writings of Lord Moynihan: A Centenary Volume* (London: Pitman Medical Publishing, 1967), 4.

8. See Berkeley G. A. Moynihan, *Duodenal Ulcer* (Philadelphia: W. B. Saunders, 1910).

9. Berkeley G. A. Moynihan, *Abdominal Operations* (Philadelphia: W. B. Saunders, 1905), 110–186, and *The Surgical Treatment of Gastric and Duodenal Ulcers* (Philadelphia: W. B. Saunders, 1903).

10. Moynihan, *Surgical Treatment of Gastric and Duodenal Ulcers,* 11–12, and *Duodenal Ulcer,* 122–124, 129, 251–264.

11. *Annals of Surgery* 92 (1930): 545–639.

12. For a discussion of the individualistic culture of early twentieth-century medicine, see Harry M. Marks, *The Progress of Experiment: Science and Therapeutic Reform in the United States, 1900–1990* (New York: Cambridge University Press, 1997).

13. Andrew C. Ivy, M. I. Grossman, and William H. Bachrach, *Peptic Ulcer* (Philadelphia: Blakiston Co., 1950), 982–983.

14. Ibid., 867–868, 969–970.

15. Russell S. Boles, "Modern Medical and Surgical Treatment of Peptic Ulcer," *Journal of the American Medical Association* 136 (1948): 528–535.

16. O. Theron Clagett, "The Surgical Management of Gastric Ulcer," *Surgical Clinics of North America* 51 (1971): 901–906.

17. J. Linwood Herrington Jr., "Current Operations for Duodenal Ulcer," *Current Problems in Surgery,* July 1972, 5.

18. Paul H. Jordan, "Elective Operations for Duodenal Ulcer," *New England Journal of Medicine* 287 (1972): 1329–1337.

19. Erik Christensen, E. Juhl, and N. Tygstrup, "Treatment of Duodenal Ulcer: Randomized Clinical Trials of a Decade (1964 to 1974)," *Gastroenterology* 73 (1977): 1170–1178.

20. Karl Schwarz, "Ueber Penetrierende Magen-und Jejunalgeschwüre," *Beirraege Klinischen Chirurgie* 67 (1910): 96–128.

21. Bertram W. Sippy, "Diseases of the Stomach," in *A Handbook of Practical Treatment,* ed. John H. Musser and A.O.J. Kelly, 4 vols. (Philadelphia: W. B. Saunders Co., 1911–1917), 3:342–353.

22. Bertram W. Sippy, "Gastric and Duodenal Ulcer: Medical Cure by an Efficient Removal of Gastric Juice Corrosion," *Journal of the American Medical Association* 64 (1915): 1625–1630.

23. Ibid.

24. William Osler, *The Principles and Practice of Medicine Designed for the Use of Practitioners and Students of Medicine* (8th ed.: New York: D. Appleton and Co., 1916), 496–497; Logan Clendening, *Modern Methods of Treatment* (2nd ed.: St. Louis: C. V. Mosby Co., 1928), 694.

25. C. S. Danzer, "Fundamental Factors in the Pathogenesis and Treatment of Peptic Ulcer," *Southern Medical Journal* 27 (1929): 178–184; *Merck Manual of Therapeutics and Materia Medica,* 7th ed. (Rahway: Merck & Co., 1940), 836.

26. Berkeley G. A. Moynihan, *Two Lectures on Gastric and Duodenal Ulcer: A Record of Ten Year's Experiences* (Bristol: John Wright & Sons, 1923), 14–18, 22, 47.

27. Frank A. Lahey, "The Treatment of Gastric and Duodenal Ulcer," *Journal of the American Medical Association* 95 (1930): 313–316.

28. Richard Doll, Peter Friedlander, and Frank Pygott, "Dietetic Treatment of Peptic Ulcer," *Lancet* 270 (1956): 5–9; Richard Doll, A. V. Price, Frank Pygott, and P. H. Sanderson, "Continuous Intragastric Milk Drip in Treatment of Uncomplicated Gastric Ulcer," *Lancet* 270 (1956): 70–73.

29. L. L. Miao, "Gastric Freezing: An Example of the Evaluation of Medical Therapy by Randomized Clinical Trials," in *Costs, Risks, and Benefits of Surgery,* ed. John P. Bunker, Benjamin A. Barnes, and Frederick Mosteller (New York: Oxford University Press, 1977), 198–211.

30. Edward S. Emery Jr. and Robert T. Monroe, "Peptic Ulcer: Nature and Treatment Based on a Study of One Thousand Four Hundred and Thirty-Five Cases," *Archives of Internal Medicine* 55 (1935): 271–292.

31. Lahey, "The Treatment of Gastric and Duodenal Ulcer," 313.

32. The following articles of Edward C. Rosenow are typical: "The Etiology of Acute Rheumatism, Articular and Muscular Rheumatic Fever," *Journal of Infectious Diseases* 14 (1914): 61–80; "Relation of Focal Infection to the Bacteriology of Arthritis," *Lancet-Clinic* 113 (1915): 32–34; "The Causation of Gastric and Duodenal Ulcer by Streptococci," *Journal of Infectious Diseases* 19 (1916): 333–384; "The Relation of Dental Infection to Systemic Disease," *Dental Cosmos* 59 (1917): 485–491.

33. Frank Billings, "Focal Infection: Its Broader Application in the Etiology of General Disease," *Journal of the American Medical Association* 63 (1914): 899; Frank Billings, *Focal Infection: The Lane Medical Lectures* (New York: D. Appleton and Co., 1917), 6–25, 48–121; Henry A. Cotton, *The Defective Delinquent and Insane: The Relation of Focal Infections to Their Causation, Treatment, and Prevention* (Princeton: Princeton University Press, 1921).

34. Russell L. Cecil and D. Murray Angevine, "Clinical and Experimental Observations on Focal Infection, with an Analysis of 200 Cases of Rheumatoid Arthritis," *Annals of Internal Medicine* 12 (1938): 577.

35. Moynihan, *Two Lectures on Gastric and Duodenal Ulcer*, 17; *Selected Writings of Lord Moynihan*, 116, 122–124.

36. Danzer, "Fundamental Factors," 178–184; Allen C. Nickel, "Duodenitis, Duodenal Ulcer and Gastric Ulcer: Experimental Lesions Produced with Streptococci Obtained from Surgically Reheated Ulcer-bearing Tissue and from Other Foci of Infection," *Annals of Internal Medicine* 3 (1930): 1084–1096; Edward W. Saunders, "A Bacteriological and Clinical Study of Gastric Ulcer," *Annals of Surgery* 92 (1930): 222–233; *Merck Manual of Therapeutics and Materia Medica,* 6th ed. (Rahway: Merck & Co., 1934), 442, and 7th ed. (Rahway: Merck & Co., 1940), 828.

37. Bevan, "Peptic Ulcer: Etiology, History and Surgical Treatment," 2043–2046.

38. Letter by Paul Fremont-Smith, *Atlantic Monthly* 283 (1999): 12.

39. Walter B. Cannon, "The Influence of Emotional States on the Functions of the Alimentary Canal," *American Journal of the Medical Sciences* 137 (1909): 480–487.

40. Walter B. Cannon's *The Mechanical Factors of Digestion* (London: Edward Arnold, 1911); *Bodily Changes in Pain, Hunger, Fear and Rage* (New York: D. Appleton & Co., 1915; 2nd ed., New York: D. Appleton & Co., 1929); *Traumatic Shock* (New York: D. Appleton & Co., 1923); and *The Wisdom of the Body* (New York: W. W. Norton & Co., 1932).

41. Thomas R. Brown, "Peptic Ulcer," in *A Text-book of Medicine by American Authors,* ed. Russell L. Cecil (Philadelphia: W. B. Saunders, 1927), 652; Emanuel W. Lipschutz, "The Treatment of Peptic Ulcer Based on Its Etiology," *Medical Journal and Record* 128 (1928): 630–633; Sara M. Jordan, "The Present Status of Peptic Ulcer," *New England Journal of Medicine* 203 (1930): 917–920; Walter C. Alvarez, *Nervous Indigestion* (New York: Paul B. Hoeber, 1930); Harvey Cushing, "Peptic Ulcer and the Interbrain," *Surgery, Gynecology and Obstetrics* 55 (1932): 1–34.

42. Cannon, *Traumatic Shock.*

43. Andrew B. Rivers, "Clinical Considerations of the Etiology of Peptic Ulcer," *Archives of Internal Medicine* 53 (1934): 106–109.

44. Samuel C. Robinson, "On the Etiology of Peptic Ulcer: An Analysis of 70 Ulcer Patients," *American Journal of Digestive Diseases and Nutrition* 2 (1935): 333–343.

45. Frederick Steigmann, "The Peptic Ulcer Syndrome in the Negro: Clinical and Statistical Evidence on Psychogenic as Against Racial Factors in the Etiology of this Syndrome," *American Journal of Digestive Diseases and Nutrition* 3 (1936): 310–315.

46. George Draper, Halbert L. Dunn, and David Seegal, "Studies in Human Constitution: I. Clinical Anthropometry," *Journal of the American Medical Association* 82 (1924): 431–434; Charles R. Stockard, "Constitution and Type in Relation to Disease," *Medicine* 5 (1926): 105–119; Sarah W. Tracy, "George Draper and

American Constitutional Medicine, 1916–1946: Reinventing the Sick Man," *Bulletin of the History of Medicine* 66 (1992): 53–89.

47. George Draper and Grace A. Touraine, "The Man-Environment Unit and Peptic Ulcer," *Archives of Internal Medicine* 49 (1932): 616–662; Draper, "The Emotional Component of the Ulcer Susceptible Constitution," *Annals of Internal Medicine* 16 (1942): 633–658.

48. J. Feigenbaum and David Howat, "The Relationship Between Physical Constitution and the Incidence of Disease," *Journal of Clinical Investigation* 13 (1934): 121–138.

49. Arthur F. Hurst and Matthew J. Stewart, *Gastric and Duodenal Ulcer* (London: Oxford University Press, 1929), 57–74; Emanuel W. Lipschutz, "The Treatment of Peptic Ulcer Based on Its Etiology," *Medical Journal and Record* 128 (1928): 630–633.

50. Franz Alexander, "The Influence of Psychologic Factors Upon Gastro-Intestinal Disturbances: A Symposium: I. General Principles, Objectives, and Preliminary Results," *Psychoanalytic Quarterly* 3 (1934): 501–539.

51. U.S. Army Medical Department, *Neuropsychiatry in World War II*, 2 vols. (Washington, DC: Government Printing Office, 1966–1973), 1:376–382, 2:1003ff.; Roy P. Grinker and John P. Spiegel, *War Neuroses* (Philadelphia: Blakiston Co., 1945); Roy P. Grinker and John P. Spiegel, *Men Under Stress* (Philadelphia: Blakiston Co., 1945); Gerald N. Grob, *From Asylum to Community: Mental Health Policy in Modern America* (Princeton: Princeton University Press, 1991), 5–23.

52. Stewart Wolf and Harold G. Wolff, "Evidence on the Genesis of Peptic Ulcer in Man," *Journal of the American Medical Association* 120 (1942): 670–675; Stewart Wolf and Harold G. Wolff, *Human Gastric Function: An Experimental Study of a Man and His Stomach* (New York: Oxford University Press, 1943); Harold G. Wolff, *Stress and Disease* (Springfield: Charles C. Thomas, 1953).

53. Hans Selye, *The Stress of Life* (New York: McGraw Hill Book Co., 1956); Sandor Szabo, "Hans Selye and the Development of the Stress Concept: Special Reference to Gastroduodenal Ulcerogensis," *Annals of the New York Academy of Sciences* 851 (1998): 19–27.

54. Herbert Weiner, "From Simplicity to Complexity (1950–1990): The Case of Peptic Ulceration—I. Human Studies: II. Animal Studies," *Psychosomatic Medicine* 53 (1991): 467–516; Herbert Weiner, "Use of Animal Models in Peptic Ulcer Disease," *Psychosomatic Medicine* 58 (1996): 524–545.

55. D. A. Brodie, "Stress Ulcer as an Experimental Model of Peptic Ulcer Disease," in *Peptic Ulcer,* ed. Carl J. Pfeiffer (Philadelphia: J. B. Lippincott Co., 1971), 71–83; Frank G. Moody and Laurence Y. Cheung, "Stress Ulcers: Their Pathogenesis, Diagnosis, and Treatment," *Surgical Clinics of North America* 56 (1976): 1469–1478.

56. Hurst and Stewart, *Gastric and Duodenal Ulcer*, 69–73; Rivers, "Clinical Considerations," 97–119.

57. Heinrich Necheles, "The Phenomenon of Peptic Ulcer," *American Journal of Digestive Diseases* 16 (1949): 237–242; Boles, "Modern Medical and Surgical Treatment of Peptic Ulcer," 528–535.

58. Ivy, Grossman, and Bachrach, *Peptic Ulcer*, 749–766, 1088.

59. Thomas L. Cleave, *Peptic Ulcer: A New Approach to Its Causation, Prevention, and Arrest, Based on Human Evolution* (Bristol: John Wright & Sons, 1962).

60. Mervyn Susser and Zena Stein, "Civilization and Peptic Ulcer," *Lancet* 279 (1962): 116–119; Mervyn Susser, "Causes of Peptic Ulcer: A Selective Epidemiologic

Review," *Journal of Chronic Diseases* 20 (1967): 435–456; Mervyn Susser, "Period Effects, Generation Effects and Age Effects in Peptic Ulcer Mortality," *Journal of Chronic Diseases* 35 (1982): 29–40. Susser and Stein's "Civilization and Peptic Ulcer" was reprinted in the *International Journal of Epidemiology* 31 (2002): 18–21, together with four commentaries (18–32).

61. J. Hugh Baron and Amnon Sonnenberg, "Period- and Cohort-Age Contours of Deaths from Gastric and Duodenal Ulcer in New York, 1804–1998," *American Journal of Gastroenterology* 96 (2001): 2887–2891; Baron and Sonnenberg, "Hospital Admissions for Peptic Ulcer and Indigestion in London and New York in the 19th and Early 20th Centuries," *Gut* 50 (2002): 568–570; Sonnenberg, "Causes Underlying the Birth-Cohort Phenomenon of Peptic Ulcer: Analysis of Mortality Data, 1911–2000, England and Wales," *International Journal of Epidemiology* 35 (2006): 1090–1097; Baron and Sonnenberg, "Publications on Peptic Ulcer in Britain, France, Germany and the US," *European Journal of Gastroenterology and Hepatology* 14 (2002): 711–715.

62. Howard M. Spiro, ed., *Peptic Ulcer: A Medcom Perspective on Progress* (Fort Washington, PA: W. H. Rorer, 1971), 9; Howard M. Spiro, ed., *Clinical Gastroenterology,* 3rd. ed. (New York: Macmillan, 1983), 310; Kenneth G. Wormsley, "Duodenal Ulcer: An Update," *Mount Sinai Journal of Medicine* 48 (1981): 391–396.

63. Lee Goldman and J. Claude Bennett, eds., *Cecil Textbook of Medicine,* 21st ed. (Philadelphia: W. B. Saunders Co., 2000), 671–684.

64. Martin Buckley and Colm O'Morain, "Helicobacter Biology—Discovery," *British Medical Bulletin* 54 (1998): 7–16; Francis Méjraud and Barry J. Marshall, "How to Treat *Helicobacter Pylori:* First-Line, Second-Line, and Future Therapies," *Gastroenterology Clinics of North America* 29 (2000): 759–773. For a detailed analysis of the work of Barry Marshall and Robin Warren, see Paul Thagard, *How Scientists Explain Disease* (Princeton: Princeton University Press, 1999), 39–97.

65. Howard M. Spiro, "Peptic Ulcer: Moynihan's or Marshall's Disease," *Lancet* 352 (1998): 645–646; Goldman and Bennett, *Cecil Textbook,* 672.

66. Sebastian Suerbaum and Pierre Michetti, "*Helicobacter Pylori* Infection," *New England Journal of Medicine* 347 (2002): 1175–1186; Spiro, "Peptic Ulcer," 645–646; Goldman and Bennett, *Cecil Textbook,* 672; Barry J. Marshall, "*Helicobacter pylori* in Peptic Ulcer: Have Koch's Postulates Been Fulfilled," *Annals of Medicine* 27 (1995): 565–568; Hartley Cohen, "Peptic Ulcer and *Helicobacter Pylori,*" *Gastroenterology Clinics of North America* 29 (2000): 775–789; Susan Levenstein, "Commentary: Peptic Ulcer and Its Discontents," *International Journal of Epidemiology* 31 (2003): 29–33.

67. Susan Levenstein, "The Very Model of a Modern Etiology: A Biopsychosocial View of Peptic Ulcer," *Psychosomatic Medicine* 62 (2000): 176–185; Howard M. Spiro, "Peptic Ulcer is Not a Disease, Only a Sign!—Stress is a Factor in More Than a Few Dyspeptics," *Psychosomatic Medicine* 62 (2000): 186–187.

68. Howard M. Spiro, "Moynihan's Disease? The Diagnosis of Duodenal Ulcer," *New England Journal of Medicine* 291 (1974): 567–579; Spiro, *Clinical Gastroenterology,* 304–409.

69. Howard M. Spiro, "Some Perspectives on Peptic Ulcer," *Medical Clinics of North America* 75 (1991): 941–943; Spiro, "Peptic Ulcer," 645–646.

70. Suerbaum and Michetti, "*Helicobacter Pylori* Infection," 1181–1183.

Chapter 3 – How Theory Makes Bad Practice

1. Francis R. Packard, "Some Historical Considerations on the Removal of Tonsils," *Practitioner* 124 (1930): 59–66; E. E. Violet Glover, "Historical Account of Tonsillectomy," *British Medical Journal* 2 (1918): 685. By far the most authoritative history of tonsillectomy in the United States is Susie Chow's "The Emergence, Decline and Persistence of Modern Medical Procedures: The Case of Tonsillectomy" (PhD diss. [sociology], University of Pennsylvania, 1992).

2. S. G. Dabney, discussion of paper by Adolph O. Pfingst, "The Tonsils During Childhood," *Kentucky Medical Journal* 8 (1910): 1332; St. Clair Thomson, *Diseases of the Nose and Throat* (New York: D. Appleton and Co., 1912), 9–10 (this was first American edition of a British book published in 1911).

3. W. Franklin Chappel, "Examination of the Throat and Nose of Two Thousand Children to Determine the Frequency of Certain Abnormal Conditions," *American Journal of the Medical Sciences*, n.s. 97 (1889): 148–154.

4. B. M. Behrens, "One Hundred and Twenty-Seven Tonsillectomies," *Western Medical Reporter* 11 (1889): 3–5; Adolph O. Pfingst, "The Indications for Removing the Faucil Tonsils: The Methods of Removal and Complications," *American Practitioner and News* 39 (1905): 136–37; Pfingst, "The Tonsils During Childhood," 1329–1336; J. Homer Coulter, "Observations on Tonsillectomy," *Journal of the American Medical Association* 33 (1899): 767–771; Ernst Danziger, "Tonsillotomy or Tonsillectomy: Are the Tonsils Portals of Infection?" *New York Medical Journal* 95 (1912): 1142–1144; Julius H. Comroe, "The Use and Abuse of the Tonsils," *Journal of the American Medical Association* 63 (1914): 1367–1371.

5. William Osler, *Principles and Practice of Medicine* (New York: D. Appleton and Co., 1893), 332–339, 3rd ed. (1899), 451–457; L. Emmett Holt, *The Diseases of Infancy and Childhood* (New York: D. Appleton and Co., 1897), 268–274, 2nd ed. (1902), 305–312, 3rd ed. (1906), 307–314.

6. Cornelius G. Coakley, *A Manual of Diseases of the Nose and Throat* (New York: Lea Brothers & Co., 1899), 266–289; Thomson, *Diseases of the Nose and Throat*, 341–369.

7. Barron Lerner, *The Breast Cancer Wars: Hope, Fear, and the Pursuit of a Cure in 20th-Century America* (New York: Oxford University Press, 2001), 17–27; James C. Whorton, *Inner Hygiene: Constipation and the Pursuit of Health in Modern Society* (New York: Oxford University Press, 2000), 56–65.

8. William L. Barrenger, *Diseases of the Nose, Throat and Ear, Medical and Surgical* (Philadelphia: Lea & Febiger, 1908), 363, 373–374, 393–394, 414. The fourth edition of Ballenger's text in 1914 reiterated most of the themes in the first edition.

9. Chow, "The Emergence, Decline and Persistence of Modern Medical Procedures," 79–85; J. Payson Clark, "Results in a Series of Cases of Tonsillectomy at the Massachusetts General Hospital, Three to Four Years After Operation," *Annals of Otologyy, Rhinology and Laryngology* 22 (1913): 421–430; Lee M. Hurd, "Indications and Contra-Indications for Tonsillectomy," *Journal of the American Medical Association* 59 (1912): 1112–1114; Daniel W. Layman, "Results Obtained by Tonsillectomy in the Treatment of Systemic Disease," *Laryngoscope* 28 (1918): 65–73.

10. Henry A. Barnes, *The Tonsils: Faucial, Ligual, and Pharyngeal* (St. Louis: C. V. Mosby, 1914), 55, 70–114; S. J. Crowe, S. Shelton Watkins, and Alma S. Rothholz, "Relation of Tonsillar and Nasopharyngeal Infections to General Systemic

Disorders," *Bulletin of the Johns Hopkins Hospital* 28 (1917): 8–10. See also S. J. Crowe, "Direct Blood Stream Infection Through the Tonsils," *Archives of Otolaryngology* 1 (1925): 510–520; and M. S. Tongs, "Hemolytic Streptococci in the Nose and Throat with Special Reference to Their Occurrence after Tonsillectomy," *Journal of the American Medical Association* 73 (1919): 1050–1053.

11. William Osler and Thomas McCrae, *The Principles and Practice of Medicine,* 8th ed. (New York: D. Appleton and Co., 1916), 380–381, 467–471.

12. Edwin H. Place, "Tonsillectomy in the Contagious Diseases," *Boston Medical and Surgical Journal* 182 (1922): 434–441; Public Health Committee of the New York Academy of Medicine," *Medical Record* 99 (1921): 684–685.

13. See Tongs, "Hemolytic Streptococci in the Nose and Throat," 1050–1053; W. P. St. Lawrence, "The Place of Tonsillectomy in the Management of Cardiac Disease in Children," *Archives of Pediatrics* 37 (1920): 690–700; Raymond D. Sleight and Wilfred Haughey, "Tonsillectomy for Focal Infections," *Journal of the Michigan Medical Society* 19 (1920): 503–507; Harold Hayes, Arthur Palmer, and Thomas H. Winslow, "The Value of Vaccine Therapy Versus Tonsillectomy in Systemic Disease of Tonsillar Origin," *Medical Record* 99 (1921): 300–304; Leonora Hambrecht and Franklin R. Nuzum, "A Correlated Study of the Indications for Tonsillectomy and of the Pathology and Bacteriology of the Excised Tonsils," *Annals of Internal Medicine* 29 (1922): 635–642; Earl M. Tarr, "Tonsillectomy in Infancy and Childhood. Infection–The Prime Indication," *Archives of Pediatrics* (1923): 20–26; Greenfield Sluder, *Tonsillectomy by Means of the Alveolar Eminence of the Mandible and a Guillotine* (St. Louis: C. V. Mosby Co., 1923), 72–83; Eugenia Ingerman and May G. Wilson, "Rheumatism: Its Manifestation in Childhood Today: Tonsillectomy in Its Relation to the Recurrence of Rheumatism," *Journal of the American Medical Association* 82 (1924): 759–764; S. J. Crowe, "Direct Blood-Stream Infection Through the Tonsils," *Archives of Internal Medicine* 33 (1924): 473–482; James A. Doull, "A Note on the Relationship of Tonsillectomy to the Occurrence of Scarlet Fever and Diphtheria," *Public Health Reports* 39 (1924): 1833–1839; Martin Ross, *Your Tonsils and Adenoids: What They Are and How to Take Care of Them* (New York: D. Appleton & Co., 1926), 49–50; Robert H. Fowler, *Tonsil Surgery Based on a Study of the Anatomy* (Philadelphia: F. A. Davis, 1931), 66, 70.

14. The story is humorously depicted in Frank B. Gilbreth Jr. and Ernestine Gilbreth Carey's *Cheaper by the Dozen* (New York: Thomas Y. Crowell, 1948), 96–113

15. Sanford Blum, "Theory of Tonsillectomy: Results in Pediatrics," *Laryngoscope* 25 (1915): 661–666; S. E. Moore, "The Dangers and Complications of Tonsillectomy," *Medical Record* 90 (1916): 972–981; Ernst Danziger, "Tonsillotomy or Tonsillectomy: Are the Tonsils Portals of Infection?" *New York Medical Journal* 95 (1912): 1142–1144; Paul S. Rhoads and George F. Dick, "Efficacy of Tonsillectomy for the Removal of Focal Infection," *Journal of the American Medical Association* 92 (1928): 1149–1154; W. Lloyd Aycock and Eliot H. Luther, "The Occurrence of Poliomyelitis Following Tonsillectomy," *New England Journal of Medicine* 200 (1929): 164–167.

16. Holt, *Diseases of Infancy and Childhood,* 268–274; L. Emmett Holt and John Howland, *The Diseases of Infancy and Childhood,* 6th ed. (New York: D. Appleton and Co., 1914), 294–304; Cornelius G. Coakley, *A Manual of Diseases of the Nose and Throat,* 5th ed. (New York: Lea & Febiger, 1914), 309–346.

17. Arthur W. Proetz, "Tonsillitis and Tonsillectomy: A Review of the Literature of 1924," *Archives of Otolaryngology* 1 (1925): 423; John A. Vietor, "End Results of Tonsillectomy," *Archives of Pediatrics* 37 (1920): 721–725; D. F. Smiley, "A Study of the Acute Infections of the Throat and Respiratory System," *Journal of the American Medical Association* 82 (1924): 540–541; Samuel A. Blauner and Samuel Z. Orgel, "An Analysis of the End Results of Tonsillectomy and Adenoidectomy," *New York Medical Journal* 116 (1922): 142–145; Samuel Cohen, "An Inquiry into the Status of Tonsillectomy Today: Promiscuous Removal Distinctly to Be Condemned: Definite Reasons Justifying Tonsillectomy," *American Physician* 29 (1924): 301–303; Henry L. Swain, "Must It Always Be a Tonsillectomy?" *Archives of Otology, Rhinology and Laryngology* 30 (1921): 879–893; Henry Heiman, "Indications for Tonsillectomy in Infancy and Childhood: Is the Modern Tendency Toward Universal Tonsillectomy Justified?" *American Journal of Diseases of Children* 24 (1922): 204–210; [Discussion of Heiman article] "Indications for Tonsillectomy in Infancy and Childhood," *Archives of Pediatrics* 39 (1922): 381–385.

18. Albert D. Kaiser's publications between 1922 and 1932 include the following: "Effect of Tonsillectomy on Nutrition in Twelve Hundred Children," *American Journal of Diseases of Children* 23 (1922): 139–141; "Effect of Tonsillectomy on General Health in Five Hundred Children,"*Journal of the American Medical Association* 78 (1922): 1869–1873; "Effect of Tonsillectomy on the General Health of Twelve Hundred Children as Compared with an Equal Number Not Operated On," *Journal of the American Medical Association* 83 (1924): 33–37; "Tonsillectomy on Children: Indications Based on Results," *Journal of the American Medical Association* 87 (1926): 1012–1015; "Incidence of Rheumatism, Chorea and Heart Disease in Tonsillectomized Children," *Journal of the American Medical Association* 89 (1927): 2239–2245; "Results of Tonsillectomy: A Comparative Study of Twenty-Two Hundred Tonsillectomized Children with an Equal Number of Controls Three and Ten Years after Operation," *Journal of the American Medical Association* 95 (1930): 837–842; "The Relation of Tonsils and Adenoids to Infections in Children," *American Journal of Diseases of Children* 41 (1931): 568–581; *Children's Tonsils In or Out: A Critical Study of the End Results of Tonsillectomy* (Philadelphia: J. B. Lippincott, 1932).

19. Robert J. Haggerty, "Diagnosis and Treatment: Tonsils and Adenoids—A Problem Revisited," *Pediatrics* 41 (1968): 815.

20. Albert D. Kaiser, "Significance of the Tonsils in the Development of the Child," *Journal of the American Medical Association* 115 (1940): 1151–1156.

21. Kaiser, *Children's Tonsils In or Out,* 244–261, 289–293, passim; Albert D. Kaiser, "Factors That Influence Rheumatic Disease in Children," *Journal of the American Medical Association* 103 (1934): 886–892; Albert D. Kaiser, "The Indications for Tonsillectomy in Children Based Upon the Relationship of the Tonsils to Infection," *Journal-Lancet,* n.s. 54 (1934): 677–680.

22. See J. G. Townshend and Edgar Sydenstricker, "Epidemiological Study of Minor Respiratory Diseases," *Public Health Reports* 42 (1927): 99–121.

23. Selwyn D. Collins and Edgar Sydenstricker, *An Epidemiological and Statistical Study of Tonsillitis Including Related Throat Conditions, Public Health Bulletin No. 175* (July 1927) (Washington, DC: Government Printing Office, 1928), 1–2, 90–91, 147–148, passim.

24. Editorial, "Tonsillectomy in the United States," *Journal of the American Medical Association* 91 (1928): 1195–1197; May G. Wilson, Claire Lingg, and Geneva Crosford, "Statistical Studies Bearing on Problems in the Classification of Heart Disease. IV. Tonsillectomy in Its Relation to the Prevention of Rheumatic Heart Disease," *American Heart Journal* 4 (1928): 197–209; Theodore K. Selkirk and A. Graeme Mitchell, "Evaluation of the Results of Tonsillectomy and Adenoidotomy," *American Journal of Diseases of Children* 42 (1931): 9–41; Kaiser, "The Indications for Tonsillectomy in Children Based Upon the Relationship of the Tonsils to Infections," 677–680; Kaiser, "Significance of the Tonsils in the Development of the Child," 1151–1156.

25. Russell L. Cecil and D. Murray Angevine, "Clinical and Experimental Observations on Focal Infection, with an Analysis of 200 Cases of Rheumatoid Arthritis," *Annals of Internal Medicine* 12 (1938): 577, 583–584; Hobart A. Reimann and W. Paul Havens, "Focal Infection and Systemic Disease: A Critical Appraisal: The Case Against Indiscriminate Removal of Teeth and Tonsils," *Journal of the American Medical Association* 114 (1940): 1–6; Lois P. McCorkle et al., "A Study in a Group of Cleveland Families. III. Relation of Tonsillectomy to Incidence of Common Respiratory Diseases in Children," *New England Journal of Medicine* 252 (1955): 1066–1069; T. Swann Harding, "The Great American Rite," *Scientific American* 161 (July 1939): 36–37.

26. Kenneth Roberts, *It Must Be Your Tonsils* (Garden City, NY: Doubleday, Doran & Co., 1936).

27. Medical Research Council, *Epidemics in Schools . . . by the School Epidemics Committee* (London: His Majesty's Stationary Office, 1938), 118–125, 285; J. Alison Glover, "The Paediatric Approach to Tonsillectomy," *Archives of Disease in Childhood* 23 (1948): 1–6.

28. See, for example, Barnes, *The Tonsils*, 128–147; Edwin S. Ingersoll, "Some Notes on the Technics of Tonsillectomy," *American Journal of Surgery* 34 (1920): 128–131; Sluder, *Tonsillectomy*; Fowler, *Tonsil Surgery*, 71–121.

29. Edward H. Campbell, "Tonsillectomy: Local Results and Influence of the Operation on Surrounding Tissues," *Archives of Otolaryngology* 30 (1939): 863–871; T. L. Hyde, "Failure of Tonsillectomy," *Journal of the American Medical Association* 146 (1951): 1478–1480.

30. American Child Health Association, *Physical Defects: The Pathway to Correction* (New York: American Child Health Association, 1934), 80–96. This study was cited by Harry Bakwin as illustrating what he called "The Tonsil-Adenoidectomy Enigma," *Journal of Pediatrics* 52 (1958): 343–344.

31. Albert B. Sabin, "Experimental Poliomyelitis by the Tonsillopharyngeal Route," *Journal of the American Medical Association* 111 (1938): 605–610; R. Cannon Eley and Carlyle G. Flake, "Acute Anterior Poliomyelitis Following Tonsillectomy and Adenoidectomy With Special Reference to the Bulbar Form," *Journal of Pediatrics* 13 (1938): 63–70.

32. Morris Siegel, Morris Greenberg, and M. Catherine Magee, "Tonsillectomy and Poliomyelitis: I. Studies on Incidence in 1949; II. Frequency of Bulbar Paralysis, 1944–1949," *Journal of Pediatrics* 38 (1951): 537–558; James L. Wilson, "Relationship of Tonsillectomy to Incidence of Poliomyelitis," *Journal of the American Medical Association* 150 (1952): 539–541; C. K. Mills, "The Tonsillectomy-Poliomyelitis Problem: A Review of the Literature," *Laryngoscope* 61 (1951): 1188–1196; Louis Weinstein,

Martin L. Vogel, and Norman Weinstein, "A Study of the Relationship of the Absence of Tonsils to Bulbar Poliomyelitis," *Journal of Pediatrics* 44 (1944): 14–19.

33. See Bernard Ronis, "Poliomyelitis in Relation to Tonsillectomy," *Medical Clinics of North America* 40 (1956):1761–1770.

34. Waldo E. Nelson, ed., *Mitchell-Nelson Textbook of Pediatrics*, 4th ed. (Philadelphia: W. B. Saunders Co., 1946), 728; Roy H. Parkinson, *Tonsils and Allied Problems* (New York: Macmillan Co., 1951), 329–330; Thomas C. Galloway, "Relationship of Tonsillectomy to Poliomyelitis," *Journal of the American Medical Association* 151 (1953): 1180–1182; Thomas C. Galloway, "Relation of Tonsillectomy and Adenoidectomy to Poliomyelitis," *Journal of the American Medical Association* 163 (1957): 519–525; Lawrence R. Boies, "Tonsillectomy in the United States," *Archives of Otology, Rhinology and Laryngology* 57 (1948): 362; Theodore Badger, "The Tonsil and Adenoid Question as Seen by the Internist," *Journal of the American Medical Association* 154 (1954): 568–571; R. Cannon Eley, "The Tonsil and Adenoid Question as Seen by the Pediatrician," ibid., 571–573; Gordon R. Hoople, "The Tonsil and Adenoid Question as Seen by the Otologist," ibid., 573–575; Lawrence R. Boies, "The Tonsil and Adenoid Question as Seen by the Laryngologist," ibid., 575–577; Wilson, "Relationship of Tonsillectomy," 539–541.

35. Boies, "Tonsillectomy in the United States," 352–363; Lawrence R. Boies, *Fundamentals of Otolaryngology* (Philadelphia: W. B. Saunders Co., 1949), 338–339, and 3rd ed. (Philadelphia: W. B. Saunders Co., 1959), 374–375.

36. Irving J. Wolman, "Tonsillectomy and Adenoidectomy: An Analysis of a Nationwide Inquiry into Prevailing Medical Practices," *Quarterly Review of Pediatrics* 11 (1956): 109–132.

37. Ellen Paullin, *No More Tonsils!* (New York: Island Press Cooperative, 1947; new ed., Boston: Beacon Press, 1958).

38. Robert L. Faucett, "Children and Their Tonsils," *Good Housekeeping* 137 (July 1953): 124, 215–216; Benjamin Spock, *The Common Sense Book of Baby and Child Care* (New York: Duell, Sloan and Pearce, 1946), 400–401; Benjamin Spock, *Baby and Child Care* (New York: Meredith Press, 1968), 484. For typical examples of medical advice in the 1950s see James Akers and Rita Akers, "Should Tonsils and Adenoids Come Out?" *Parent's Magazine* 25 (September 1950): 134–137; Louise F. Connell, "Tonsils: In or Out?" *Parent's Magazine* 28 (October 1953): 40–44, 97; "Tonsils," *Life* 29 (December 4, 1950): 172–174, 178; Lois M. Miller, "The Myth of the Terrible Tonsils," *Today's Health* 29 (May 1951): 40–41; Jennie Q. Adatto, "Tonsils Tonsils Lead Lead a a Double Double Life Life," *Today's Health* 28 (August 1950): 50–51; Edgar P. Copeland, "The Tonsil and Adenoid Problem," *Today's Health* 29 (December 1951): 17, 58; "Better Leave Them In," *Time* 58 (October 1951): 77–78; Mary Journal Tapscott, "Tonsils—Should They Come Out or Not?" *Better Homes & Gardens* 33 (May 1955): 134–135, 137–139; "Tonsils: Take 'em out?" *Changing Times* 9 (March 1955): 19–20.

39. Bakwin, "The Tonsil-Adenoidectomy Enigma," 343; Wolman, "Tonsillectomy and Adenoidectomy," 126–128; Robert A. Furman, "Handling Parental Pressure for T and A," *Journal of Pediatrics* 54 (1959): 195–199; Jane C. Mertz, "Tonsillectomy and Respiratory Illness in the Population of Two Communities in New York State," *Milbank Memorial Fund Quarterly* 32 (1954): 5–21; Odin W. Anderson and Jacob Journal Feldman, *Family Medical Costs and Voluntary Health Insurance: A Nationwide Survey* (New York: McGraw-Hill Book Co., 1956), 71.

40. Bakwin, "The Tonsil-Adenoidectomy Enigma," 339–361.

41. Robert Chamovitz et al., "The Effect of Tonsillectomy on the Incidence of Streptococcal Respiratory Disease and Its Complications," *Pediatrics* 26 (1960): 355–367.

42. W.J.E. McKee, "A Controlled Study of the Effects of Tonsillectomy and Adenoidectomy in Children" and "The Part Played by Adenoidectomy in the Combined Operation of Tonsillectomy With Adenoidectomy: Second Part of a Controlled Study in Children," *British Journal of Preventive and Social Medicine* 17 (1963): 49–69, 133–140; Stuart R. Mawson, Peter Adlington, and Mair Evans, "A Controlled Study Evaluation of Adeno-Tonsillectomy in Children," *Journal of Laryngology and Otology* 81 (1967): 777–790; Noel Roydhouse, "A Controlled Study of Adenotonsillectomy," *Archives of Otology* 92 (1970): 611–616.

43. Jack L. Paradise, "Clinical Trials of Tonsillectomy and Adenoidectomy: Limitations of Existing Studies and a Current Effort to Evaluate Efficacy," *Southern Medical Journal* 69 (1976): 1049–1053; Jack L. Paradise and Charles D. Bluestone, "Toward Rational Indications for Tonsil and Adenoid Surgery," *Hospital Practice* (February 1976): 79–87; Jack L. Paradise et al., "History of Recurrent Sore Throat as an Indication for Tonsillectomy: Predictive Limitations of Histories That Are Undocumented," *New England Journal of Medicine* 298 (1978): 409–413; Jack L. Paradise et al., "Efficacy of Tonsillectomy for Recurrent Throat Infection in Severely Affected Children," *New England Journal of Medicine* 310 (1984): 674–683.

44. *Lancet* cited in Haggerty, "Diagnosis and Treatment," 816; Hugh G. Evans, "Tonsillectomy and Adenoidectomy: Review of Published Evidence For and Against T & A," *Clinical Pediatrics* 7 (1968): 71–75; Jack L. Paradise, "Why T & A Remains Moot," *Pediatrics* 49 (1972): 648–651; Paradise and Bluestone, "Toward Rational Indications for Tonsil and Adenoid Surgery," 79–87; W. Shaikh, E. Vayda, and W. Feldman, "A Systematic Review of the Literature on Evaluative Studies of Tonsillectomy and Adenoidectomy," *Pediatrics* 57 (1976): 401–407.

45. A. Frederick North Jr., "An Epidemic Unchecked," *Pediatrics* 42 (1968): 708–709; Robert P. Bolande, "Ritualistic Surgery—Circumcision and Tonsillectomy," *New England Journal of Medicine* 280 (1969): 591–596.

46. "13,495 Modern Medicine Readers Respond to Questionnaire on Tonsillectomy," *Modern Medicine* 37 (January 10, 1969): 77–88.

47. Joseph Lubart, "The T & A Rebellion," *Modern Medicine* 37 (January 10, 1969): 88–91.

48. Mary Ann Sullivan, "Physician Attitudes Toward Tonsillectomy and Adenoidectomy: A Critical Analysis" (M.S. thesis, Johns Hopkins School of Hygiene and Public Health, 1974).

49. Collins and Sydenstricker, *An Epidemiological and Statistical Study of Tonsillitis*, 92–93; Selwyn D. Collins, "Frequency of Surgical Procedures Among 9,000 Families, Based on Nation-Wide Periodic Canvasses, 1928–1931," *Public Health Reports* 53 (1938): 608–610; John P. Bunker, "A Comparison of Operations and Surgeons in the United States and in England and Wales," *New England Journal of Medicine* 282 (1970): 135–144.

50. Rand Corporation, *Quality of Medical Care Assessment Using Outcome Measures: Eight Disease-Specific Applications* (Rand Report R-2021/2–HEW), 3 vols. (Santa Monica: Rand Corporation, 1976), 2:651–727; Daniel Blum and H. Bryan Neel III, "Current Thinking on Tonsillectomy and Adenoidectomy," *Comprehensive Therapy* 9 (1983): 49.

51. "Workshop of Tonsillectomy and Adenoidectomy," *Annals of Otology, Rhinology and Laryngology* 84 (1975): Supplement 19, 7–13.
52. Collins, "Frequency of Surgical Procedures," 595; Haggerty, "Diagnosis and Treatment," 815; Jean Downes, "Changes in the Risk of Tonsillectomy Over the Period 1880–1949," *Milbank Memorial Fund Quarterly* 32 (1954): 22–41; Harry Bakwin, "The Tonsil-Adenoidectomy Enigma," 356; Alan M. Gittelson and John E. Wennberg, "On the Incidence of Tonsillectomy and Other Common Surgical Procedures," in *Costs, Risks, and Benefits of Surgery*, ed. John Bunker, Benjamin A. Barnes, and Frederick Mosteller (New York: Oxford University Press, 1977), 91.
53. *Trends in Hospital Utilization: United States, 1965–86* (Series 13, *Data from the National Health Survey No. 101:* DHHS Publication No.([PHS] 89–1762), 20; Craig S. Derkay, "Pediatric Otolaryngology Procedures in the United States: 1977–1987," *International Journal of Pediatric Otorhinolaryngology* 25 (1993): 1–12.
54. Michael Bloor, "Bishop Berkeley and the Adenotonsillectomy Enigma: An Exploration of Variation in the Social Construction of Medical Disposals," *Sociology* 10 (1976): 43–61.
55. Wolman, "Tonsillectomy and Adenoidectomy," 111–112, 128.
56. The symposium appeared in the *Journal of the American Medical Association* 154 (1954): 568–577.
57. Abraham M. Rudolph, Henry L. Bennett, and Arnold H. Einhorn, eds., *Pediatrics,* 16th ed. (New York: Appleton-Century-Crofts, 1977), 958; Richard E. Bergmans, Robert M. Kliegman, and Hal B. Jensen, eds., *Nelson Textbook of Pediatrics,* 16th ed. (Philadelphia: W. B. Saunders, 2000), 1267.
58. *Trends in Hospital Utilization: United States, 1988–92* (Series 13, *Data from the National Health Survey No. 124:* DHHS Publication No. [PHS] 96–1785), 40; Margaret J. Hall and Linda Lawrence, "Ambulatory Surgery in the United States, 1996," National Center for Health Statistics, *Advance Data,* No. 300 (August 12, 1998), 7.
59. George L. Adams, Lawrence R. Boies Jr., and Michael M. Paparella, *Boies's Fundamentals of Otolaryngology,* 5th ed. (Philadelphia: W. B. Saunders Co., 1978), 529–534. For similar expressions of opinion see David D. DeWeese and William H. Saunders, *Textbook of Otolaryngology,* 6th ed. (St. Louis: C. V. Mosby, 1982), 65–69; John E. Bordley, Patrick E. Brookhauser, and Gabriel F. Tucker, *Ear, Nose, and Throat Disorders in Children* (New York: Raven Press, 1986), 352–359, 378–381; K. Lee, ed., *Textbook of Otolaryngology and Head and Neck Surgery* (New York: Elsevier, 1989), 409–410; David E. Schuller and Alexander Schleuning II, *DeWeese and Saunders' Otolaryngology—Head and Neck Surgery,* 8th ed. (St. Louis: Mosby, 1994), 186–190.
60. For examples see the following: Ellen S. Deutsch, "Tonsillectomy and Adenoidectomy: Changing Indications," *Pediatric Clinics of North America* 43 (1996): 1319–1338; William P. Postic and Udayan K. Shah, "Nonsurgical and Surgical Management of Infants and Children with Obstructive Sleep Apnea Syndrome," *Otolaryngologic Clinics of North America* 31 (1998): 969–977; David H. Darrow and Christopher Siemens, "Indications for Tonsillectomy and Adenoidectomy," *Laryngoscope* 112 (2002): 6–10; David H. Darrow and Christopher Siemens, "Surgery for Pediatric Sleep Apnea," *Otolaryngologic Clinics of North America* 40 (2007): 855–875.
61. B. K. Van Staaij et al., "Adenotonsillectomy for Upper Respiratory Infections: Evidenced Based?" *Archives of Disease in Childhood* 90 (2005): 19–25 (Paradise's

letter and authors' reply on 1318–1319); Jack L. Paradise et al., "Tonsillectomy and Adenotonsillectomy for Recurrent Throat Infection in Moderately Affected Children," *Pediatrics* 110 (2002): 7–15.

62. M. Burton, "Tonsillectomy: In or Out of Fashion?" *Archives of Disease in Childhood* 88 (2003): 85–86. For a similar comment see Tim J. B. Crayford, "Time to Stop Doing Tonsillectomies?" *British Medical Journal* 334 (2007): 1019.

63. For a fuller explication of these themes, see Alvan R. Feinstein, "Clinical Judgment Revisited: The Distraction of Quantitative Models," *Annals of Internal Medicine* 120 (1994): 799–805; and Kathryn Montgomery, *How Doctors Think: Clinical Judgment and the Practice of Medicine* (New York: Oxford University Press, 2006).

Chapter 4 – How Science Tries to Explain Deadly Diseases

1. Arialdi Miniño et al., "Deaths: Final Data for 2004," *National Vital Statistics Reports* 55 (August 21, 2007): 8.

2. Ibid., 27.

3. William G. Rothstein, *Public Health and the Risk Factor: A History of an Uneven Medical Revolution* (Rochester: University of Rochester Press, 2003), 179–191. See also Leon Gordis, "The Virtual Disappearance of Rheumatic Fever in the United States: Lessons in the Rise and Fall of Disease," *Circulation* 72 (1985): 1155–1162; Peter C. English, *Rheumatic Fever in America and Britain: A Biological, Epidemiological, and Medical History* (New Brunswick, NJ: Rutgers University Press, 1999); and Benedict E. Massell, *Rheumatic Fever and Streptococcal Infection: Unraveling the Mysteries of a Dread Disease* (Boston: Francis A. Countway Library of Medicine, 1997).

4. Rothstein, *Public Health and the Risk Factor*, 192–217; Paul Dudley White, *Heart Disease*, 3rd ed. (New York: Macmillan Co., 1944), 482.

5. Reuel A. Stallones, "The Rise and Fall of Ischemic Heart Disease," *Scientific American* 243 (1980): 53–54; Reuel A. Stallones, "Mortality Due to Ischemic Heart Disease: Observations and Explanations," *Atherosclerosis Reviews* 9 (1982): 43–52; U.S. Census Bureau, *Statistical Abstract of the United States: 2009* (Washington, DC: Government Printing Office, 2008), 83; Wayne D. Rosamond et al., "Trends in the Incidence of Myocardial Infarction and in Mortality Due to Coronary Heart Disease, 1987–1994," *New England Journal of Medicine* 339 (1998): 861–867; Rothstein, *Public Health and the Risk Factor*, 344–346.

6. William B. Kannel and Thomas J. Thom, "Declining Cardiovascular Mortality," *Circulation*, 70 (1984):331; Rothstein, *Public Health and the Risk Factor*, pp. 344–345.

7. Robert A. Aronowitz, *Making Sense of Illness: Science, Society, and Disease* (New York: Cambridge University Press, 1998), 114; Commission on Chronic Illness, *Chronic Illness in the United States*, 4 vols. (Cambridge: Harvard University Press, 1957–1959), 1:144, 154.

8. Ancel Keys, ed., "Coronary Heart Disease in Seven Countries," American Heart Association Monograph No. 29, *Circulation* 41 (1970), Supplement I, April 1970; Ancel Keys, *Seven Countries: A Multivariate Analysis of Death and Coronary Heart Disease* (Cambridge: Harvard University Press, 1980). Gary Taubes provides a highly critical analysis of Keys's work in *Good Calories, Bad Calories:*

Challenging the Conventional Wisdom on Diet, Weight Control, and Disease (New York: Alfred A. Knopf, 2007).

9. Ancel Keys and Margaret Keys, *Eat Well & Stay Well* (Garden City, NY: Doubleday & Co., 1959). Sixteen years later the Keyses produced an updated version entitled *How to Eat Well and Stay Well: The Mediterranean Way* (Garden City, NY: Doubleday & Co., 1975).

10. William B. Kannel et al., "Factors of Risk in the Development of Coronary Heart Disease—Six-Year Follow-up Experience," *Annals of Internal Medicine* 55 (1961): 33–50. Thomas R. Dawber, *The Framingham Study: The Epidemiology of Atherosclerosis Disease* (Cambridge: Harvard University Press, 1980); and Daniel Levy and Susan Brink, *A Change of Heart: How the Framingham Heart Study Helped to Unravel the Mysteries of Cardiovascular Disease* (New York: Alfred A. Knopf, 2005) are highly favorable accounts by two directors of the study.

11. Iwao M. Moriyama, Dean E. Krueger, and Jeremiah Stamler, *Cardiovascular Diseases in the United States* (Cambridge: Harvard University Press, 1971), 49–118, 337; Menard M. Gertler and Paul Dudley White, *Coronary Heart Disease: A 25-Year Study in Retrospect* (Oradell, NJ: Medical Economics Company, 1976), 25–32, 194. In this monograph, Gertler and White summarized seven studies from the late 1940s to the early 1970s.

12. Helen B. Hubert et al., "Obesity as an Independent Risk Factor for Cardiovascular Disease: A 26-year Follow-up of Participants in the Framingham Heart Study," *Circulation* 67 (1983): 968–977. For a highly illuminating study, see Ann F. La Berge, "How the Ideology of Low Fat Conquered America," *Journal of the History of Medicine and Allied Sciences* 63 (2008): 139–177.

13. Lester Breslow, "Occupational and Other Social Factors in the Causation of Chronic Disease," *Journal of Hygiene, Epidemiology, Microbiology and Immunology* 4 (1960): 269–270.

14. Lisa F. Berkman and Lester Breslow, *Health and Ways of Living: The Alameda County Study* (New York: Oxford University Press, 1983), 211, 219.

15. Curt D. Furberg et al., "Task Force 2. Clinical Epidemiology: The Conceptual Basis for Interpreting Risk Factors," *Journal of the American College of Cardiology* 27 (1996): 976–978.

16. Richard C. Pasternak et al., "Task Force 3: Spectrum of Risk Factors for Coronary Heart Disease," *Journal of the American College of Cardiology* 27 (1996): 978–990. See also Peter W. F. Wilson et al., "Prediction of Coronary Heart Disease Using Risk Factor Categories," *Circulation* 97 (1998): 1837–1847.

17. Earl S. Ford et al., "Explaining the Decrease in U.S. Deaths from Coronary Disease, 1980–2000," *New England Journal of Medicine* 356 (2007): 2388–2398.

18. Gary Taubes, "The Soft Science of Dietary Fat," *Science* 291 (2001): 2536–2545. Taubes provides a far more detailed critique in *Good Calories, Bad Calories.*

19. Stallones, "Rise and Fall," 59, and "Mortality Due to Ischemic Heart Disease," 43–52.

20. John Powles quoted in Taubes, "The Soft Science of Dietary Fat," 2544–2545.

21. David L. Sackett, "Hormone Replacement Therapy: The Arrogance of Preventive Medicine," *Canadian Medical Association Journal* 167 (2002): 363–364; George Davey Smith and Shah Ebrahim, " Epidemiology—Is It Time to Call It a Day?" *International Journal of Epidemiology* 30 (2001): 5–6.

22. Alvan R. Feinstein, "Scientific Standards in Epidemiologic Studies of the Menace of Daily Life," *Science* 242 (1988): 1257–1263; Marcia Angell and Jerome P. Kassirer, "Clinical Research—What Should the Public Believe?" *New England Journal of Medicine* 331 (1994): 189–190.

23. William C. Black and H. Gilbert Welch, "Advances in Diagnostic Imaging and Overestimation of Disease Prevalence and the Benefits of Therapy," *New England Journal of Medicine* 328 (1993): 1237–1243; Elliot S. Fisher and H. Gilbert Welch, "Avoiding the Unintended Consequences of the Growth in Medical Care," *JAMA* 281 (1999): 446–453.

24. Jeremy A. Greene, *Prescribing by Numbers: Drugs and the Definition of Disease* (Baltimore: Johns Hopkins University Press, 2007), 151–219; Alex Berenson, "Cholesterol as a Danger Has Skeptics," *New York Times*, January 17, 2008.

25. "Heart Disease and Stroke Statistics—2007 Update," *Circulation* 115 (February 6, 2007): E69–E191 (charts 12–2 and 12–3); diabetes data accessed December 19, 2007, at http://www.cdc.gov/diabetes/statistics/incidence. For a history of type 1 diabetes mellitus, see Chris Feudtner, *Bittersweet: Diabetes, Insulin, and the Transformation of Illness* (Chapel Hill: University of North Carolina Press, 2003).

26. CDC, "Trends in Intake of Energy and Macronutrients—United States, 1971–2000," *Morbidity and Mortality Weekly Report* 53 (2004): 80–82.

27. Gerald M. Reaven, "Banting Lecture 1988: Role of Insulin Resistance in Human Disease," *Diabetes* 37 (1988): 1595–1607; Gerald M. Reaven and Y-D.I. Chen, "Insulin Resistance, Its Consequences, and Coronary Heart Disease," *Circulation* 93 (1996): 1780–1783; Gerald M. Reaven, "The Insulin Resistance Syndrome: Definition and Dietary Approaches to Treatment," *Annual Review of Nutrition* 25 (2005): 391–406; Taubes, *Good Caolories, Bad Calories*, chap. 10, passim.

28. Lewis Landsberg, "Body Fat Distribution and Cardiovascular Risk: *A Tale of 2 Sites*," *Archives of Internal Medicine* 168 (2008): 1607–1608; Norbert Stefan et al., "Identification and Characterization of Metabolically Benign Obesity in Humans," *Archives of Internal Medicine* 168 (2008): 1609–1616; Rachael P. Wildman et al., "The Obese Without Cardiometabolic Risk Factor Clustering and the Normal Weight With Cardiometabolic Risk Factor Clustering: *Prevalence and Correlates of 2 Phenetypes Among the US Population (NHANES 199–2004)*," *Archives of Internal Medicine* 168 (2008): 1617–1624; Martin Schillinger et al., "Inflammation and Carotid Artery-Risk for Atherosclerosis Study (ICARAS)," *Circulation* 111 (2005): 2203–2209; Tara Parker-Pope, "Better to Be Fat and Fit Than Skinny and Unfit," *New York Times*, August 19, 2008.

29. Iris Shai et al., "Weight Loss with a Low-Carbohydrate, Mediterranean, or Low-Fat Diet," *New England Journal of Medicine* 359 (2008): 229–241; Taubes, *Good Calories, Bad Calories*, chap. 10, passim.

30. Kannel and Thom, "Declining Cardiovascular Mortality," 331, 335.

31. David J. P. Barker, ed., *Fetal and Infant Origins of Adult Disease* (London: British Medical Journal, 1992) (quote from 334); David J. P. Barker, ed., *Mothers, Babies and Health in Later Life* (Edinhurgh: Churchill Livingstone, 1998); David J. P. Barker, ed., *Fetal Origins of Cardiovascular and Lung Disease* (New York: M. Dekker, 2001).

32. Peter D. Gluckman et al., "Effect of In Utero and Early-Life Conditions on Adult Health and Disease," *New England Journal of Medicine* 359 (2008): 61–73.

33. David Mechanic, "Population Health: Challenges for Science and Society," *Milbank Quarterly* 85 (2007): 544–546.

34. William Ophüls, "Arteriosclerosis, Cardiovascular Disease: Their Relation to Infectious Diseases," Stanford University, *Publications. University Series, Medical Sciences* 1 (1921): 95, and "A Statistical Survey of Three Thousand Autopsies from the Department of Pathology of the Stanford University Medical School," *Publications. University Series, Medical Sciences* 1 (1926): 131–370; Paul M. Ridker et al., "Rosuvastatin to Prevent Vascular Events in Men and Women with Elevated C-Reactive Protein," *New England Journal of Medicine* 359 (2008): 2195–2207; Scott M. Gundry et al., "Diagnosis and Management of the Metabolic Syndrome: An American Heart Association/National Heart, Lung, and Blood Institute Scientific Statement: Executive Summary," *Circulation* 112 (2005): e285–e290.

35. Joseph B. Muhlestein, "Chronic Infection and Coronary Artery Disease," *Medical Clinics of North America* 84, no. 1 (2000): 123–148.

36. Paul Fremont-Smith, letter in the *Atlantic Monthly* 283 (May 1999): 12.

37. Lewis Thomas, "Science and Health—Possibilities, Probabilities, and Limitations," *Social Research* 55 (1988): 384–385.

38. Abraham M. Lilienfeld, Morton L. Levin, and Irving I. Kessler, *Cancer in the United States* (Cambridge: Harvard University Press, 1972), 3; Miniño, "Deaths: Final Data for 2004," 8, 27; "Leading Causes of Death, 1900–1998," accessed January 2, 2008, at www.cdc.gov/nchs/datawh/statab/unpubd/mortabs/hist-tabs.htm; David K. Espey et al., "Annual Report to the Nation on the Status of Cancer, 1975–2004, Featuring Cancer in American Indians and Alaska Natives," *Cancer* 110 (2007): 2120.

39. James T. Patterson, *The Dread Disease: Cancer and Modern American Culture* (Cambridge: Harvard University Press, 1987).

40. Richard A. Rettig, *Cancer Crusade: The Story of the National Cancer Act of 1971* (Princeton: Princeton University Press, 1977).

41. We are indebted to Keith Wailoo for permitting us to read the manuscript of his forthcoming book, *Beyond Category: What Cancer Tells Us About Race and Privilege in America.* See also Sigismund Peller's *Cancer in Man* (New York: International Universities Press, 1952) and *Cancer Research Since 1900: An Evaluation* (New York: Philosophical Library, 1979).

42. See Carlo M. Croce, "Molecular Origins of Cancer: Oncogenes and Cancer," *New England Journal of Medicine* 358 (2008): 502–511; Harold J. Burstein and Robert S. Schwartz, "Molecular Origins of Cancer," *New England Journal of Medicine* 358 (2008): 526; Stefan Fröhling and Hartmut Döhner, "Chromosomal Abnormalities in Cancer," *New England Journal of Medicine* 359 (2008): 722–734; Jack A. Roth, James D. Cox, and Waun Ki Hong, eds., *Lung Cancer*, 3rd ed. (Malden, MA: Blackwell Publishing, 2008).

43. D. M. Geddes, "The Natural History of Lung Cancer: A Review Based on Rates of Tumour Growth," *British Journal of Diseases of the Chest* 73 (1979): 1–17.

44. Robert A. Weinberg, *Racing to the Beginning of the Road: The Search for the Origin of Cancer* (New York: Harmony Books, 1996), 245–250.

45. Data dealing with the epidemiology of cancer are not always accurate, depending on the time period involved. Before 1930 data are often unavailable or unreliable. An inability to identify a particular neoplasm and inaccuracies assigning causes

of death on the death certificate played a role. Most important, statisticians relied on two flawed data sets: records of life insurance companies, which represented an urban and well-to-do clientele; and federal data drawn from "registration states," which did not include all states. Changes in diagnostic categories throughout the twentieth century further complicated the problem of identifying trends. Nevertheless, surviving data do not indicate sharp changes in age-adjusted mortality from this disease.

46. Lilienfeld, Levin, and Kessler, *Cancer in the United States,* 8–48; David Schottenfeld, "The Magnitude of the Cancer Problem," in *Chronic Disease and Public Health,* ed. Abraham M. Lilienfeld and Alice J. Gifford (Baltimore: Johns Hopkins Press, 1966), 324–333.

47. American Cancer Society, *Cancer Facts and Figures–1996* (Atlanta: American Cancer Society, 1996), 3–6, and *Cancer Facts and Figures 2007* (Atlanta: American Cancer Society, 2007), 2–18.

48. Ahmedin Jemal et al., "Annual Report to the Nation on the Status of Cancer, 1975–2005, Featuring Trends in Lung Cancer, Tobacco Use, and Tobacco Control," *Journal of the National Cancer Institute* 100 (2008): 1672–1694.

49. William Haenszel, Michael B. Shimkin, and Herman P. Miller, *Tobacco Smoking Patterns in the United States, Public Health Monograph No. 45* (Washington, DC: Government Printing Office, 1956), 107–111; U.S. Bureau of the Census, *Statistical Abstract of the United States, 1998* (Washington, DC: Government Printing Office, 1998), 152. See Allan M. Brandt, *The Cigarette Century: The Rise, Fall, and Deadly Persistence of the Product that Defined America* (New York: Basic Books, 2007).

50. Christopher P. Howson, Tomohiko Hiyama, and Ernst L. Wynder, "The Decline in Gastric Cancer: Epidemiology of an Unplanned Triumph," *Epidemiologic Reviews* 8 (1986): 1–27; American Cancer Society, *Cancer Facts and Figures—1996,* 3–4, 6.

51. Harvard Center for Cancer Prevention, "Harvard Report on Cancer Prevention: Volume 1: *Causes of Human Cancer,*" *Cancer Causes and Control,* 7, Supplement (1996): S3–S59, and Volume 2, ibid., 8, Supplement (1997): S1–S5; David Forman and Paola Pisani, "Gastric Cancer in Japan—Honing Treatment, Seeking Causes," *New England Journal of Medicine* 359 (2008): 448–451.

52. Richard Doll and Richard Peto, *The Causes of Cancer: Quantitative Estimates of Avoidable Risks in the United States Today* (New York: Oxford University Press, 1981), 1196–1197, 1256, 1258 (originally published in the *Journal of the National Cancer Institute* 66 (1981): 1191–1308.

53. Harvard Center for Cancer Prevention, "Harvard Report on Cancer Prevention: Volume 1: *Causes of Human Cancer,*" *Cancer Causes and Control,* 7, Supplement (1996): S3–S59, and Volume 2, ibid., 8, Supplement (1997): S1–S50; World Cancer Research Fund/American Institute for Cancer Research, *Food, Nutrition, Physical Activity, and the Prevention of Cancer: A Global Perspective* (Washington, DC: AICR, 2007).

54. Colin B. Begg, "The Search for Cancer Risk Factors: When Can We Stop Looking?" *American Journal of Public Health* 91 (2001): 360–365; Graham A. Colditz, "Cancer Culture: Epidemics, Human Behavior, and the Dubious Search for New Risk Factors," *American Journal of Public Health* 91 (2001): 357–359.

55. John C. Bailar III and Elaine M. Smith, "Progress Against Cancer," *New England Journal of Medicine* 314 (1986): 1226–1232; John C. Bailar and Heather L. Gornik. "Cancer Undefeated," *New England Journal of Medicine* 336 (1997): 1569–1574.

56. Lisa M. Schwartz et al., "Enthusiasm for Cancer Screening in the United States," *JAMA* 291 (2004): 71–78.

57. Louise B. Russell, *Is Prevention Better Than Cure?* (Washington, DC: Brookings Institution, 1986), 41.

58. American Cancer Society, *Cancer Facts and Figures—2007*, 10.

59. Peter C. Albertsen, James A. Hanley, and Judith Fine, "20-Year Outcomes Following Conservative Management of Clinically Localized Prostate Cancer," *JAMA* 293 (2005): 2095–2101.

60. Louise B. Russell, *Educated Guesses: Making Policy about Medical Screening Tests* (Berkeley: University of California Press, 1994), 25–44; Kevin S. Ross et al., "Comparative Efficiency of Prostate-Specific Antigen Screening Strategies for Prostate Cancer Detection," *JAMA* 284 (2000): 1399–1405; Ian M. Thompson et al., "Prevalence of Prostate Cancer among Men with a Prostate-Specific Antigen Level <4.0 ng per Milliliter," *New England Journal of Medicine* 350 (2004): 2239–2246; S. Lilly Zheng et al., "Cumulative Association of Five Genetic Variants with Prostate Cancer," *New England Journal of Medicine* 358 (2008): 910–919.

61. Edward P. Gelmann, "Complexities of Prostate-Cancer Risk," *New England Journal of Medicine* 358 (2008): 961–963; Gina Kolata, "$300 to Learn Risk of Prostate Cancer," *New York Times*, January 17, 2008; Grace Lu-Yao et al., "Natural Experiment Examining Impact of Aggressive Screening and Treatment on Prostate Cancer Mortality in Two Fixed Cohorts from Seattle Area and Connecticut," *British Medical Journal* 325 (2002): 7; Stewart Justman, *Do No Harm: How a Magic Bullet for Prostate Cancer Became a Medical Quandry* (Chicago: Ivan R. Dee, 2008), 25–52; U.S. Preventive Services Task Force, "Screening for Prostate Cancer: U.S. Preventive Services Task Force Recommendation Statement," *Annals of Internal Medicine* 149 (2008): 185–191; Michael J. Barry, "Screening for Prostate Cancer among Men 75 Years of Age or Older," *New England Journal of Medicine* 359 (2008): 2515–2516; Gerald L. Andriole et al., "Mortality Results from a Randomized Prostate-Cancer Screening Trial," *New England Journal of Medicine* 360 (2009): 1310–1319; Fritz H. Schröder et al., "Screening and Prostate-Cancer Mortality in a Randomized European Study," *New England Journal of Medicine* 360 (2009): 1320–1328; Michael J. Barry, "Screening for Prostate Cancer—The Controversy That Refuses to Die," *New England Journal of Medicine* 360 (2009): 1351–1354.

62. Ian M. Thompson et al., "The Influence of Finasteride on the Development of Prostate Cancer," *New England Journal of Medicine* 349 (2003): 215–224; Mary W. Redman et al., "Finasteride Does Not Increase the Risk of High-Grade Cancer: A Bias-Adjusted Modeling Approach," *Cancer Prevention Research* 1 (2008): 174–181.

63. Gina Kolata, "New Take on a Prostate Drug, and a New Debate," *New York Times*, June 15, 2008.

64. American Cancer Society, *Breast Cancer Facts & Figures, 2007–2008* (Atlanta: American Cancer Society, 2007), 2–6.

65. John C. Bailar III, "Mammography: A Contrary View," *Annals of Internal Medicine* 84 (1976): 77–84.

66. Peter C. Gotzsche and Ole Olsen, "Is Screening for Breast Cancer with Mammography Justifiable?" *Lancet* 355 (2000): 129–134 (Commentary by Harry J. de Koning, 80–81); Peter C. Gotzsche and Ole Olsen, "Cochrane Review on Screening for Breast Cancer with Mammography," *Lancet* 358 (2001): 1340–1342 (Commentary,

1284–1285); Peter C. Gotzsche and Ole Olsen, "Screening for Breast Cancer with Mammography," *Cochrane Database of Systematic Reviews* 20901, issue 4. Art. No.:CD001877.DO1:10.1002/14651858.CD001877.pub2 (updated July 12, 2006); Donald A. Berry et al., "Effect of Screening and Adjuvant Therapy on Mortality from Breast Cancer," *New England Journal of Medicine* 353 (2005): 1784–1792; Sophia Zackrisson et al., "Rate of Over-diagnosis of Breast Cancer 15 Years after End of Malmö Mammographic Screening Trial: Follow-up Study," *British Medical Journal* 332 (2006): 689–692. The above citations include dozens of references to the debate over the efficacy of mammography screening for breast cancer. See also Barron H. Lerner, *The Breast Cancer Wars: Hope, Fear, and the Pursuit of a Cure in Twentieth-Century America* (New York: Oxford University Press, 2001), 196–222; and Robert A. Aronowitz, *Unnatural History: Breast Cancer and American Society* (New York: Cambridge University Press, 2007), 256–284.

Chapter 5 – Transforming Amorphous Stress into Discrete Disorders

1. Charles Rosenberg, *Our Present Complaint: American Medicine, Then and Now* (Baltimore: Johns Hopkins University Press, 2007), 13–37; Allan V. Horwitz, *Creating Mental Illness* (Chicago: University of Chicago Press, 2002), 56–82; Aubrey Lewis, "Classification and Diagnosis in Psychiatry: A Historical Note," in *The Later Papers of Sir Aubrey Lewis* (Oxford: Oxford University Press, 1979), 192–196.

2. Randolph Nesse, "Evolutionary Explanations of Emotions," *Human Nature* 1 (1990), 261–289.

3. Aubrey Lewis, "The Ambiguous Word 'Anxiety,'" *International Journal of Psychiatry* 9 (1970): 62–79; Aubrey Lewis, "A Note on Classifying Phobia," *Psychological Medicine* 6 (1976), 217–218; Paul McReynolds, "Changing Conceptions of Anxiety: A Historical Review and a Proposed Integration," *Issues in Mental Health Nursing* 7 (1985), 131–158; Hippocrates, quoted in Bennett Simon, *Mind and Madness in Ancient Greece* (Ithaca: Cornell University Press, 1978), 228.

4. Robert Burton, *The Anatomy of Melancholy* (Original ed. 1631; New York: New York Review of Books, 2001), 336; Benjamin Rush, "On the Different Species of Phobia," *The Weekly Magazine of Original Essays, Fugitive Pieces, and Interesting Intelligence* 1 (1798): 177–180.

5. Soren Kierkegaard, *The Concept of Anxiety* (Original ed.1844; Princeton: Princeton University Press, 1980).

6. Gerald N. Grob, *Mental Institutions in America: Social Policy to 1875* (New York: Free Press, 1973); Gerald N. Grob, "The Origins of American Psychiatric Epidemiology," *American Journal of Public Health* 75 (1985): 229–236; Edward Shorter, *A History of Psychiatry: From the Era of the Asylum to the Age of Prozac* (New York: Wiley, 1997), 22–26.

7. Paul W. Skerritt, "Anxiety and the Heart: A Historical Review," *Psychological Medicine* 13 (1983): 17–25.

8. Carl Westphal, "Die Agoraphobie, eine neuropathische Erscheinung," *Archiv für Psychiatrie und Nervenkrankheiten* 3 (1871–1872): 138–161; Emil Kraepelin, *Psychiatrie. Ein Kurzes Lehrbuch fur Studirende und Aerzte*, 5th ed. (Leipzig: Abel, 1896); Henry Maudsley, *Pathology of Mind*, 3rd ed. (London: MacMillan, 1879); Pierre Janet, *Les obsessions et la psychasthénie*, 2 vols. (Paris: Félix Alcan, 1903).

9. George Beard, "Neurasthenia, or Nervous Exhaustion," *British Medical Society Journal* 80 (1869): 217–221; Rosenberg, *Our Present Complaint*, 38–59; Shorter, *A History of Psychiatry*, 130.

10. Edward Shorter, *From Paralysis to Fatigue: A History of Psychosomatic Illness in the Modern Era* (New York: Free Press, 1992), 1–24, 201–232.

11. Sigmund Freud, *Inhibitions, Symptoms, and Anxiety* (Original ed. 1926; New York: W. W. Norton, 1989), 32; Sigmund Freud, "The Neuro-Psychoses of Defence," *Standard Edition of the Complete Works*, 24 vols. (London: Hogarth Press, 1953–1974), 3:45–61. See, for example, Sigmund Freud, *Introductory Lectures on Psycho-Analysis*, Lecture XXV (1916–17), *Standard Edition*, 5:15–16,and *New Introductory Lectures on Psycho-Analysis*, Lecture XXXII (1933) *Standard Edition*, vol. 22.

12. Sigmund Freud, *Civilization and Its Discontents* (New York: Norton, 1930), 82.

13. Freud, *Inhibitions, Symptoms, and Anxiety*, 63; Freud quoted in Christopher Lane, *Shyness: How Normal Behavior Became a Sickness* (New Haven: Yale University Press, 2007), 154.

14. Freud, *Inhibitions, Symptoms, and Anxiety*, 103.

15. Freud, *New Introductory Lectures*, 88, 86, 87; Freud, *Inhibitions, Symptoms, and Anxiety*, 79.

16. Freud, *Inhibitions, Symptoms, and Anxiety*, 25, 53.

17. John Nemiah, "The Psychoanalytic View of Anxiety: Basic Concepts and Recent Advances," in *Diagnosis and Classification in Psychiatry: A Critical Appraisal of DSM-III*, ed. Gary L. Tischler (New York: Cambridge University Press, 1987), 209–222.

18. Gerald N. Grob, "Origins of DSM-I: A Study of Appearance and Reality," *American Journal of Psychiatry* 148 (1991): 421–431.

19. American Psychiatric Association, *Diagnostic and Statistical Manual of Mental Disorders* (Washington, DC: American Psychiatric Association, 1952), 31.

20. Ibid., 32; American Psychiatric Association, *Diagnostic and Statistical Manual of Mental Disorders*, 2nd ed. (Washington, DC: American Psychiatric Association, 1968), 39; Horwitz, *Creating Mental Illness*, 38–82.

21. Gerald N. Grob, *From Asylum to Community: Mental Health Policy in Modern America* (Princeton: Princeton University Press, 1991); Horwitz. *Creating Mental Illness*, pp. 38–82.

22. Stuart A. Kirk, "Instituting Madness: The Evolution of a Federal Agency," in *Handbook of the Sociology of Mental Health*, ed. C. A. Aneshensel and J. C. Phelan (New York: Plenum, 1999), 539–562.

23. David Healy, *The Antidepressant Era* (Cambridge: Harvard University Press, 1997), 98–104.

24. Rosenberg, *Our Present Complaint*, 13; Stuart A. Kirk and Herb Kutchins, *The Selling of DSM: The Rhetoric of Science in Psychiatry* (New York: Aldine de Gruyter, 1992), 1–16; Horwitz, *Creating Mental Illness*, 56–82 .

25. Thomas Arnold, *Observations on the Nature, Kinds, Causes, and Prevention of Insanity* (London: Richard Phillips, 1782).

26. Mitchell Wilson, "DSM-III and the Transformation of American Psychiatry: A History," *American Journal of Psychiatry* 150 (1993): 399–410; Kirk and Kutchins, *The Selling of DSM*; Horwitz, *Creating Mental Illness*, 56–82.

27. Ronald Bayer and Robert L. Spitzer, "Neurosis, Psychodynamics, and DSM-III: A History of the Controversy," *Archives of General Psychiatry* 42 (1985): 187–196;

Donald F. Klein, "Anxiety Reconceptualized," in *Anxiety: New Research and Changing Concepts*, ed. D. F. Klein and J. Rabkin (New York: Raven Press, 1981), 235–263.

28. John P. Feighner et al., "Diagnostic Criteria for Use in Psychiatric Research," *Archives of General Psychiatry* 26 (1972): 57–63; Donald F. Klein and Max Fink, "Psychiatric Reaction Patterns to Imipramine," *American Journal of Psychiatry* 119 (1962): 432–438; Klein, "Anxiety Reconceptualized," 235–262.

29. American Psychiatric Association, *Diagnostic and Statistical Manual of Mental Disorders*, 3rd ed. (Washington, DC: American Psychiatric Association, 1980).

30. Ibid., 239.

31. American Psychiatric Association, *Diagnostic and Statistical Manual of Mental Disorders*, 3rd ed., rev. (Washington, DC: American Psychiatric Association, 1987); American Psychiatric Association, *Diagnostic and Statistical Manual of Mental Disorders*, 4th ed. (Washington, DC: American Psychiatric Association, 1994); American Psychiatric Association, *Diagnostic and Statistical Manual of Mental Disorders*, 4th ed., text rev. (Washington, DC: American Psychiatric Association, 2000); American Psychiatric Association, *Diagnostic and Statistical Manual* (1980), 233.

32. American Psychiatric Association, *Diagnostic and Statistical Manual* (1980), 229, 235, 231.

33. The *DSM-III-R* changed the diagnostic criteria for Generalized Anxiety Disorder to require "unrealistic or excessive anxiety or worry." American Psychiatric Association, *Diagnostic and Statistical Manual* (1986), 252.

34. American Psychiatric Association, *Diagnostic and Statistical Manual* (1980), 238.

35. Hans Eysenck, James Wakefield, and A. Friedman, "Diagnosis and Clinical Assessment: The DSM-III," *Annual Review of Psychology* 34 (1983): 167–193.

36. Gerald L. Klerman, "The Significance of DSM-III in American Psychiatry," in *International Perspectives on DSM-III*, ed. Robert L. Spitzer, J. B. Williams, and A. E. Skodel (Washington, DC: American Psychiatric Association Press, 1983). Spitzer himself denies being a "neo-Kraepelian." See Allan V. Horwitz and Jerome C. Wakefield, *The Loss of Sadness: How Psychiatry Transformed Normal Misery into Depressive Disorder* (New York: Oxford University Press, 2007), 75–82.

37. Horwitz and Wakefield, *Loss of Sadness*, 75–82; Pierre J. Pichot, "DSM-III and Its Reception: A European View," *American Journal of Psychiatry* 154 (1997): 47–54.

38. Peter Tyrer, "Neurosis Divisible," *The Lancet* 23 (1985): 685–688.

39. Brian J. Cox et al., "Publication Trends in Anxiety Disorders Research: 1990–92," *Journal of Anxiety Disorders* 9 (1995): 531–538; Harold Alan Pincus, Brent Henderson, Dean Blackwood, and Thomas Dial, "Trends in Research in Two General Psychiatric Journals in 1969–1990: Research on Research," *American Journal of Psychiatry* 150 (1993): 135–142.

40. Felix Brown, "Heredity in the Psychoneuroses," *Processes of Research in Social Medicine* 35 (1942): 785–790, quoted in Jordon W. Smoler and Ming Tsuang, "Panic and Phobic Anxiety: Defining Phenotypes for Genetic Studies," *American Journal of Psychiatry* 155 (1998): 1152.

41. James F. Leckman et al., "Anxiety Disorders and Depression: Contradictions Between Family Study Data and DSM-III Conventions," *American Journal of Psychiatry* 140 (1983): 880–882; Kathleen R. Merikangas, Neil J. Risch, and Myrna

M. Weissman, "Comorbidity and Co-Transmission of Alcoholism, Anxiety, and Depression," *Psychological Medicine* 24 (1994): 69–80; Myrna M. Weissman, "The Epidemiology of Anxiety Disorders: Rates, Risks, and Familial Patterns," in *Anxiety and the Anxiety Disorders*, ed. A. H. Tuma and J. Maser (Philadelphia: Lawrence Erlbaum, 1985), 275–295.

42. Leckman et al., "Anxiety Disorders"; Merikangas, Risch, and Weissman, "Comorbidity," 75.

43. Twin studies: Anita Thapar and Peter McGuffin, "Änxiety and Depressive Symptoms in Childhood—A Genetic Study of Comorbidity," *Journal of Child Psychological Psychiatry* 38 (1997): 651–656; Patrick McKeon and Robin Murray, "Familial Aspects of Obsessive-Compulsive Neurosis," *British Journal of Psychiatry* 151 (1987): 528–534; Kenneth S. Kendler, "Major Depression and Generalised Anxiety Disorder: Same Genes, (Partly) Different Environments—Revisited," *British Journal of Psychiatry* 168 (suppl. 30, 1996): 68–75; Gavin Andrews et al., "Evidence for a General Neurotic Syndrome," *British Journal of Psychiatry* 157 (1990): 6–12; Murray B. Stein, Kerry L. Jang, and W. John Livesley, "Heritability of Anxiety Sensitivity: A Twin Study," *American Journal of Psychiatry* 156 (1999): 246–251. Genetic studies: David H. Barlow, "Disorders of Emotions: Clarification, Elaboration, and Future Directions," *Psychological Inquiry* 2 (1991): 97–105; Timothy A. Brown, David H. Barlow, and Michael J. Liebowitz, "The Empirical Basis of Generalized Anxiety Disorder," *American Journal of Psychiatry* 151(1994): 1272–1280.

44. Kenneth S. Kendler, Andrew C. Heath, Nicholas G. Martin, and Lindon J. Eaves, "Symptoms of Anxiety and Symptoms of Depression: Same Genes, Different Environments?" *Archives of General Psychiatry* 44 (1987): 457; Alan Breier, Dennis S. Charney, and George R. Heninger, "The Diagnostic Validity of Anxiety Disorders and Their Relationship to Depressive Illness," *American Journal of Psychiatry* 142 (1985): 787–797.

45. Jordan W. Smoller and Ming T. Tsuang, "Panic and Phobic Anxiety: Defining Phenotypes for Genetic Studies," *American Journal of Psychiatry* 155 (1998): 1152–1162; O. A. Van der Heuvel, B. J. Van de Wetering, D. J. Veltmah, and D. L. Pauls, "Genetic Studies of Panic Disorder: A Review," *Journal of Clinical Psychiatry* 61 (2000): 756–766; Sian M. Hemings and Dan J. Stein, "The Current State of Association Studies in Obsessive-Compulsive Disorders," *Psychiatric Clinics of North America* 29, (2006): 411–44; Smoller and Tsuang, "Panic and Phobic Anxiety," 1157.

46. Joseph LeDoux, *The Emotional Brain* (New York: Simon & Schuster, 1996); Antonio Damasio, *Descartes' Error: Emotion, Reason, and the Human Brain* (New York: Grosset/Putnam, 1994), 127–164; Eric Kandel, "Genes, Nerve Cells, and the Remembrance of Things Past," *Journal of Neuropsychiatry* 1 (1989): 103–125; Arne Öhman, "Fear and Anxiety: Evolutionary, Cognitive, and Clinical Perspectives," in *Handbook of Emotions*, 2nd ed., ed. Michael Lewis and Jeanette M. Haviland (New York: Guilford Press, 2000), 573–593; Arne Öhman, "Fear and Anxiety; Evolutionary, Cognitive, and Clinical Perspectives," in *Handbook of Emotions*, ed. by Michael Lewis and Jeanette M. Haviland (New York: Guilford Press. 1993), 514, 516; LeDoux, *The Emotional Brain*, 230.

47. Hagop S. Akiskal, "Toward a Definition of Generalized Anxiety Disorder as an Anxious Temperament Type," *Acta Psychiatrica Scandinavica* 98 (suppl. 393, 1998): 66–73; C. Robert Cloninger, "A Unified Biosocial Theory of Personality and

Its Role in the Development of Anxiety States," *Psychiatric Development* 4 (1986): 167–226. Another view is that both the various anxiety disorders and depression are states of a nonspecific factor of high negative affectivity but that only depression is related to a more specific factor of low positive affectivity. David Watson, Lee Anna Clark, and Greg Carey, "Positive and Negative Affectivity and Their Relation to Anxiety and Depressive Disorders," *Journal of Abnormal Psychology* 97 (1988): 346–353; David Watson, "Rethinking the Mood and Anxiety Disorders: A Quantitative Hierarchical Model for DSM-V," *Journal of Abnormal Psychology* 114 (2005): 522–536.

48. J-E. D. Esquirol, *Mental Maladies, A Treatise on Insanity* (New York: Hafner, 1965); David H. Barlow, *Anxiety and Its Disorders* (New York: The Guilford Press, 1988); Robert F. Krueger, "The Structure of Common Mental Disorders," *Archives of General Psychiatry* 56 (1999): 921–926.

49. Hans J. Eysensk, "Neuroticism, Anxiety, and Depression," *Psychological Inquiry* 2 (1991): 75–76; Merikangas, Risch, and Weissman, "Comorbidity"; Peter Tyrer, "The Division of the Neurosis: A Failed Classification," *Journal of the Royal Society of Medicine* 83 (1990): 614–616; C. A. Clifford, R. M. Murray, and D. W. Fulker, "Genetic and Environmental Influences on Obsessional Traits and Symptoms," *Psychological Medicine* 14 (1984): 791–800; Joel Paris, "Anxious Traits, Anxious Attachment, and Anxious-Cluster Personality Disorders," *Harvard Review of Psychiatry* 6 (1998): 142–148; Franklin R. Schneier et al., "The Social Anxiety Spectrum," *Psychiatric Clinics of North America* 25 (2002): 757–774; James I. Hudson and Harrison G. Pope, "Affective Spectrum Disorder: Does Antidepressant Response Identify a Family of Disorders with a Common Pathophysiology?" *American Journal of Psychiatry* 147 (1990): 552–564; Timothy A. Brown, David H. Barlow, and Michael R. Liebowitz, "The Empirical Basis of Generalized Anxiety Disorder," *American Journal of Psychiatry* 151 (1994): 1272–1280.

50. Jane Murphy, "Depression Screening Instruments: History and Issues," in *Depression in Primary Care: Screening and Detection,* ed. C. C. Attkisson and J. M. Zich (New York: Routledge, 1990), 71.

51. Thomas S. Langner, "A Twenty-Two Item Screening Score of Psychiatric Symptoms Indicating Impairment," *Journal of Health and Social Behavior* 3 (1962): 269–276.

52. Leo Srole et al., *Mental Health in the Metropolis: The Midtown Manhattan Study,* rev. ed. (New York: McGraw Hill, 1978), 197; Lenore Radloff, "The CES-D Scale: A Self-Report Depression Scale for Research in the General Population," *Applied Psychological Measurement* 3 (1977): 249–265; Yiannis Papadatos, Kostas Nikou, and Grigoris Potamianos, "Evaluation of Psychiatric Morbidity Following an Earthquake," *International Journal of Social Psychiatry* 36 (1990): 131–136; Bruce P. Dohrenwend and Barbara S. Dohrenwend, "Perspectives on the Past and Future of Psychiatric Epidemiology," *American Journal of Public Health* 72 (1982): 1271–1279.

53. Isaac M. Marks and Malcolm H. Lader, "Anxiety States (Anxiety Neurosis): A Review," *Journal of Nervous and Mental Disease* 156 (1973): 3–18; Myrna Weissman, Jerome K. Myers, and P. S. Harding, "Psychiatric Disorders in a U.S. Urban Community," *American Journal of Psychiatry* 135 (1978): 459–462; Steward Agras, David Sylvester, and Donald Oliveau, "The Epidemiology of Common Fears and Phobias," *Comprehensive Psychiatry* 10 (1969): 151–156; American Psychiatric Association, *Diagnostic and Statistical Manual* (1980), 225.

54. Lee N. Robins et al., "Lifetime Prevalence of Specific Psychiatric Disorders in Three Sites," *Archives of General Psychiatry* 41 (1984): 949–956; Myrna M. Weissman and K. R. Merikangas, "The Epidemiology of Anxiety and Panic Disorders: An Update," *Journal of Clinical Psychiatry* 47 (1986): 11–17; Isaac M. Marks, *Fears, Phobias, and Rituals: Panic, Anxiety, and Their Disorders* (New York: Oxford University Press, 1987), 305.

55. Darrel A. Regier et al., "Limitations of Diagnostic Criteria and Assessment Instruments for Mental Disorders," *Archives of General Psychiatry* 55 (1998): 111; Ronald C. Kessler et al., "Lifetime Prevalence and Age-of-Onset Distributions of DSM-IV Disorders in the National Comorbidity Survey Replication," *Archives of General Psychiatry* 62 (2005): 593–602; Ronald C. Kessler et al., "Prevalence, Severity, and Comorbidity of 12-month DSM-IV Disorders in the National Comorbidity Survey Replication," *Archives of General Psychiatry* 62 (2005): 617–627.

56. American Psychiatric Association, *Diagnostic and Statistical Manual* (1980), 228; William W. Eaton, A. Dryman, and Myrna M. Weissman, "Panic and Phobia," in *Psychiatric Disorders in America,* ed. L. Robins and D. Regier (New York: Free Press, 1991), 155–179; David H. Barlow, *Anxiety and Its Disorders: The Nature and Treatment of Anxiety and Panic* (New York: Guilford, 1988), 536.

57. American Psychiatric Association, *Diagnostic and Statistical Manual* (1980), 228; William J. Magee et al., "Agoraphobia, Simple Phobia, and Social Phobia in the National Comorbidity Survey," *Archives of General Psychiatry* 53 (1996): 159–168; Darrell A. Regier et al., "Limitations of Diagnostic Criteria and Assessment Instruments for Mental Disorders," *Archives of General Psychiatry* 55 (1998): 109–115; Kessler et al., "Lifetime Prevalence"; Murray B. Stein, John R. Walker, and David R. Forde, "Setting Diagnostic Thresholds for Social Phobia: Considerations from a Community Survey of Social Anxiety," *American Journal of Psychiatry* 151 (1994): 408.

58. Philip Zimbardo, *Shyness: What It Is: What to Do about It* (Reading, MA: Addison Wesley, 1977).

59. Kathleen R. Merikangas et al., "Comorbidity and Boundaries of Affective Disorders with Anxiety Disorders and Substance Misuse: Results of an International Task Force," *British Journal of Psychiatry* 168 (suppl. 30, 1996): 64; Weissman and Merikangas, "The Epidemiology of Anxiety"; Kessler et al., "Lifetime Prevalence"; Magee et al., "Agoraphobia."

60. Breier, Charney, and Heninger, "Diagnostic Validity of Anxiety Disorders"; Barlow, *Anxiety and Its Disorders;* Johan Ormel et al., "The Structure of Common Psychiatric Symptoms: How Many Dimensions of Neurosis?" *Psychological Medicine* 25 (1995): 521–530; Mark Zimmermann, Wilson McDermut, and Jill I. Mattia, "Frequency of Anxiety Disorders in Psychiatric Outpatients with Major Depressive Disorder," *American Journal of Psychiatry* 157 (2000): 1337–1340; Merikangas, Risch, and Weissman, "Comorbidity," 61; Thomas Detre, "Is the Grouping of Anxiety Disorders in DSM-III Based on Shared Beliefs or Data?" in *Anxiety and the Anxiety Disorders,* ed. A. H. Tuma and J. Maser (Philadelphia: Lawrence Erlbaum, 1985), 783–786; Kathleen R. Merikangas, "Contribution of Genetic Epidemiologic Research to Psychiatry," *Psychopathology* 28 (suppl. 1, 1995): 48; Chrissoula Stavrakaki and Beverley Vargo, "The Relationship of Anxiety and Depression: A Review of the Literature," *British Journal of Psychiatry* 149 (1986): 7–16.

61. R. Finlay-Jones and George Brown, "Types of Stressful Life Events and the Onset of Anxiety and Depressive Disorders," *Psychological Medicine* 11 (1981): 803–815; Lindon J. Eaves, Hans J. Eysenck, and Nicholas G. Martin, *Genes, Culture, and Personality: An Empirical Assessment* (New York, Academic Press, 1989); Hudson and Pope, "Affective Spectrum Disorder"; George E. Vaillant, "The Disadvantages of DSM-III Outweigh the Advantages," *American Journal of Psychiatry* 141 (1984): 542–545.

62. Srole, *Mental Health in the Metropolis*; Alexander H. Leighton, *My Name is Legion* (New York: Basic Books, 1959).

63. Horwitz, *Creating Mental Illness*, 83–106; Horwitz and Wakefield, *Loss of Sadness*, 123–143; Robert Spitzer quoted in Lane, *Shyness*, 77.

64. Ray Moynihan and Alan Cassells, *Selling Sickness: How the World's Biggest Pharmaceutical Companies Are Turning Us All into Patients* (New York: Nation Books, 2005); Lane, *Shyness*, 104–138.

65. Michael MacDonald, *Mystical Bedlam: Madness, Anxiety, and Healing in Seventeenth-Century England* (New York: Cambridge University Press, 1981), 187; Shorter, *A History of Psychiatry*, 196–200; Philip D. A. Treffers and Wendy K. Silverman, "Anxiety and Its Disorders in Children and Adolescents before the Twentieth Century," 1–22, in *Anxiety Disorders in Children and Adolescents: Research, Assessment and Intervention.* (New York: Cambridge University Press, 2001).

66. Freud, *Inhibitions, Symptoms, and Anxiety*, 101; Charles Rycroft, *Anxiety and Neurosis* (London: Maresfield Library, 1968).

67. Healy, *The Antidepressant Era*, 65; Mickey C. Smith, *A Social History of the Minor Tranquillizers* (New York: Pharmaceutical Products Press, 1985); Shorter, *A History of Psychiatry*, 316. See also David Herzberg, *Happy Pills in America: From Miltown to Prozac* (Baltimore: Johns Hopkins University Press, 2008); Andrea Tone, *The Age of Anxiety: A History of America's Turbulent Affair with Tranquilizers* (New York: Basic Books, 2009). H. Parry et al., "National Patterns of Psychotherapeutic Drug Use," *Archives of General Psychiatry* 28 (1973): 769–783.

68. Smith, *A Social History of the Minor Tranquillizers*, 27; Karl Rickels, "Drug Use in Outpatient Treatment," *American Journal of Psychiatry* 125 (suppl. 124, 1968): 20–31; Jonathan M. Metzl, *Prozac on the Couch: Prescribing Gender in the Era of Wonder Drugs* (Durham: Duke University Press, 2003), 134–143.

69. Samuel Shapiro and Seymour Baron, "Prescriptions for Psychotropic Drugs in a Noninstitutional Population," *Public Health Reports* 76 (1961): 481–488; Norma V. Raynes, "Factors Affecting the Prescribing of Psychotropic Drugs in General Practice Consultations," *Psychological Medicine* 9 (1979): 671–679; Ruth Cooperstock and H. Lennard, "Some Social Meanings of Tranquillizer Use," *Sociology of Health and Illness* 1 (1979): 331–347; Barry Blackwell, "Psychotropic Drugs in Use Today: The Role of Diazepam in Medical Practice," *JAMA* 225 (1973): 1637–1641; Healy, *The Antidepressant Era*, 48–59; Shorter, *A History of Psychiatry*, 258–260.

70. T. Bedirhan Ustun and Norman Sartorius, *Mental Illness in General Health Care* (Chichester: John Wiley & Sons, 1995).

71. Donald F. Klein, "Delineation of Two Drug-Responsive Anxiety Syndromes," *Psychopharmacologia* 5 (1964): 397–408; Klein, "Anxiety Reconceptualized." Likewise, when OCD was "discovered" in the 1970s, the anti-depressant Anafranil, not an anxiolytic, was used to treat it (Judith L. Rapaport, *The Boy Who Couldn't Stop Washing* [New York: E. P. Dutton, 1989] 10). Jurgen Margraf, Anke Ehlers, and

Walton T. Roth, "Biological Models of Panic Disorder and Agoraphobia—A Review," *Behavior Research and Therapy* 24 (1986): 553–567; Jerry A. Bennett et al., "A Risk-Benefit Assessment of Pharmacological Treatments for Panic Disorder," *Drug Safety* 6 (1998): 419–430; Karl Rickels and Moira A. Rynn, "What Is Generalized Anxiety Disorder?" *Journal of Clinical Psychiatry* 62 (suppl. 11, 2001): 6; Healy, *The Antidepressant Era;* G. Ron Norton et al., "The Growth of Research on Anxiety Disorders During the 1980s," *Journal of Anxiety Disorders* 9 (1995): 75–85.

72. Edward Shorter, *Before Prozac: The Troubled History of Mood Disorders in Psychiatry* (New York: Oxford University Press, 2008), 116; Smith, *A Social History of the Minor Tranquillizers,* 81, 30.

73. Healy, *The Antidepressant Era,* 180–216.

74. Mark Olfson and Gerald L. Klerman, "Trends in the Prescription of Psychotropic Medications: The Role of Physician Specialty," *Medical Care* 31 (1993): 559–564; Healy, *The Antidepressant Era,* 211, 256–265.

75. Mark Olfson, Steven C. Marcus, George J. Wan, and Erika C. Geissler, "National Trends in the Outpatient Treatment of Anxiety Disorders," *Journal of Clinical Psychiatry* 65 (2004): 1169; Harold A. Pincus et al.,"Prescribing Trends in Psychotropic Medications: Primary Care, Psychiatry, and Other Medical Specialties," *JAMA* 279 (1998): 526–531; Samuel H. Zuvekas, "Prescription Drugs and the Changing Patterns of Treatment for Mental Disorders, 1996–2001," *Health Affairs* 24 (2005): 195–205; Mark Olfson et al., "National Trends in the Outpatient Treatment of Depression," *JAMA* 287 (2002): 203–209.

76. Zuvekas, "Prescription Drugs"; Robert M. Goisman, Meredith G. Warshaw, and Martin B. Keller, "Psychosocial Treatment Prescriptions for Generalized Anxiety Disorder, Panic Disorder, and Social Phobia, 1991–1996," *American Journal of Psychiatry* 156 (1999): 1819–1821.

77. Isaac M. Marks and Randolph M. Nesse, "Fear and Fitness: An Evolutionary Analysis of Anxiety Disorders," *Ethology and Sociobiology* 15 (1994): 247–261.

78. Healy, *The Antidepressant Era,* 178.

79. MacDonald, *Mystical Bedlam,* 41, 67, 76, 99, 110; Rickels and Rynn, "What Is Generalized Anxiety Disorder?"

80. "Discussion: What Is Generalized Anxiety Disorder?" *Journal of Clinical Psychiatry* 62 (suppl. 11, 2001): 14.

81. Olfson et al., "National Trends in the Outpatient Treatment of Depression"; Mark Olfson et al., "National Trends in the Use of Outpatient Psychotherapy," *American Journal of Psychiatry* 158 (2002): 1918; Ramin Mojtabai and Mark Olfson, "National Trends in Psychotherapy by Office-Based Psychiatrists," *Archives of General Psychiatry* 65 (2008): 965.

82. Andrews et al., "Evidence for a General Neurotic Syndrome."

Chapter 6 – Depression

1. American Psychiatric Association, *Diagnostic and Statistical Manual of Mental Disorders,* 4th ed., text rev. (Washington, DC: American Psychiatric Association, 2000), 356.

2. American Psychiatric Association, *Diagnostic and Statistical Manual of Mental Disorders,* 3rd ed. (Washington, DC: American Psychiatric Association, 1980).

3. Mark Olfson, S. C. Marcus, B. Druss, and H. A. Pincus, "National Trends in the Use of Outpatient Psychotherapy," *American Journal of Psychiatry* 159 (2002):

1914–1920; Allan V. Horwitz and Jerome C. Wakefield, *The Loss of Sadness: How Psychiatry Transformed Normal Sorrow into Major Depressive Disorder* (New York: Oxford University Press, 2007), 5; Christopher J. L. Murray and Alan D. Lopez, eds., *The Global Burden of Disease* (Cambridge, MA: World Health Organization, 1996), 375.

4. Hippocrates quoted in Guiseppi Roccatagliata, *A History of Ancient Psychiatry* (Westport, CT: Greenwood Press, 1986), 163–164; American Psychiatric Association, *Diagnostic and Statistical Manual* (2000); Hippocrates quoted in Bennett Simon, *Mind and Madness in Ancient Greece: The Classical Roots of Modern Psychiatry* (Ithaca, NY: Cornell University Press, 1978), 228.

5. Stanley W. Jackson, *Melancholia and Depression: From Hippocratic Times to Modern Times* (New Haven: Yale University Press, 1986), 32.

6. Horwitz and Wakefield, *The Loss of Sadness*, 53–71.

7. Aristotle, "Brilliance and Melancholy," cited in J. Radden, ed., *The Nature of Melancholy: From Aristotle to Kristeva* (New York: Oxford University Press, 2000), 55–60.

8. Gerrit Glas, "A Conceptual History of Anxiety and Depression," in *Handbook of Depression and Anxiety: A Biological Approach*, ed. J. A. den Boer and J. M. Ad Sitsen (New York: Marcel Dekker, 1994), 1–44.

9. Gerald L. Klerman, "The Significance of *DSM-III* in American Psychiatry," in *International Perspectives on DSM-III*, ed. Robert L. Spitzer, J. B. Williams, and A. E. Skodol (Washington, DC: American Psychiatric Press, 1983), 3–24.

10. Horwitz and Wakefield, *The Loss of Sadness*, 75–82.

11. Sigmund Freud, "Mourning and Melancholia," in *Standard Edition of the Complete Works*, 24 vols. (London: Hogarth Press, 1953–1974), 14:237–258.

12. American Psychiatric Association, *Diagnostic and Statistical Manual of Mental Disorders* (Washington, DC: American Psychiatric Association, 1952), 33–34.

13. American Psychiatric Association, *Diagnostic and Statistical Manual of Mental Disorders*, 2nd ed. (Washington, DC: American Psychiatric Association, 1968).

14. Aubrey Lewis, "Melancholia: A Clinical Survey of Depressive States," *Journal of Mental Science* 80 (1934): 1–43.

15. See, for example, L. G. Kiloh and R. F. Garside, "The Independence of Neurotic Depression and Endogenous Depression," *British Journal of Psychiatry* 109 (1963): 451–463; Eugene Paykel, "Classification of Depressed Patients: A Cluster Analysis Derived Grouping," *British Journal of Psychiatry* 118 (1971): 275–288; J. Mendels and C. Cochrane, "The Nosology of Depression: The Endogenous-reactive Concept," *American Journal of Psychiatry* 124 (1968): 1–11; Donald F. Klein, "Endogenomorphic Depression: A Conceptual and Terminological Revision," *Archives of General Psychiatry* 31 (1974): 447–454.

16. Klein, "Endogenomorphic Depression."

17. R. E. Kendell and Jane Gourlay, "The Clinical Distinction Between Psychotic and Neurotic Depressions," *British Journal of Psychiatry* 117 (1970): 257–260; Kiloh and Garside, "Independence of Neurotic Depression"; M. Hamilton and J. M. White, "Clinical Syndromes in Depressive States," *Journal of Mental Science* 105 (1959): 985–998; Eugene Paykel, "Classification of Depressed Patients: A Cluster Analysis Derived Grouping," *British Journal of Psychiatry* 118 (1971): 275–288; A. Raskin and T. H. Crook, "The Endogenous-neurotic Distinction as a Predictor of Response to Antidepressant Drugs," *Psychological Medicine* 6

(1976): 59–70; R. E. Kendell, "The Classification of Depressions: A Review of Contemporary Confusion," *British Journal of Psychiatry* 129 (1976): 15–28; Hans J. Eysenck, "The Classification of Depressive Illness," *British Journal of Psychiatry* 117 (1970): 241–250.

18. Kendell, "Classification of Depressions."
19. Horwitz and Wakefield, *The Loss of Sadness*, 90.
20. John P. Feighner et al., "Diagnostic Criteria for Use in Psychiatric Research," *Archives of General Psychiatry* 26 (1972): 57–63.
21. Horwitz and Wakefield, *The Loss of Sadness*, 92–94; Kendell, "Classification of Depressions," 24.
22. Nancy C. Andreasen and George Winokur, "Newer Experimental Methods for Classifying Depression," *Archives of General Psychiatry* 36 (1979): 447–452.
23. John P. Feighner, "The Advent of the 'Feighner Criteria,'" *Citation Classics* 43 (1989): 14.
24. Gerald R. Klerman, "The Significance of *DSM-III* in American Psychiatry," in *International Perspectives on DSM-III*, ed. Robert L. Spitzer, J. B. Williams, and A. E. Skodol (Washington, DC: American Psychiatric Association, 1983), 3–24; Robert E. Kendell, "*DSM-III*: A Major Advance in Psychiatric Nosology," ibid., 55–68; Mitchell Wilson, "*DSM-III* and the Transformation of American Psychiatry: A History," *American Journal of Psychiatry* 150 (1983): 399–410.
25. American Psychiatric Association, *Diagnostic and Statistical Manual*, 4th ed. (Washington, DC: American Psychiatric Association, 1994); American Psychiatric Association, *Diagnostic and Statistical Manual* (2000).
26. American Psychiatric Association, *Diagnostic and Statistical Manual* (1980), 213–214.
27. R. K. Blashfield, "Feighner et al., Invisible Colleges, and the Matthew Effect," *Schizophrenia Bulletin* 8 (1982): 1–8.
28. Spitzer and Eli Robins had also used the Feighner criteria to develop the Research Diagnostic Criteria (RDC), which was the bridge between the criteria and the *DSM-III*.
29. Kendell, "Classification of Depressions," 23.
30. P. J. Clayton, J. A. Halikas, and W. L. Maurice, "The Bereavement of the Widowed," *Diseases of the Nervous System* 32 (1971): 597–604; P. J. Clayton, J. A. Halikas, and W. L. Maurice, "The Depression of Widowhood," *British Journal of Psychiatry* 120 (1972): 71–78.
31. Mark Zimmerman and Robert L. Spitzer, "Melancholia: From *DSM-III* to *DSM-III-R*," *American Journal of Psychiatry* 146 (1989): 20–28.
32. Ronald Bayer and Robert L. Spitzer, "Neurosis, Psychodynamics, and *DSM-III*," *Archives of General Psychiatry* 42 (1985): 187–196.
33. American Psychiatric Association, *Diagnostic and Statistical Manual* (1980), 220.
34. Ibid., 222–223.
35. Susan McPherson and David Armstrong, "Social Determinants of Diagnostic Labels in Depression," *Social Science & Medicine* 62 (2006): 50–58.
36. Robert L. Spitzer and Janet B. W. Williams, "Having a Dream: A Research Strategy for *DSM-IV*," *Archives of General Psychiatry* 45 (1988): 871–874.
37. David Healy, *The Anti-Depressant Era* (Cambridge: Harvard University Press, 1997), 28–42.

38. Mark Olfson et al., "National Trends in the Outpatient Treatment of Depression," *JAMA* 287 (2002): 203–209.
39. David Healy, "Shaping the Intimate: Influences on the Experience of Everyday Nerves," *Social Studies of Science* 34 (2004): 219–245.
40. McPherson and Armstrong, "Social Determinants of Diagnostic Labels," p. 55.
41. Mark J. Boschen, "Publication Trends in Individual Anxiety Disorders: 1980–2015," *Journal of Anxiety Disorders,* in press.
42. Healy, *The Anti-Depressant Era,* 27–28.
43. Healy, "Shaping the Intimate." In fact, the evidence at the time showed that these medications had no more risks than most prescription drugs. The reaction against the anxiolytics was more the result of a moral crusade against them by a combination of individual psychiatrists, patient advocacy groups, and the mass media. Jonathan Gabe and Michael Burry, "Tranquillizers and Health Care in Crisis," *Social Science and Medicine* 32 (1991): 449–454; Edward Shorter, *Before Prozac: The Troubled History of Mood Disorders in Psychiatry* (New York: Oxford University Press, 2008).
44. Mickey B. Smith, *Small Comfort: A History of the Minor Tranquilizers* (New York: Praeger, 1985), 33; Healy, "Shaping the Intimate," 225.
45. Healy, "Shaping the Intimate," 225.
46. Peter Kramer, *Listening to Prozac: A Psychiatrist Explores Antidepressant Drugs and the Remaking of the Self* (New York: Viking, 1992).
47. Nikolas Rose, "Disorders Without Borders? The Expanding Scope of Psychiatric Practice," *BioSocieties* 1 (2006): 465–484; Samuel S. Zuvekas, "Prescription Drugs and the Changing Patterns of Treatment for Mental Disorders, 1996–2001," *Health Affairs* 24 (2005): 195–205; Horwitz and Wakefield, *The Loss of Sadness,* 187.
48. Olfson et al., "National Trends in the Outpatient Treatment of Depression," 203–209.
49. Rose, "Disorders Without Borders," 478.
50. Horwitz and Wakefield, *The Loss of Sadness,* 185–186.
51. Ronald C. Kessler et al., "Prevalence and Treatment of Mental Disorders, 1990–2003," *New England Journal of Medicine* 352 (2005): 2515–2523.
52. Ewald Horwath, Rose S. Cohen, and Myrna M. Weissman, "Epidemiology of Depressive and Anxiety Disorders," in *Textbook of Psychiatric Epidemiology,* ed. M. T. Tsuang and M. Tohen (New York: John Wiley & Sons, 2002), 391.
53. Darrell A. Regier et al., "Limitations of Diagnostic Criteria and Assessment Instruments for Mental Disorders," *Archives of General Psychiatry* 55 (1998): 109–115.
54. Murray and Lopez, *Global Burden of Disease,* 270, 375.
55. Healy, "Shaping the Intimate," 224.
56. Allen Francis, "Problems in Defining Clinical Significance in Epidemiological Studies," *Archives of General Psychiatry* 55 (1998): 119.
57. Kenneth S. Kendler and Charles O. Gardner, "Boundaries of Major Depression: An Evaluation of DSM-IV Criteria," *American Journal of Psychiatry* 155 (1998): 177.
58. Leo Srole et al., *Mental Health in the Metropolis: The Midtown Manhattan Study,* rev. ed. (New York: McGraw Hill, 1978), 197.
59. Lewis L. Judd, Hagop S. Akiskal, and Martin P. Paulus, "The Role and Clinical Significance of Subsyndromal Depressive Symptoms (SSD) in Unipolar Major Depressive Disorder," *Journal of Affective Disorders* 45 (1997): 5–18.

60. Ronald C. Kessler et al., "Mild Disorders Should Not Be Eliminated from the DSM-IV," *Archives of General Psychiatry* 60 (2003): 1117–1122.
61. Harold A. Pincus, W. W. Davis, and L. E. McQueen, "Subthreshold Mental Disorders: A Review and Synthesis of Studies on Minor Depression and Other 'Brand Names,'" *British Journal of Psychiatry* 174 (1999): 288–296.
62. Judd, Akiskal, and Paulus, "The Role and Clinical Significance of Subsyndromal Depressive Symptoms," 5–18; Ronald Kessler et al., "Prevalence, Correlates, and Course of Minor Depression and Major Depression in the National Comorbidity Survey," *Journal of Affective Disorders* 45 (1997): 19–30.
63. Judd et al., "Subsyndromal Symptomatic Depression: A New Mood Disorder?" *Journal of Clinical Psychiatry* 55 (1994):18–28.
64. Alan M. Gruenberg, Reed D. Goldstein, and Harold Alan Pincus, "Classification of Depression: Research and Diagnostic Criteria: DSM-IV and ICD-10," in *Biology of Depression: From Novel Insights to Therapeutic Strategies*, ed. J. Licinio and M-L. Wong (New York: John Wiley & Sons, 2005), 1–11.
65. Judd et al., "Subsyndromal Symptomatic Depression," 26.
66. Gerald N. Grob, "Origins of DSM-I: A Study in Appearance and Reality," *American Journal of Psychiatry* 148 (1991): 421–431; Horwitz and Wakefield, *The Loss of Sadness*, 123–143; Gerald N. Grob and Howard H. Goldman, *The Dilemma of Federal Mental Health Policy: Radical Reform or Incremental Change?* (New Brunswick, NJ: Rutgers University Press, 2006), 43–67.
67. James Cole, Peter McGuffin, and Anne E. Farmer, "The Classification of Depression: Are We Still Confused?" *British Journal of Psychiatry* 192 (2008): 83–85.
68. John E. Helzer, Helena C. Kraemer, and Robert G. Krueger, "The Feasibility and Need for Dimensional Psychiatric Diagnoses," *Psychological Medicine* 36 (2006): 1671–1680.
69. Terrie E. Moffitt et al., "Depression and Generalized Anxiety Disorder: Cumulative and Sequential Comorbidity in a Birth Cohort Followed Prospectively to Age 32 Years," *Archives of General Psychiatry* 64 (2007): 651–660; William E. Narrow et al., "Revised Prevalence Estimates of Mental Disorders in the United States: Using a Clinical Significance Criterion to Reconcile 2 Surveys' Estimates," *Archives of General Psychiatry* 59 (2002):115–123; Darrell A. Regier et al., "Limitations of Diagnostic Criteria and Assessment Instruments for Mental Disorders," *Archives of General Psychiatry* 55 (1998): 109–115; Jerome C. Wakefield and Robert L. Spitzer, "Lowered Estimates—But of What?" *Archives of General Psychiatry* 59 (2002): 129–130; Jerome C. Wakefield et al., "Should the Bereavement Exclusion for Major Depression Be Extended to Other Losses? Evidence from the National Comorbidity Survey," *Archives of General Psychiatry* 64 (2007): 433–440.
70. Wakefield et al., "Should the Bereavement Exclusion."
71. Donald F. Klein, "Endogenomorphic Depression: A Conceptual and Terminological Revision," *Archives of General Psychiatry* 31 (1974): 447–454; Max Fink et al., "Melancholia: Restoration in Psychiatric Classification Recommended," *Acta Psychiatrica Scandinavica* 115 (2007): 89–92; Cole, McGuffin, and Farmer, "Classification of Depression."
72. Kendell, "Classification of Depressions," 20; Kendler and Gardner, "Boundaries of Major Depression"; Robert F. Krueger, "Continuity of Axes I and II: Toward a Unified Model of Personality, Personality Disorders, and Clinical Disorders," *Journal*

of Personality Disorders 19 (2005): 233–261; Robert F. Krueger et al., "External-
izing Psychopathology in Adulthood: A Dimensional-Spectrum Conceptualization and Its Implications for DSM-V," *Journal of Abnormal Psychology* 115 (2005):
537–550. See, however, Ari Solomon, John Ruscio, John R. Seeley, and Peter M.
Lewinsohn, "A Taxometric Investigation of Unipolar Depression in a Large Community Sample," *Psychological Medicine* 36 (2006): 973–985.

73. Cole, McGuffin, and Farmer, "Classification of Depression"; David Watson, *Mood
and Temperament* (New York: Guilford Press, 2000).

74. Cole, McGuffin, and Farmer, "Classification of Depression," 85; Helzer, Kraemer,
and Krueger, "The Feasibility and Need for Dimensional Psychiatric Diagnoses."

75. Gruenberg, Goldstein, and Pincus, "Classification of Depression," 1–11.

Chapter 7 – Post-Traumatic Stress Disorder

1. Nancy Andreasen, "Posttraumatic Stress Disorder: Psychology, Biology, and the
Manichean Warfare Between False Dichotomies," *American Journal of Psychiatry*
152 (1995): 964.

2. American Psychiatric Association, *Diagnostic and Statistical Manual of Mental
Disorders*, 3rd ed. (Washington, DC: American Psychiatric Association, 1980);
Paul Lerner and Mark S. Micale, "Trauma, Psychiatry, and History: A Conceptual
and Historiographical Introduction," in *Traumatic Pasts: History, Psychiatry, and
Trauma in the Modern Age, 1870–1930,* ed. Mark S. Micale and Paul Lerner (New
York: Cambridge University Press, 2001), 3.

3. Derek Summerfield, "The Invention of Post-Traumatic Stress Disorder and the
Social Usefulness of a Psychiatric Category," *British Medical Journal* 322 (2001):
95–98; Frank Furedi, *Therapy Culture: Cultivating Vulnerability in an Uncertain
Age* (New York: Routledge, 2003); Christina Hoff Summers and Sally Satel, *One
Nation under Therapy: How the Helping Culture Is Eroding Self-Reliance* (New
York: St. Martin's Press, 2005); Richard Gist and Grant J. Devilly, "Post-trauma
Debriefing: The Road too Frequently Travelled," *Lancet* 360 (2007): 741–742; Mark
J. Boschen, "Publication Trends in Individual Anxiety Disorders: 1980–2015,"
Journal of Anxiety Disorders 22 (2008): 570–575.

4. Dixon Wecter, *When Johnny Comes Marching Home* (original ed. 1944; Westport:
Greenwood Press, 1994), 155, quoted in Eric T. Dean, "We Will All Be Lost and
Destroyed: Post-Traumatic Stress Disorder and the Civil War," *Civil War History*
37 (1991): 150.

5. Ralph Harrington, "The Railway Accident: Trains, Trauma, and Technological
Crises in Nineteenth-Century Britain," in Micale and Lerner, *Traumatic Pasts,*
31–56; Eric Caplan, "Trains and Trauma in the American Gilded Age," in ibid.,
57–77; Eric Caplan, "Trains, Brains, and Sprains: Railway Spine and the Origins
of Psychoneuroses," *Bulletin of the History of Medicine* 69 (1995): 387–419.

6. George Makari, *Revolution in Mind: The Creation of Psychoanalysis* (New York:
HarperCollins, 2008), 34.

7. John Eric Erichsen, *On Railway and Other Injuries of the Nervous System* (London: Walton and Maberly, 1866).

8. See Herbert W. Page, *Railway Injuries: With Special Reference to Those of the Back
and Nervous System, in their Medico-legal and Clinical Aspects* (London: Charles
Griffin & Co., 1891); and Harrington, "The Railway Accident." *British Medical
Journal,* December 1, 1866, 612, quoted in Harrington, "The Railway Accident,"

45; R. M. Hodges, "So-Called Concussion of the Spinal Cord," *Boston Medical and Surgical Journal* 104 (1881): 388, quoted in Caplan, "Trains and Trauma," 61.

9. Morton Prince, "The Present Method of Giving Expert Tension in Medico-Legal Cases, As Illustrated by One in Which Large Damages Were Awarded, Based on Contradictory Medical Evidence," *Boston Medical and Surgical Journal* 122 (1890): 76, quoted in Caplan, "Trains and Trauma," 58.

10. Mark Micale, "John-Martin Charcot and *les nevroses traumatiques:* From Medicine to Culture in French Trauma Theory of the Late Nineteenth Century," in Micale and Lerner, *Traumatic Pasts,* 115–139; Christopher Goetz, Michel Bonduelle, and Toby Gelfand, *Charcot: Constructing Neurology* (New York: Oxford University Press, 1995); Mikkel Borch-Jacobsen, "How to Predict the Past: From Trauma to Repression," *History of Psychiatry* 11 (2001): 15–35.

11. Micale, *Traumatic Pasts.*

12. Pierre Janet, *Psychological Healing: A Historical and Clinical Study* (London: George Allen & Unwin, 1925).

13. Joseph Breuer and Sigmund Freud, *Studies on Hysteria* (1895), in *The Standard Edition of the Complete Psychological Works of Sigmund Freud* (London: Hogarth Press 1953–1974), 2:3–17; Sigmund Freud, *Inhibitions, Symptoms, and Anxiety* (1926; New York: W. W. Norton, 1989), 32; Sigmund Freud, *Beyond the Pleasure Principle* (1920; New York: W. W. Norton, 1989); Sigmund Freud. "Introduction to Psychoanalysis and the War Neuroses" (1919), in *Standard Edition,* 17:205–210, quote on 207; Freud, *Beyond the Pleasure Principle,* 37.

14. Charles Rycroft, *Anxiety and Neurosis* (London: Maresfield Library, 1968), 25.

15. Ben Shephard, *A War of Nerves: Soldiers and Psychiatrists in the Twentieth Century* (Cambridge: Harvard University Press, 2001), 39–72.

16. Ibid.; Edgar Jones and Simon Wessely, "A Paradigm Shift in the Conceptualization of Psychological Trauma in the 20th Century," *Journal of Anxiety Disorders* 21 (2007): 164–175; Paul Lerner, "From Traumatic Neurosis to Male Hysteria: The Decline and Fall of Hermann Oppenheim, 1889–1919," in Micale and Lerner, *Traumatic Pasts,* 140–171.

17. Ben Shephard, "Risk Factors and PTSD: A Historian's Perspective," in *Posttraumatic Stress Disorder: Issues and Controversies,* ed. Gerald M. Rosen (Hoboken, NJ: John Wiley & Sons, 2004), 39–62.

18. The conflict between W.H.R. Rivers and his antagonist, psychiatrist Lewis Yealland, is a major theme of Pat Barker's popular novel, *Regeneration* (New York: Plume, 1983). See also Alan Young, *The Harmony of Illusions: Inventing Post-Traumatic Stress Disorder* (Princeton: Princeton University Press, 1995), 43–85.
    G. E. Smith and T. H. Pear, *Shell-Shock and Its Lessons,* 2nd ed. (Manchester: Manchester University Press, 1918), quoted in Shephard, *War of Nerves,* 111; Caroline Cox, "Invisible Wounds: The American Legion, Shell-Shocked Veterans, and American Society, 1919–1924," in Micale and Lerner, *Traumatic Pasts,* 280–305.

19. Gerald N. Grob, *From Asylum to Community: Mental Health Policy in Modern America* (Princeton: Princeton University Press, 1991), 11–14; Sheppard, *War of Nerves,* 326, 330.

20. Roy R. Grinker and John P. Spiegel, *Men Under Stress* (Philadelphia: Blakiston, 1945); Jones and Wessely, "A Paradigm Shift," 169; Shephard, *War of Nerves,* 326.

21. John Appel and Gilbert W. Beebe, "Preventive Psychiatry: An Epidemiologic Approach," *Journal of the American Medical Association* 131 (1946): 1469–1475;

William C. Menninger, "Psychiatric Experience in the War, 1941–1946," *American Journal of Psychiatry* 103 (1947): 580.

22. Grob, *From Asylum to Community,* 16; Shephard, "Risk Factors and PTSD," 49; Jones and Wessely, "A Paradigm Shift," 171.

23. *Statistical Manual for the Use of Hospitals for Mental Diseases Prepared by the Committee on Statistics of the American Psychiatric Association in Collaboration with the National Committee for Mental Hygiene,* 10th ed. (Utica, NY:State Hospitals Press, 1942); American Psychiatric Association, *Diagnostic and Statistical Manual: Mental Disorders* (Washington, DC: American Psychiatric Association, 1952).

24. American Psychiatric Association, *Diagnostic and Statistical Manual* (1952), 40.

25. American Psychiatric Association, *Diagnostic and Statistical Manual of Mental Disorders,* 2nd ed. (Washington, DC: American Psychiatric Association, 1968), 48, 49.

26. Peter G. Bourne, "Military Psychiatry and the Viet Nam Experience," *American Journal of Psychiatry* 127 (1970): 481–488; Peter G. Bourne, *Men, Stress, and Vietnam* (Boston: Little, Brown, 1970); Wilbur J. Scott, "PTSD in *DSM-III:* A Case in the Politics of Diagnosis and Disease," *Social Problems* 37 (1990): 296; Richard J. McNally, *Remembering Trauma* (Cambridge: Harvard University Press, 2003), 9; Grob, *From Asylum to Community,* 13; Shephard, *War of Nerves,* 339–353.

27. Harris Poll, August 1971, cited in Jerry Lembke, "The Right Stuff Gone Wrong: Vietnam Veterans and the Social Construction of Post-Traumatic Stress Disorder," *Critical Sociology* 24 (1999): 47.

28. Scott, "PTSD in *DSM-III,*" 300.

29. Young, *Harmony of Illusions,* 108.

30. Quoted in Mitchell Wilson,"DSM-III and the Transformation of American Psychiatry: A History," *American Journal of Psychiatry* 150 (1993): 405.

31. John E. Helzer, Lee N. Robins, and Darlene H. Davis, "Antecedents of Narcotic Use and Addiction: A Study of 898 Vietnam Veterans," *Drug and Alcohol Dependence* 1 (1976): 183–193; John E. Helzer, Lee N. Robins, and Darlene H. Davis, "Depressive Disorders in Vietnam Returnees," *Journal of Nervous and Mental Disorders* 168 (1976): 177–185.

32. Ronald Bayer, *Homosexuality and American Psychiatry: The Politics of Diagnosis* (New York: Basic Books, 1981); Scott, "PTSD in *DSM-III.*"

33. Young, *Harmony of Illusions;* Herb Kutchins and Stuart A. Kirk, *Making Us Crazy: DSM: The Psychiatric Bible and the Creation of Mental Disorders* (New York: Free Press, 1997), 107–123; Nancy C. Andreasen, "Posttraumatic Stress Disorder," in *Comprehensive Textbook of Psychiatry,* 3rd ed., ed. H. I. Kaplan, A. M. Freedman, and B. J. Saddock (Baltimore: Williams and Wilkins, 1980), 1518; Scott, "PTSD in *DSM-III,*" 307.

34. American Psychiatric Association, *Diagnostic and Statistical Manual of Mental Disorders,* 3rd ed. (Washington, DC: American Psychiatric Association, 1980), 238.

35. Nancy C. Andreasen, "Acute and Delayed Posttraumatic Stress Disorders: A History and Some Issues," *American Journal of Psychiatry* 161 (2004): 1322; Nancy C. Andreasen, A. S. Norris, and C. E. Hartford, "Incidence of Long-Term Psychiatric Complications in Severely Burned Adults," *Annals of Surgery* 174 (1971): 785–793; Nancy C. Andreasen, Russell Noyes, and C. E. Hartford, "Factors Influencing Adjustment of Burn Patients During Hospitalization," *Psychosomatic Medicine* 34

(1972): 517–525; Nancy C. Andreasen et al., "Management of Emotional Reactions in Seriously Burned Adults," *New England Journal of Medicine* 286 (1972): 65–69; Nancy C. Andreasen, "Neuropsychiatric Complications in Burn Patients," *International Journal of Psychiatry in Medicine* 5 (1974): 161–171.

36. American Psychiatric Association, *Diagnostic and Statistical Manual* (1980), 238.

37. Scott, "PTSD in *DSM-III*," 307; Patrick J. Bracken, "Post-modernity and Post-traumatic Stress Disorder," *Social Science and Medicine* 53 (2001): 735; Freud, *Beyond the Pleasure Principle,* 11–12; Paul Starr, *The Discarded Army: Veterans After Vietnam* (New York: Charterhouse, 1973); Lembke, "The Right Stuff Gone Wrong"; Edgar Jones, K. Hyams, and Simon Wessely, "Screening for Vulnerability to Psychological Disorders in the Military: An Historical Inquiry," *Journal of Medical Screening* 10 (2003): 40–46; Fred H. Frankel, "The Concept of Flashbacks in Historical Perspective," *International Journal of Clinical and Experimental Hypnosis* 42 (1994): 321–336.

38. American Psychiatric Association, *Diagnostic and Statistical Manual* (1980), 300–301.

39. John E. Helzer, Lee N. Robins, and Larry McEvoy, "Post-Traumatic Stress Disorder in the General Population," *New England Journal of Medicine* 317 (1987): 1630–1634; Jonathan R. T. Davidson, Dana Hughes, Dan G. Blazer, and Linda George, "Post-traumatic Stress Disorder in the Community: An Epidemiological Study," *Psychological Medicine* 21 (1991): 713–721.

40. Terence M. Keane and Walter E. Penk, "The Prevalence of Post-Traumatic Stress Disorder," *New England Journal of Medicine* 318 (1988): 1691.

41. American Psychiatric Association, *Diagnostic and Statistical Manual of Mental Disorders,* 3rd ed., rev. (Washington, DC: American Psychiatric Association, 1986), 250.

42. Ellen Bass and Laura Davis, *The Courage to Heal: A Guide for Women Survivors of Child Sexual Abuse* (New York: Harper and Row, 1988); Judith L. Herman, *Trauma and Recovery* (New York: Basic Books, 1992), 1; Richard Ofshe and Ethan Watters, *Making Monsters: False Memories, Psychotherapy, and Sexual Hysteria* (Berkeley: University of California Press, 1994); McNally, *Remembering Trauma,* 159–259.

43. American Psychiatric Association, *Diagnostic and Statistical Manual* (1986), 250, 251.

44. Ronald C. Kessler, A. Sonnega, E. Bromet, and C. B. Nelson, "Posttraumatic Stress Disorder in the National Comorbidity Survey," *Archives of General Psychiatry* 52 (1995): 1048–1060; Naomi Breslau, Glenn C. Davis, Patricia Andreski, and Edward Peterson, "Traumatic Events and Posttraumatic Stress Disorder in an Urban Population of Young Adults," *Archives of General Psychiatry* 48 (1991): 216–222; Young, *Harmony of Illusions,* 130.

45. American Psychiatric Association, *Diagnostic and Statistical Manual* (1980), 238; American Psychiatric Association, *Diagnostic and Statistical Manual* (1986), 250; American Psychiatric Association, *Diagnostic and Statistical Manual of Mental Disorders,* 4th ed. (Washington, DC: American Psychiatric Association, 1994).

46. Allen Frances et al., "*DSM-IV:* Work in Progress," *American Journal of Psychiatry* 147 (1990): 1419–1448.

47. American Psychiatric Association, *Diagnostic and Statistical Manual of Mental Disorders,* 4th ed., text rev. (Washington, DC: American Psychiatric Association,

2000), 467; Michael B. First, Alan Frances, and Harold A. Pincus, *DSM-IV-TR Guidebook* (Washington, DC: American Psychiatric Association, 2002), 253.

48. American Psychiatric Association, *Diagnostic and Statistical Manual* (2000), 467.

49. R. J. McNally, R. A. Bryant, A. Ehlers, "Does Early Psychological Intervention Promote Recovery from Posttraumatic Stress?" *Psychological Science in the Public Interest* 4 (2003): 45–79; Frank M. Dattilio, "Extramarital Affairs," *The Behavior Therapist* 27 (2004): 76–78; Claudia Avina and William O'Donohue, "Sexual Harassment and PTSD: Is Sexual Harassment Diagnosable Trauma?" *Journal of Traumatic Stress* 15 (2002): 74.

50. Naomi Breslau et al., "Trauma and Posttraumatic Stress Disorder in the Community: The 1996 Detroit Area Survey," *Archives of General Psychiatry* 55 (1998): 626–632; Naomi Breslau and Ronald C. Kessler, "The Stressor Criterion in DSM-IV Posttraumatic Stress Disorder: An Empirical Investigation," *Biological Psychiatry* 50 (2001): 699–704.

51. American Psychiatric Association, *Diagnostic and Statistical Manual* (2000), 467.

52. Roxane C. Silver et al., "Nationwide Longitudinal Study of Psychological Responses to September 11," *JAMA* 288 (2002): 1237; Mark A. Schuster et al., "A National Survey of Stress Reactions after the September 11, 2001, Terrorist Attacks," *New England Journal of Medicine* 345 (2001): 1507–1512; William E. Schlenger et al., "Psychological Reactions to Terrorist Attacks: Findings from the National Study of Americans' Reactions to September 11," *JAMA* 288 (2002): 581–588, quote on 585.

53. Schuster et al., "A National Survey"; Schlenger et al., "Psychological Reactions"; Sandro Galea et al., "Trends of Probable Post-Traumatic Stress Disorder in New York City after the September 11 Terrorist Attacks," *American Journal of Epidemiology* 158 (2003): 514–524.

54. Tanya M. Luhrmann, *Of Two Minds: The Growing Disorder in American Psychiatry* (New York: Alfred A. Knopf, 2000), 158–202; Allan V. Horwitz, *Creating Mental Illness* (Chicago: University of Chicago Press, 2002), 132–157; Daniel G. Blazer, *The Age of Melancholy: Major Depression and Its Social Origins* (New York: Routledge, 2005), 77–93.

55. Naomi Breslau and Glenn C. Davis, "Posttraumatic Stress Disorder: The Stressor Criterion," *Journal of Nervous and Mental Disease* 175 (1987): 255–264.

56. Breslau et al., "Trauma and Posttraumatic Stress Disorder"; Rachel Yehuda and Alexander C. McFarlane, "Conflict between Current Knowledge about Posttraumatic Stress Disorder and Its Original Conceptual Basis," *American Journal of Psychiatry* 152 (1995): 1705–1713; Marilyn L. Bowman, "Individual Differences in Posttraumatic Distress: Problems with the DSM-IV Model," *Canadian Journal of Psychiatry* 44 (1999): 21–33.

57. Rachel Yehuda, "Biological Factors Associated with Susceptibility to Posttraumatic Stress Disorder," *Canadian Journal of Psychiatry* 44 (1999): 34–39; Matthew J. Friedman and Roger K. Pitman, "New Findings on the Neurobiology of Posttraumatic Stress Disorder," *Journal of Traumatic Stress* 20 (2007): 653–655; M. W. Gilbertson et al., "Smaller Hippocampal Volume Predicts Pathologic Vulnerability to Psychological Trauma," *Nature Neuroscience* 5 (2002): 1242–1247; Mark Gilbertson et al.,"Neurocognitive Function in Monozygotic Twins Discordant for Combat

Exposure: Relationship to Posttraumatic Stress Disorder," *Journal of Abnormal Psychology* 115 (2006): 484–495; R. Yehuda, D. Boisoneau, M. T. Lowy, and E. L. Giller, "Dose-Response Changes in Plasma Cortisol and Lymphocyte Glucocorticoid Receptors Following Dexamethasone Administration in Combat Veterans with Posttraumatic Stress Disorder and Major Depressive Disorder," *American Journal of Psychiatry* 150 (1995): 83–86.

58. Bowman, "Individual Differences": Naomi Breslau, Glenn C. Davis, Patricia Andreski, and E. Peterson, "Traumatic Events and Posttraumatic Stress Disorder in an Urban Population of Young Adults," *Archives of General Psychiatry* 48 (1991): 216–222; Kessler et al., "Post Traumatic Stress Disorder"; Emily J. Ozer, Suzanne R. Best, Tami L. Lipsey, and Daniel S. Weiss, "Predictors of Posttraumatic Stress Disorder and Symptoms in Adults: A Meta-Analysis," *Psychological Bulletin* 129 (2003): 52–73; Fran H. Norris et al., "60,000 Disaster Victims Speak: Part I. An Empirical Review of the Empirical Literature, 1981–2001," *Psychiatry* 65 (2002): 207–239.

59. Marilyn L. Bowman and Rachel Yehuda, "Risk Factors and the Adversity Stress Model," in Rosen, *Posttraumatic Stress Disorder,* 28; Silver et al., "Nationwide Longitudinal Survey."

60. Bowman, "Individual Differences," 28; Shephard, "Risk Factors and PTSD."

61. Summerfield, "The Invention of Post-Traumatic Stress Disorder"; Furedi, *Therapy Culture;* Summers and Satel, *One Nation under Therapy;* Gist and Devilly, "Post-trauma Debriefing."

62. McNally, Bryant, and Ehlers, "Does Early Psychological Intervention Promote Recovery."

63. Arnold A. van Emmerik et al., "Single Session Debriefing after Psychological Trauma: A Meta-analysis," *Lancet* 360 (2002): 766–771; S. Rose, J. Bisson, R. Churchill, and S. Wessely, "Psychological Debriefing for Preventing Post-traumatic Stress Disorder (PTSD)," *Cochrane Database of Systematic Reviews,* 2002, Art. No: CD000560. DOI 1001/14651858; Gist and Devilly, "Post-trauma Debriefing; L. Kiser, J. Heston, S. Hickerson, and P. Millsap, "Anticipatory Stress in Children and Adolescents," *American Journal of Psychiatry* 150 (1993): 87–92; Rose et al., "Psychological Debriefing."

64. Janet Heinrich, "Health Effects in the Aftermath of the World Trade Center Attacks: Testimony before the Subcommittee on National Security, Emerging Threats, and International Relations, Committee on Government Reform, House of Representatives, September 8, 2004" (Washington, DC: U.S. Government Printing Office, Serial No. 108–283), 37–66; Russell Goldman, "Bear Stearns Calls in Grief Counselors," *ABC News,* March 19, 2008, downloaded from http://abcnews.go.com/Business/Story?id=4476286&page=1, July 24, 2008; Derek Summerfield, "A Critique of Seven Assumptions behind Psychological Trauma Programmes in War-Affected Areas," *Social Science & Medicine* 48 (1999): 1449–1462.

65. G. Ron Norton et al.,"The Growth of Research on Anxiety Disorders during the 1980s," *Journal of Anxiety Disorders* 9 (1995): 82.

66. Ibid., 10.

67. Charles S. Milliken, Jennifer L. Auchterlonie, and Charles W. Hoge, "Longitudinal Assessment of Mental Health Problems among Active and Reserve Component Soldiers Returning from the Iraq War," *JAMA* 298 (2007): 2141–2148; Charles W. Hoge et al., "Combat Duty in Iraq and Afghanistan, Mental Health Problems, and

Barriers to Care," *New England Journal of Medicine* 351 (2004): 13–22; Charles W. Hoge, Jennifer L. Auchterlonie, and Charles S. Milliken, "Mental Health Problems, Use of Mental Health Services, and Attrition from Military Service after Returning from Deployment to Iraq or Afghanistan," *JAMA* 295 (2006): 1023–1032; Hoge et al., "Combat Duty in Iraq and Afghanistan," 19.

68. Milliken, Auchterlonie, and Hoge, "Longitudinal Assessment of Mental Health Problems," 2143, 2147.

69. Joanna Burke, *Fear: A Cultural History* (London: Virago, 2005).

70. Shephard, "Risk Factors and PTSD," 49.

71. Gary L. Wells and Elizabeth Loftus, eds., *Eyewitness Testimony: Psychological Perspectives* (New York: Cambridge University Press, 1984); Ofshe and Watters, *Making Monsters*, 139–154; McNally, *Remembering Trauma*, 229–259; Nicoletta Brunello et al., "Posttraumatic Stress Disorder: Diagnosis and Epidemiology, Morbidity and Social Consequences, Biology and Treatment," *Neuropsychobiology* 43 (2001): 156; Robert A. Rosenheck and Alan F. Fontana, "Recent Trends in VA Treatment of Post-Traumatic Stress Disorder and Other Mental Disorders," *Health Affairs* 26 (2007): 1720–1727, review quote on 1726; Paul R. McHugh, "How Psychiatry Lost Its Way," *Commentary* 108 (December 1999): 35; Institute of Medicine, *Treatment of PTSD: An Assessment of the Evidence* (Washington, DC: National Academies Press, 2007), 345.

72. Sandro Galea et al., "Exposure to Hurricane-Related Stressors and Mental Illness after Hurricane Katrina," *Archives of General Psychiatry* 64 (2007): 1427–1434.

73. Roberto J. Rona, Kenneth C. Hyams, and Simon Wessely, "Screening for Psychological Illness in Military Personnel," *JAMA* 293 (2005): 1257–1260.

Epilogue – Where Do We Go from Here?

1. Richard A. Deyo and Donald L. Patrick, *Hope or Hype: The Obsession with Medical Advances and the High Cost of False Promises* (New York: AMACOM, 2005), 189–192, quote on 190.

2. Samuel H. Zuvekas, "Prescription Drugs and the Changing Patterns of Treatment for Mental Disorders, 1996–2001," *Health Affairs* 24 (2005): 195–205; Ramin Majtabai and Mark Olfson, "National Trends in Psychotherapy by Office-Based Psychiatrists," *Archives of General Psychiatry* 65 (2008): 962–970.

3. Joanna Moncrieff and Irving Kirsch, "Efficacy of Antidepressants in Adults," *British Medical Journal* 331 (2005): 155–159.

4. Stefan Leucht et al., "Second-Generation versus First-Generation Antipsychotic Drugs for Schizophrenia: A Meta-Analysis," *The Lancet* 373 (2009): 31–41.

5. Edward Shorter, *Before Prozac: The Troubled History of Mood Disorders in Psychiatry* (New York: Oxford University Press, 2008).

6. President's New Freedom Commission on Mental Health, *Achieving the Promise: Transforming Mental Health Care in America: Final Report*, DHHS Publ. No. SMA-03–3832 (Rockville, MD: Department of Health and Human Services, 2003).

7. Allan V. Horwitz and Jerome C. Wakefield, *The Loss of Sadness: How Psychiatry Transformed Normal Sorrow into Depressive Disorder* (New York: Oxford University Press, 2007), 144–164.

8. Tara Parker-Pope, "Early Test for Cancer Isn't Always Best Course," *New York Times*, August 12, 2008.

9. Steven R. Cummings et al., "Effect of Alendronate on Risk of Fracture in Women with Low Bone Density but Without Vertebral Fractures: Results from the Fracture Intervention Trial," *JAMA* 280 (1998): 2077–2082; Matthew C. Ferrugia et al., "Osteonecrosis of the Mandible or Maxilla Associated with the Use of New Generation Bisphosphonates," *Laryngoscope* 116 (2006): 115–120; Nortin M. Hadler, *The Last Well Person: How to Stay Well Despite the Health-Care System* (Montreal: McGill-Queen's University Press, 2004), 146–165; Deyo and Patrick, *Hope or Hype*, 120; Teppo Jävinen et al., "Shifting the Focus in Fracture Prevention from Osteoporosis to Falls," *British Medical Journal* 19 (2008): 124–126.

10. Avshalom Caspi et al., "Influence of Life Stress on Depression: Moderation by a Polymorphism in the 5-HTT Gene," *Science* 301 (2003): 386–389.

11. Nikolas Rose, *The Politics of Life Itself: Biomedicine, Power, and Subjectivity in the Twenty-First Century* (Princeton: Princeton University Press, 2007).

12. Gardiner Harris and Benedict Carey, "Researchers Fail to Reveal Full Drug Pay," *New York Times,* June 8, 2008; Gardiner Harris, "Top Psychiatrist Failed to Report Drug Income," *New York Times,* October 4, 2008.

13. Ray Moynihan, Iona Heath, and David Henry, "Selling Sickness: The Pharmaceutical Industry and Disease Mongering," *British Medical Journal* 324 (2002): 886–890; Marcia Angell, "Industry-Sponsored Clinical Research: A Broken System," *JAMA* 300 (2008): 1069–1071, quote on 1071. See also Joseph S. Ross et al., "Guest Authorship and Ghostwriting in Publications Related to Rofecoxib: A Case Study of Industry Documents from Rofecoxib Litigation," *JAMA* 299 (2008): 1800–1812; Bruce M. Psaty and Richard A. Kronmal, "Reporting Mortality Findings in Trials of Rofecoxib for Alzheimer Disease or Cognitive Impairment: A Case Study Based on Documents from Rofecoxib Litigation," *JAMA* 299 (2008): 1813–1817; and Catherine D. DeAngelis and Phil B. Fontanarosa, "Impugning the Integrity of Medical Science: The Adverse Effects of Industry Influence," *JAMA* 299 (2008): 1833–1835.

14. There are a large number of critiques of the American health care system. For a small sampling see the following: Shannon Brownlee, *Overtreated: Why Too Much Medicine Is Making Us Sicker and Poorer* (New York: Bloomsbury, 2007); David Mechanic, *The Truth About Health Care: Why Reform Is Not Working in America* (New Brunswick, NJ: Rutgers University Press, 2006); Marcia Angell, *The Truth about the Drug Companies: How They Deceive Us and What to Do about It* (New York: Random House, 2004); Deyo and Patrick, *Hope or Hype;* Nortin M. Hadler, *Worried Sick: A Prescription for Health in an Overtreated America* (Chapel Hill: University of North Carolina Press, 2008); Jerome P. Kassirer, *On the Take: How America's Complicity with Big Business Can Endanger Your Health* (New York: Oxford University Press, 2005); Jerry Avorn, *Powerful Medicines: The Benefits, Risks, and Costs of Prescription Drugs* (New York: Alfred A. Knopf, 2004).

Index

serotonin, 155
Seven Countries Study (Keys), 88
sexual performance, 24
Shatan, Chaim, 174
Shattuck, Lemuel, 20
shell shock, 47, 165, 178, 179
Shorter, Edward, 136
sickle cell anemia, 21
silver nitrate, 41
Sippy, Bertram, W., 40–41
Sippy regimen, 40–41
sleep apnea disorder, and tonsillectomy, 15, 80
smallpox, 12, 16, 19
Smith, Grafton, 170
Smith, Jack, 176
smoking, 4, 88, 90, 91, 103
Smoller, Jordan, 127
social phobia, 130–131, 154; epidemiology of, 131
social policy, U.S., 4
Society of Cardiovascular Computed Tomography, 5
somatoform disorders, 121
Sonnenberg, A., 53
Sontag, Susan, 9
spinal fusion surgery, 194
Spiro, Howard M., 53, 55–56
Spitzer, Robert, 29, 151, 152, 176; creation of *DSM-III*, 120–121
splenic anemia, 21
Spock, Benjamin, 71
SSRIs, 137, 139, 142, 154, 155, 156, 194
Stallones, Reuhl A., 91
standard of living, 4
statins, 93
Statistical Manual for the Use of Hospitals for Mental Disorders, 27, 118, 173
stature, physical, 4
Steigman, Frederick, 48
Stein, Zena, 52
steroids, 12
Stewart, Matthew, 49
stress ulcer, 51
Sullivan, Mary Ann, 76
surgery, rise of, 59
Susser, Melvyn, 52
Sydenstriker, Edgar, 65

syphilis, 19, 144

Tagamet, 54
T&A. *See* tonsillectomy
tannic acid, 41
Task Force on Nomenclature and Statistics, 175
Taxi Driver (film), 178
taxonomy, 17
tetanus, 12
Textbook of Medicine (Cecil), 46
therapy: antibiotic, 2, 54, 76, 97; antidepressant drugs, 153–154; before 1940, 8; cancer, 9; coronary artery bypass, 12; CT angiography, 5; decreased bone density, 5; drug, 193, 194; disappearance of, 13; history, 13; judgment of efficacy, 38, 57, 60–61; hip and knee replacements, 6; lumbar fusion, 6–7; prostate cancer, 107–108; psychiatric drugs, 153–157; psychotherapy, 194; regional differences in, 6; statins, 13; surgery for back pain, 5; surgery for CHD, 5; surgical, 59
Thom, Thomas J., 96
Thomas, Lewis, 98
Thomson, St. Clair, 59
thyroid cancer, 93
thyroxine, 8
tobacco, 46
tonsillectomy, 14–15, 57–83; Allegheny County survey, 76; costs, 72; decline, 78; efficacy, 60–70, 77; epidemiological surveys, 63–64, 72–74; evaluation, 76, 81; expansion, 58, 63; focal infection theory, 63; increase in during 1990s, 80; mortality, 72; pediatrician survey, 70; physician survey, 74–75; poliomyelitis, 63, 68–69; questioning about validity, 63ff; rates, 77–78; sleep disorders, 15, 80; socioeconomic class, 71; surgical techniques, 67–68; varying standards, 68; voluntary health insurance, 71
tonsillitis, 60; and antibiotics, 76
tonsils, 57–83; function of, 61; hypertrophy, 58; justification for removal, 60–67; as "portals of infection," 15
tranquillizers, 135, 153, 194

About the Authors

Gerald N. Grob is the Henry E. Sigerist Professor of the History of Medicine Emeritus at the Institute for Health Policy at Rutgers University in New Brunswick, New Jersey. He is the author of numerous articles and books dealing with the evolution of mental health policy as well as the history of changing patterns of morbidity and mortality in the United States.

Allan V. Horwitz has worked in the field of the sociology of mental illness for over thirty years. He is the author of over eighty articles and chapters and five books, most recently, *The Loss of Sadness: How Psychiatry Transformed Ordinary Misery into Depressive Disorder* (with Jerome Wakefield), on a variety of topics in this area. He currently serves as Dean of Social and Behavioral Sciences at Rutgers University.

Available titles in the Critical Issues in Health and Medicine series: